New Insights in Pediatric Dermatopathology

New Insights in Pediatric Dermatopathology

Editor

Sylvie Fraitag

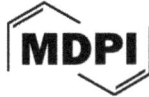

Basel • Beijing • Wuhan • Barcelona • Belgrade • Novi Sad • Cluj • Manchester

Editor
Sylvie Fraitag
Necker Hospital for Sick
Children, APHP
Paris
France

Editorial Office
MDPI AG
Grosspeteranlage 5
4052 Basel, Switzerland

This is a reprint of articles from the Special Issue published online in the open access journal *Dermatopathology* (ISSN 2296-3529) (available at: https://www.mdpi.com/journal/dermatopathology/special_issues/Pediatric_Dermatopathology).

For citation purposes, cite each article independently as indicated on the article page online and as indicated below:

Lastname, A.A.; Lastname, B.B. Article Title. *Journal Name* **Year**, *Volume Number*, Page Range.

ISBN 978-3-7258-1711-5 (Hbk)
ISBN 978-3-7258-1712-2 (PDF)
doi.org/10.3390/books978-3-7258-1712-2

© 2024 by the authors. Articles in this book are Open Access and distributed under the Creative Commons Attribution (CC BY) license. The book as a whole is distributed by MDPI under the terms and conditions of the Creative Commons Attribution-NonCommercial-NoDerivs (CC BY-NC-ND) license.

Contents

Sylvie Fraitag
New Insights in Paediatric Dermatopathology
Reprinted from: *Dermatopathology* 2021, *8*, 56, doi:10.3390/dermatopathology8040056 1

Dieter Metze, Heiko Traupe and Kira Süßmuth
Ichthyoses—A Clinical and Pathological Spectrum from Heterogeneous Cornification Disorders to Inflammation
Reprinted from: *Dermatopathology* 2021, *8*, 17, doi:10.3390/dermatopathology8020017 5

Stéphanie Leclerc-Mercier
How to Deal with Skin Biopsy in an Infant with Blisters?
Reprinted from: *Dermatopathology* 2021, *8*, 22, doi:10.3390/dermatopathology8020022 22

Athanassios Kolivras, Isabelle Meiers, Ursula Sass and Curtis T. Thompson
Histologic Patterns and Clues to Autoinflammatory Diseases in Children: What a Cutaneous Biopsy Can Tell Us
Reprinted from: *Dermatopathology* 2021, *8*, 26, doi:10.3390/dermatopathology8020026 39

Marine Cascarino and Stéphanie Leclerc-Mercier
Histological Patterns of Skin Lesions in Tuberous Sclerosis Complex: A Panorama
Reprinted from: *Dermatopathology* 2021, *8*, 29, doi:10.3390/dermatopathology8030029 58

Philippe Drabent and Sylvie Fraitag
Update on Superficial Spindle Cell Mesenchymal Tumors in Children
Reprinted from: *Dermatopathology* 2021, *8*, 35, doi:10.3390/dermatopathology8030035 75

Arnaud de la Fouchardière, Felix Boivin, Heather C. Etchevers and Nicolas Macagno
Cutaneous Melanomas Arising during Childhood: An Overview of the Main Entities
Reprinted from: *Dermatopathology* 2021, *8*, 36, doi:10.3390/dermatopathology8030036 91

Isabelle Moulonguet and Sylvie Fraitag
Panniculitis in Children
Reprinted from: *Dermatopathology* 2021, *8*, 37, doi:10.3390/dermatopathology8030037 105

Amanda Fanous, Guillaume Morcrette, Monique Fabre, Vincent Couloigner and Louise Galmiche-Rolland
Diagnostic Approach to Congenital Cystic Masses of the Neck from a Clinical and Pathological Perspective
Reprinted from: *Dermatopathology* 2021, *8*, 39, doi:10.3390/dermatopathology8030039 127

Sébastien Menzinger and Sylvie Fraitag
Pseudomalignancies in Children: Histological Clues, and Pitfalls to Be Avoided
Reprinted from: *Dermatopathology* 2021, *8*, 42, doi:10.3390/dermatopathology8030042 144

Sylvie Fraitag and Olivia Boccara
What to Look Out for in a Newborn with Multiple Papulonodular Skin Lesions at Birth
Reprinted from: *Dermatopathology* 2021, *8*, 43, doi:10.3390/dermatopathology8030043 158

Isabel Colmenero and Nicole Knöpfel
Venous Malformations in Childhood: Clinical, Histopathological and Genetics Update
Reprinted from: *Dermatopathology* 2021, *8*, 50, doi:10.3390/dermatopathology8040050 186

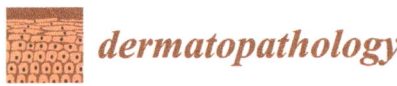

Editorial

New Insights in Paediatric Dermatopathology

Sylvie Fraitag

Paediatric Dermatopathology Unit, Department of Pathology, Hôpital Necker-Enfants Malades, APHP, 75015 Paris, France; sylvie.fraitag@aphp.fr

Keywords: paediatric dermatopathology; childhood melanoma; auto-inflammatory disorders; nodules; neonates; infants; bullous eruption in infancy; panniculitis; congenital cystic masses of the neck; congenital cysts; pseudo-malignancy; subcutaneous spindle cell neoplasms; ichthyoses; venous malformations; tuberous sclerosis complex

Citation: Fraitag, S. New Insights in Paediatric Dermatopathology. *Dermatopathology* **2021**, *8*, 531–534. https://doi.org/10.3390/dermatopathology8040056

Received: 26 November 2021
Accepted: 30 November 2021
Published: 7 December 2021

Publisher's Note: MDPI stays neutral with regard to jurisdictional claims in published maps and institutional affiliations.

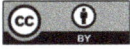

Copyright: © 2021 by the author. Licensee MDPI, Basel, Switzerland. This article is an open access article distributed under the terms and conditions of the Creative Commons Attribution (CC BY) license (https://creativecommons.org/licenses/by/4.0/).

Paediatric dermatology is an expanding subspeciality. This is well illustrated by the growing number of books and articles published on this subject in recent years [1–3].

Paediatric dermatopathology is also a relatively recent and less explored niche. There are many skin conditions common in both adults and children. However, some skin disorders are mostly observed in childhood, and some are restricted to paediatric age. Paediatric dermatopathology covers a wide range of disorders including genodermatoses, cutaneous and sub-cutaneous tumours, and inflammatory disorders.

Over the last decade, I have witnessed the expansion of paediatric dermatology alongside paediatric dermatopathology. Currently, paediatricians and paediatric dermatologists are no longer reluctant to routinely perform a cutaneous biopsy in a young child, even for a vascular lesion. As a result, dermatopathologists are more and more called upon to deal with skin biopsies in neonates, infants, and children. This was certainly not the case when I started my practice in paediatric dermatopathology.

This Special Issue covers a subset of paediatric dermatological conditions in which a great deal of knowledge has been achieved in recent times, thanks to the development of new immunomarkers, the application of molecular biology, and the introduction of new classification system(s). This Special Issue is addressed to dermatologists and pathologists interested in paediatric dermatopathology.

The difficult and complex subject of ichthyoses is brilliantly covered by Metze, D. and Traupe, H. [4]. An accurate and rapid diagnosis of a hereditary keratinization disorder is important not only for the identification of associated diseases of internal organs in syndromic forms, but it can be instrumental for genetic counselling and therapy [5,6]. It is demonstrated well in this article that these cornification disorders have different histological patterns that can allow their better recognition before genetic testing.

The onset of blisters in infancy is always a source of great concern for both parents and physicians. These blistering rashes can be caused by a wide range of benign or severe life-threatening disorders of different aetiologies, including infections, genetics, or autoimmune conditions. The underlying cause has to be determined urgently and a skin biopsy is often required and effective in achieving a rapid and precise diagnosis, and to guide the appropriate management of the baby. In this article, Leclerc-Mercier, S. illustrates in detail the different causes of blistering rashes in the neonatal period [7]. In her review, the author also provides practical instructions to the readers on how to deal with skin biopsy(s) in blistering disorders, e.g., choice of the lesion and site of the biopsy, choice of fixators, when to freeze the sample, and/or perform electron microscopy. This article is very well written and is a practical guide for dermatologists as well as pathologists from a very experienced physician in blistering disorders.

Autoinflammatory diseases are a group of emerging and growing entities defined by aberrant, antigen-independent activation of the innate immune signalling pathways [8].

The dermatopathologist's role is crucial as autoinflammatory disorders can be suspected upon cutaneous histopathological examination. Kolivras, A. et al. provide a very comprehensive overview of these complex disorders and offer practical clues that can help the clinicians in the differential diagnosis [9]. The authors describe three major histopathological patterns seen in autoinflammatory skin diseases, i.e., the "neutrophilic" pattern, the "vasculitic" pattern, and the "granulomatous" pattern. The recognition of these different patterns can facilitate the diagnosis of monogenic forms versus complex multigenic diseases.

Very little has been published on the histological aspect of skin lesions in Tuberous Sclerosis Complex (TSC). The gap has been filled by the excellent article published by Cascarino, M. and Leclerc-Mercier, S. [10]. The authors provide the reader with a comprehensive clinico-pathological overview of the different skin lesions observed in TSC, focusing on hypomelanotic lesions and cutaneous hamartomas. Helpful clues are given.

The diagnosis of cutaneous and subcutaneous spindle cell neoplasms in children is always challenging because of the potential therapeutic and prognostic implications. In addition to the well-known dermatofibrosarcoma protuberans and infantile fibrosarcoma, new entities have been described in the last decade, often with the help of cytogenetics. This comprehensive article from Drabent, P. focuses on these new entities, and their similarities and differences, such as lipofibromatosis and lipofibromatosis-like neural tumour, or plexiform myofibroblastoma and plexiform fibrohistiocytic tumour. In addition, the authors attempt to unify and simplify some confusing and close entities such as fibroblastic connective tissue nevus, medallion-like dermal dendrocyte hamartoma, or plaque-like CD34-positive dermal fibroma [11].

Cutaneous melanomas are very rare in children and their diagnosis is always challenging. The knowledge of the different types of melanomas in children has greatly improved over the last few years, mainly thanks to cytogenetics. This excellent review from de La Fouchardière, A. et al. illustrates with clarity the complexity of paediatric melanocytic malignant lesions and the need for an accurate histological classification to ensure the best clinical management, being the prognosis linked to the melanoma subtype [12].

The diagnostic of panniculitis is challenging at any age, especially in children. This subject is particularly difficult as panniculitis includes a wide range of diseases, with some entities being undoubtedly rare and difficult to recognize. Adults and children share some entities. However, several forms of panniculitis are mostly observed in childhood, or are even restricted to the paediatric age group and particularly the neonatal period. New entities have been recognized recently, mostly linked to auto-inflammation or autoimmunity [13], whereas others, obscure entities, such as Rothmann–Makai syndrome or Weber–Christian disease, are no longer considered to be specific entities. There are very few up-to-date reviews summarizing the different causes of panniculitis in children and detailing their clinical and pathological particularities. The article from Moulonguet, I. [14] is the most recent and comprehensive review on this difficult subject.

The term "pseudomalignancy" covers a large, heterogeneous group of diseases characterized by a benign cellular proliferation, hyperplasia, or infiltrate that resembles a true malignancy, either clinically or histologically. Several inflammatory skin diseases or benign proliferations in children can mimic malignant neoplasms. In this very comprehensive article, Menzinger, S. et al. [15] review the different entities observed in children, which are all traps into which the pathologist can fall. To my knowledge, there is no comparable review in the literature; this is why it seems important to me to have this article at hand when dealing with paediatric cutaneous biopsies.

Congenital cystic masses of the neck are very frequently encountered in paediatrics and their accurate classification may be challenging. Furthermore, this subject is very little and poorly described in dermatopathology books. The aim of these very experienced authors [16] is to describe clinical, radiological, and pathological findings of all the different entities, in order to provide the clinician and the pathologist with the relevant characteristics required for proper management.

Neonatal conditions with multiple cutaneous nodules have a poor prognosis and thus require a prompt diagnosis. A skin biopsy should always be part of the initial examination because the lesion's histology will guide the recommendations for further investigations and the patient's clinical management. This review summarizes the clinical and pathological features of the various disorders that may manifest at birth as multiple skin lesions, and provides the reader with numerous clinical and histological photos [17].

Our knowledge in vascular anomalies has greatly increased in recent years, thanks to the development of cytogenetics with the identification of signalling pathways and genetic mutations responsible for the development of vascular tumours/malformations [18,19]. Venous malformations (VM) represent a heterogeneous group of lesions presenting in the skin, soft tissue, and sometimes, the viscera. The recognition of relevant histopathological features, along with strict clinicopathological correlation, is essential to properly classify these lesions. This very comprehensive article, written by the best specialists in vascular anomalies [20], provides an overview of the clinicopathological features and molecular alterations of venous malformations (VM) in childhood. This review covers common VMs such as blue rubber bleb nevus syndrome, glomuvenous malformation, cerebral malformation, familial intraosseous vascular malformation, and verrucous venous malformation.

Funding: This research received no external funding.

Conflicts of Interest: The author declares no conflict of interest.

References

1. Paller, A.S.; Mancini, A.J. *Hurwitz Clinical Pediatric Dermatology: A Textbook of Skin Disorders of Childhood and Adolescence*; Elsevier: Amsterdam, The Netherlands, 2015.
2. Hoeger, P.; Kinsler, V.; Yan, A.; Harper, J.; Oranje, A.; Bodemer, C.; Larralde, M.; Luk, D.; Mendiratta, V.; Purvis, D. *Harper's Textbook of Pediatric Dermatology*, 4th ed.; Wiley: Hoboken, NJ, USA, 2019.
3. Cohen, B. *Pediatric Dermatology*, 4th ed.; Expert Consult—Online and Print: Amsterdam, The Netherlands, 2020.
4. Metze, D.; Traupe, H.; Süßmuth, K. Ichthyoses—A Clinical and Pathological Spectrum from Heterogeneous Cornification Disorders to Inflammation. *Dermatopathology* **2021**, *8*, 17. [CrossRef] [PubMed]
5. Krug, M.; Oji, V.; Traupe, H.; Berneburg, M. Ichthyoses—Part 1: Differential diagnosis of vulgar ichthyoses and therapeutic options. *J. Dtsch. Derm. Ges.* **2009**, *7*, 511–519, (In English and German). [CrossRef] [PubMed]
6. Krug, M.; Oji, V.; Traupe, H.; Berneburg, M. Ichthyoses—Part 2: Congenital ichthyoses. *J. Dtsch. Derm. Ges.* **2009**, *7*, 577–588, (In English and German). [CrossRef] [PubMed]
7. Leclerc-Mercier, S. How to Deal with Skin Biopsy in an Infant with Blisters? *Dermatopathology* **2021**, *4*, 22. [CrossRef] [PubMed]
8. Nigrovic, P.A.; Lee, P.Y.; Hoffman, H.M. Monogenic autoinflammatory disorders: Conceptual overview, phenotype, and clinical approach. *J. Allergy Clin. Immunol.* **2020**, *146*, 925–937. [CrossRef] [PubMed]
9. Kolivras, A.; Meiers, I.; Sass, U.; Thompson, C.T. Histologic Patterns and Clues to Autoinflammatory Diseases in Children: What a Cutaneous Biopsy Can Tell Us. *Dermatopathology* **2021**, *8*, 26. [CrossRef] [PubMed]
10. Cascarino, M.; Leclerc-Mercier, S. Histological Patterns of Skin Lesions in Tuberous Sclerosis Complex: A Panorama. *Dermatopathology* **2021**, *8*, 236–252. [CrossRef] [PubMed]
11. Drabent, P.; Fraitag, S. Update on Superficial Spindle Cell Mesenchymal Tumors in Children. *Dermatopathology* **2021**, *8*, 35. [CrossRef] [PubMed]
12. de la Fouchardière, A.; Boivin, F.; Etchevers, H.C.; Macagno, N. Cutaneous Melanomas Arising during Childhood: An Overview of the Main Entities. *Dermatopathology* **2021**, *8*, 301–314. [CrossRef] [PubMed]
13. Bader-Meunier, B.; Rieux-Laucat, F.; Touzot, F.; Frémond, M.L.; André-Schmutz, I.; Fraitag, S.; Bodemer, C. Inherited Immunodeficiency: A New Association with Early-Onset Childhood Panniculitis. *Pediatrics* **2018**, *141*, S496–S500. [CrossRef] [PubMed]
14. Moulonguet, I.; Fraitag, S. Panniculitis in Children. *Dermatopathology* **2021**, *8*, 315–336. [CrossRef] [PubMed]
15. Menzinger, S.; Fraitag, S. Comment on "Histopathologic features distinguishing secondary syphilis from its mimickers". *J. Am. Acad. Dermatol.* **2020**, *83*, e135. [CrossRef] [PubMed]
16. Fanous, A.; Morcrette, G.; Fabre, M.; Couloigner, V.; Galmiche-Rolland, L. Diagnostic Approach to Congenital Cystic Masses of the Neck from a Clinical and Pathological Perspective. *Dermatopathology* **2021**, *8*, 342–358. [CrossRef] [PubMed]
17. Fraitag, S.; Boccara, O. What to Look Out for in a Newborn with Multiple Papulonodular Skin Lesions at Birth. *Dermatopathology* **2021**, *8*, 390–417. [CrossRef] [PubMed]
18. Soblet, J.; Limaye, N.; Uebelhoer, M.; Boon, L.; Vikkula, M. Variable Somatic TIE2 Mutations in Half of Sporadic Venous Malformations. *Mol. Syndr.* **2013**, *4*, 179–183. [CrossRef] [PubMed]

19. Limaye, N.; Kangas, J.; Mendola, A.; Godfraind, C.; Schlögel, M.J.; Helaers, R.; Eklund, L.; Boon, L.M.; Vikkula, M. Somatic Activating PIK3CA Mutations Cause Venous Malformation. *Am. J. Hum. Genet.* **2015**, *97*, 914–921. [CrossRef] [PubMed]
20. Colmenero, I.; Knöpfel, N. Venous Malformations in Childhood: Clinical, Histopathological and Genetics Update. *Dermatopathology* **2021**, *8*, 477–493. [CrossRef] [PubMed]

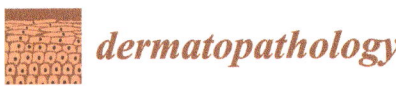

Review

Ichthyoses—A Clinical and Pathological Spectrum from Heterogeneous Cornification Disorders to Inflammation

Dieter Metze *, Heiko Traupe and Kira Süßmuth

Klinik für Hautkrankheiten, Universitätsklinik Münster, 48149 Münster, Germany; traupeh@ukmuenster.de (H.T.); Kira.Suessmuth@ukmuenster.de (K.S.)
* Correspondence: metzed@uni-muenster.de

Abstract: Ichthyoses are inborn keratinization disorders affecting the skin only (non-syndromic) or are associated with diseases of internal organs (syndromic). In newborns, they can be life-threatening. The identification of the gene defects resulted in reclassification and a better understanding of the pathophysiology. Histopathologic patterns include orthohyperkeratosis with a reduced or well-developed stratum granulosum, hyperkeratosis with ortho- and parakeratosis with preserved or prominent stratum granulosum, and epidermolytic ichthyosis. Another pattern features "perinuclear vacuoles and binucleated keratinocytes", which is associated with keratin mutations. Some ichthyoses are histologically defined by psoriasis-like features, and distinct subtypes show follicular hyperkeratosis. In addition to histological and immunohistochemical methods, these patterns allow a better histopathologic diagnosis.

Keywords: ichthyosis; hereditary keratinization disorders; dermatopathology; pattern analysis; immunohistochemistry

1. Target Readership

The article was written for dermatologists and pathologists interested in genodermatoses and dermatohistology, especially the diagnosis of ichthyoses. It is supposed to help to diagnose different types of ichthyoses when genetic analyses are not available or before genetic testing.

2. Introduction

Ichthyoses are hereditary keratinization disorders defined by universal scaling occurring over the entire body. Some forms manifest at birth ("congenital" forms), others during the first year of life ("vulgar" forms) (Table 1) [1,2].

An accurate and rapid diagnosis of a hereditary keratinization disorder is important to identify associated diseases of internal organs in syndromic forms (Table 1), to initiate genetic counseling, and to start potential therapies [1,2].

The histopathology of ichthyoses is mentioned in publications and book chapters [3] but has not been systematically studied and is often considered "nonspecific." Traditionally, therefore, the clinical picture, family history, and occasionally laboratory chemistry and electron microscopic studies have been crucial for diagnosis. Only the identification of the genetic causes has led to an understanding of the molecular mechanisms, as well as to the reclassification of these genodermatoses (Table 1) [4,5]. Assistance is provided by special networks (www.netzwerk-ichthyose.de (accessed on 3 May 2021)) and patient support-groups (https://www.ichthyose.de/ (accessed on 3 May 2021)).

In parallel, the pathological changes of the skin biopsies were characterized in more detail. Certain histological patterns could be defined. They include the following criteria: hyperkeratosis with/without parakeratosis, expression/absence of the stratum granulosum, atrophy/hyperplasia (acanthosis) of the epidermis, vacuolization/eosinophilic granules in keratinocytes, or hyperkeratosis and a degree of development of hair follicles.

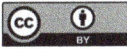

Complementary histo- and immunohistochemical methods allow for, in part, a precise diagnosis, but at least a limitation of differential diagnoses, which can then be further clarified by targeted mutation analyses [6,7].

Table 1. Clinical classification of ichthyoses.

Vulgar ichthyosis, isolated
Ichthyosis vulgaris
X-linked recessive ichthyosis
Vulgar ichthyosis, syndromic
Refsum syndrome
Multiple sulfatase deficiency
Congenital ichthyosis, isolated
Keratinopathic ichthyosis
Autosomal recessive congenital ichthyosis (ARCI)
Harlequin ichthyosis (subtype of ARCI)
Autosomal dominant lamellar ichthyosis
Congenital reticular ichthyosiform erythroderma (CRIE, Confetti ichthyosis)
Ichthyosis hystrix type Curth–Macklin
Peeling skin disease
Erythrokeratodermia
and others
Congenital ichthyosis, syndromic
HID/KID syndrome
Netherton syndrome
CHILD syndrome
SAM syndrome
Conradi–Hünermann–Happle syndrome
Sjögren–Larsson syndrome
Chanarin–Dorfmann syndrome
Trichothiodystrophy
IFAP syndrome
and others

In the following, the dermatopathological diagnosis is presented on the basis of some frequent, but also rare syndromic and life-threatening ichthyoses, which can be performed quickly, easily, and economically on sample biopsies of the skin. Hereditary keratinization disorders are also discussed. They often show a highly inflammatory, psoriasis-like picture and are therefore often misdiagnosed (Table 2) [6,8].

Table 2. Ichthyoses with a psoriasis-like picture.

Ichthyoses with Psoriasis-Like Picture
Netherton syndrome
Peeling skin disease
CHILD syndrome
Severe dermatitis, multiple allergies, metabolic wasting syndrome (SAM syndrome)
Anular epidermolytic ichthyosis

3. Ichthyosis Vulgaris

The autosomal semidominant inherited ichthyosis vulgaris is the most frequent ichthyosis (prevalence from 1:100 to 1:250) [9]. It usually develops in the course of the first year of life and manifests with dry skin or light gray fine scales (Figure 1) as well as palmoplantar hyperlinearity. The disorder is caused by loss-of-function mutations in the *filaggrin* gene (Table 3). Filaggrin is expressed in the keratohyalin granules and crosslinks the keratin filaments in the horny layer. A deficiency of filaggrin predisposes to atopic dermatitis and/or allergic rhinoconjunctivitis [8,10]. Interestingly, *filaggrin* mutations can also be observed in X-linked recessive ichthyosis underlying steroid sulfatase deficiency [10].

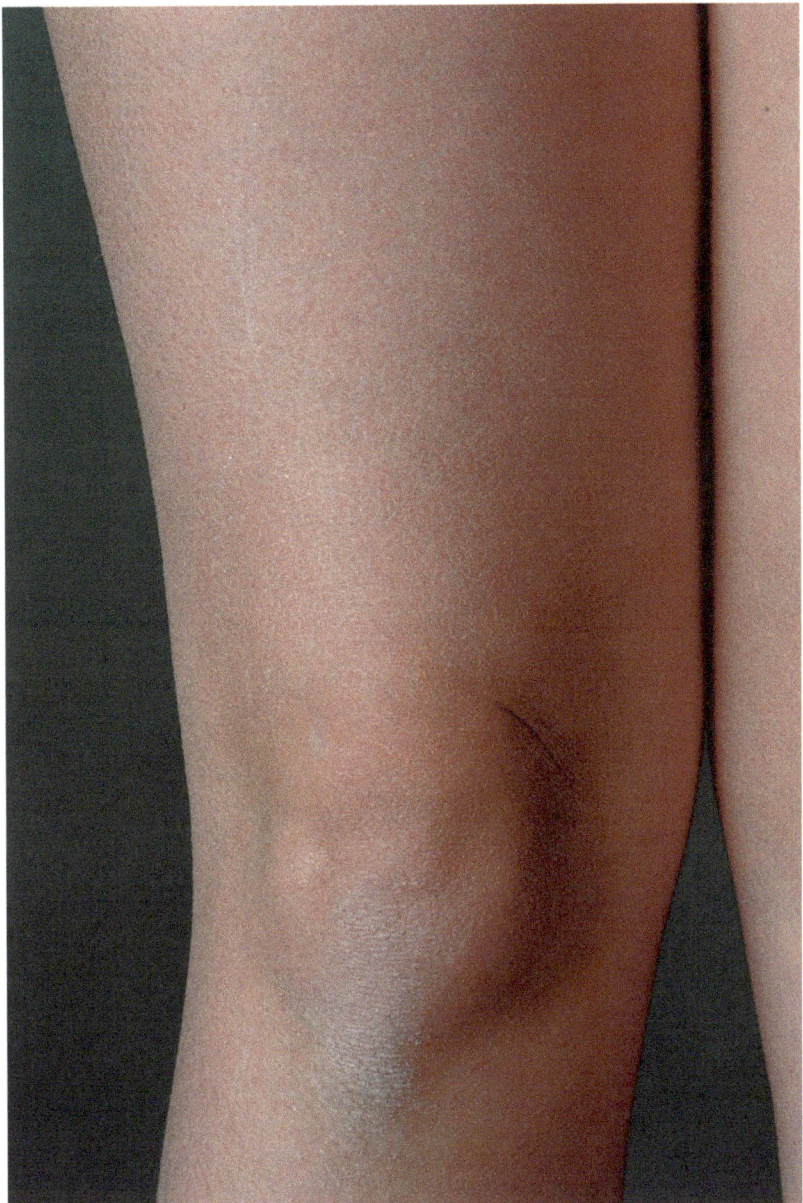

Figure 1. Ichthyosis vulgaris. Fine grey scaling on the extremities.

Table 3. Different types of ichthyosis with gene mutation and mode of inheritance.

				Gene (mode of inheritance)
		Ichthyosis		
	Common Ichthyoses	Ichthyosis Vulgaris		FLG (filaggrin) (autosomal semidominant)
		X-Linked Ichthyosis		STS (steroid sulfatase) (X-linked recessive)
Non-Syndromic Ichthyoses		Harlequin Ichthyosis		ABCA12 (ATP Binding Cassette Subfamily A Member 12) (autosomal recessive)
	ARCI and Keratinopathic Ichthyoses	Lamellar Ichthyosis, Congenital Ichthyosiform Erythroderma		TGM1 (transglutaminase−1); ALOX12B (Arachidonate 12-Lipoxygenase, 12R Type); ALOXE3 (Arachidonate Lipoxygenase 3); CYP4F22 (Cytochrome P450 Family 4 Subfamily F Member 22); NIPAL4 (Ichthyin) and others (autosomal recessive)
		Bathing Suit Ichthyosis		TGM1 (autosomal recessive)
		Keratinopathic Ichthyoses	EI	KRT1 (keratin 1); KRT10 (keratin 10) (autosomal dominant, sometimes recessive (KRT10 mutations))
			SEI	KRT2 (keratin 2) (autosomal dominant)
		Rare Variants of KPI	CRIE	KRT1 KRT10 (autosomal dominant, de novo mutations)
Further Non-Syndromic Ichthyoses		Peeling Skin Disease		CDSN (corneodesmosin) (autosomal recessive)
		Erythrokeratoderma Variabilis		GJB3 (encoding Connexin 31) GJB4 (encoding Connexin 30.3) (often autosomal dominant)
Syndromic Ichthyoses		Netherton Syndrome		SPINK5 (encoding LEKTI) (autosomal recessive)
		KID Syndrome		GJB2 (encoding Connexin 26) (autosomal dominant)
		CHILD Syndrome		NSDHL (NAD(P) Dependent Steroid Dehydrogenase-Like) (x-linked dominant)
		SAM Syndrome		DSG1 (desmoglein−1) DSP (desmoplakin) (autosomal recessive)

3.1. Histology

A characteristic feature of ichthyosis vulgaris is a markedly reduced, often completely absent stratum granulosum. The stratum corneum exhibits mild compact orthohyperkeratosis (Figure 2). Frequently, there is also hyperkeratosis of hair follicles and acrosyringia. The epidermis may be slightly widened (acanthotic) but also atrophic. Isolated mild perivascular lymphocytic infiltrates can be found in the dermis. Associated signs of spongiform dermatitis may be encountered in the setting of atopy.

Immunohistochemically, a deficiency of filaggrin can be quantified, which correlates with the number of mutations (one or two mutations in the *filaggrin* gene) and thus, the severity of ichthyosis. Ultrastructurally, there is a defect in the keratohyalin granules, which appear diminished and crumbly.

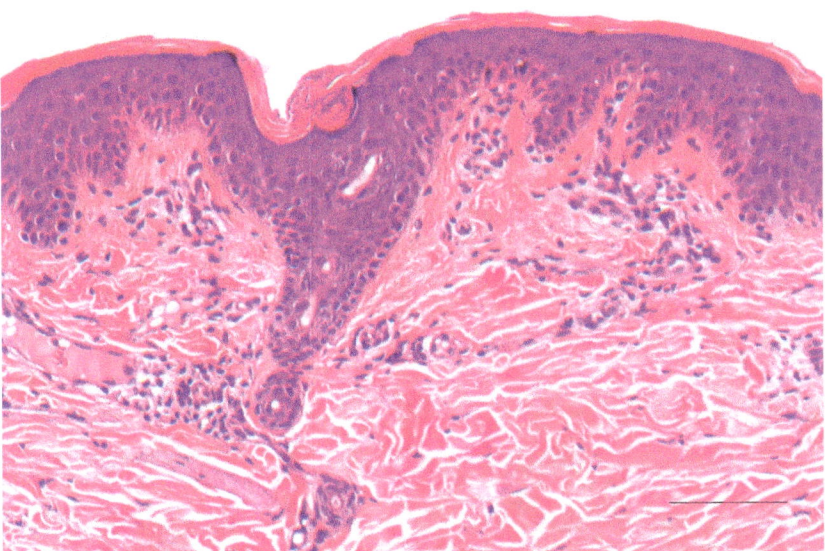

Figure 2. Ichthyosis vulgaris. Note the absent stratum granulosum and mild compact orthohyperkeratosis. Marked hyperkeratosis of the opening of the acrosyringium. Inflammatory infiltrates are almost absent. HE stain, bar = 100 µm.

3.2. Differential Diagnoses

A thinned or absent stratum granulosum with mild orthohyperkeratosis is also observed in patients with atopy and other very rare ichthyoses, such as Conradi–Hünermann–Happle syndrome [6]. It can also be found in acquired ichthyosis-like skin conditions ("acquired ichthyoses"). Causes are malignancies (lymphomas), renal insufficiency, Crohn's disease, autoimmune diseases (collagenoses), GvHD, infections (HIV, leprosy), endocrinopathies (hypothyroidism), sarcoidosis, malnutrition (vitamin A) or drugs (lipid-lowering drugs, psychotropic drugs) [11].

4. Autosomal Recessive Congenital Ichthyosis

Autosomal recessive congenital ichthyosis (ARCI) represents a genetically heterogeneous group of non-syndromic congenital ichthyoses with widely varying severity. The group comprises lamellar ichthyosis, which is most often due to tranglutaminase−1 deficiency (Table 3), congenital ichthyosiform erythroderma, and the most severe but rare subtype of harlequin ichthyosis [12]. Newborns can be born with a tight and shiny stratum corneum, which is associated with ectropion, eclabium, fluid loss, and thermal dysregulation, and resulting in potentially life-threatening complications. However, the clinical presence of a collodion membrane is also encountered in other ichthyoses [5].

Later, the collodion membrane is replaced by dark brown, adherent, plate-like scales (classic lamellar ichthyosis; Figure 3) or a whitish, poorly adherent, fine scale on reddened skin (non-bullous congenital ichthyosiform erythroderma). To varying degrees, there are associated palmoplantar keratoderma, nail dystrophies, fibrosing alopecia, and hypohidrosis with heat intolerance [5].

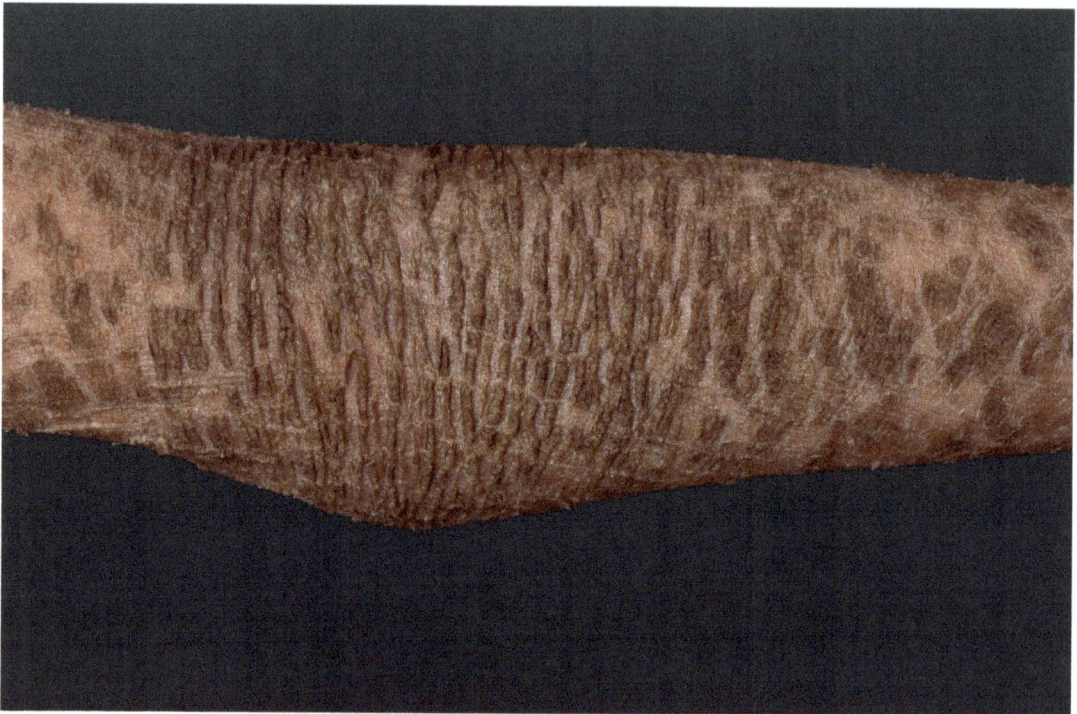

Figure 3. Lamellar ichthyosis. Dark brownish lamellar scaling in a patient with transglutaminase−1 deficiency.

The ARCI forms are caused by different mutations. In 30–40% of cases, a mutation is present in the *transglutaminase−1* gene, resulting in a disruption of protein cross-linking and the esterification of ceramides in corneocytes. Using biotinylated donor substrates, such as the amine donor monodansylcadaverine, transglutaminase activity can be visualized immediately in situ by fluorescence labeling based on the incorporation of monodansyl-cadaverine on sections of unfixed frozen biopsies [13]. Mutations are also present in the *ATB-binding cassette transporter (ABCA12)* gene, which, unlike harlequin-ichthyosis, has residual activity in milder ARCI cases. ABCA12 is required in epidermal lipid transport via the lamellar bodies. Other mutations involve the *ichthyin, lipoxygenase, or cytochrome P450 oxidase* genes *FLJ39501*. A definitive correlation of this mutation with a specific phenotype of ARCI has not been fully established [8].

4.1. Histology

Histologically, there is compact orthohyperkeratosis, a slightly widened stratum granulosum, acanthosis, and papillomatosis of the epidermis. In the papillary body, the vessels appear dilated and spiraling, and lymphocytic infiltrates are scarce or mild (Figure 4) [7].

4.2. Differential Diagnoses

The various forms of ARCI cannot be differentiated histologically, except for harlequin ichthyosis. Similarly, X-linked ichthyosis presents with almost identical pathology. Lichen simplex chronicus presents with more severe inflammation and fibrosis in the papillary body.

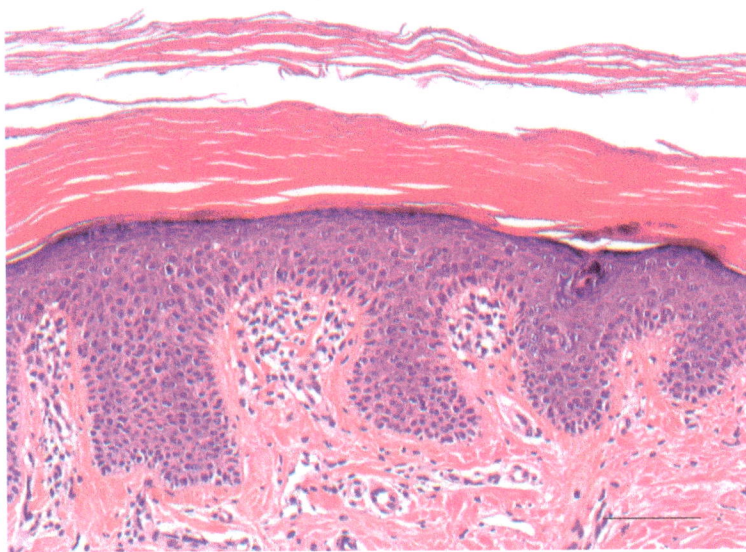

Figure 4. Autosomal recessive lamellar ichthyosis. Acanthotic epidermis with well-developed stratum granulosum and compact orthohyperkeratosis without further signs of inflammation. HE stain, original magnification, bar = 100 µm.

5. Keratinopathic Ichthyosis

Epidermolytic ichthyosis, formerly also called bullous congenital ichthyotic erythroderma Brocq, is due to a mutation of *keratin 1* or *keratin 10* and is therefore classified as keratinopathic ichthyosis (Table 3) [5]. Neonates present with erythroderma with blistering, sometimes pronounced, and later develop (spiky) keratoses, preferentially on the extremities (Figure 5). Patients with a *keratin 1* mutation also have palmoplantar keratosis, which is absent in patients with a *keratin 10* mutation because this keratin is not expressed there [14].

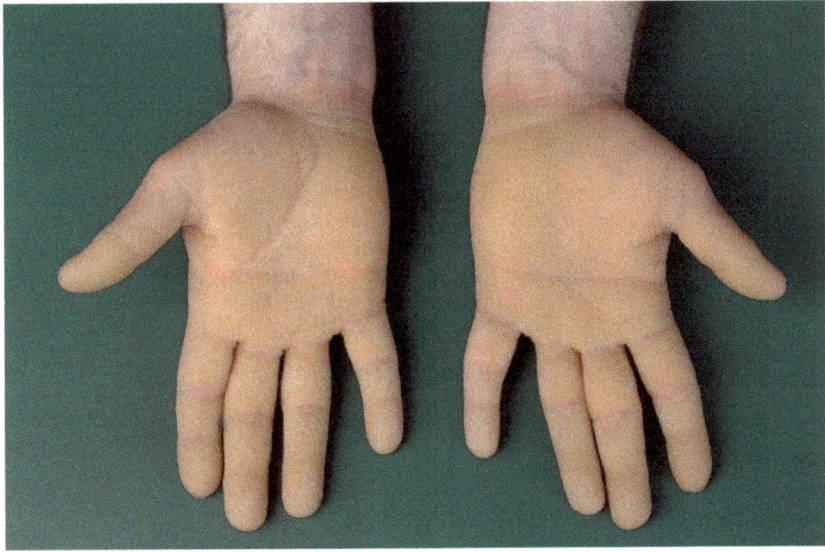

Figure 5. Epidermolytic ichthyosis. Diffuse palmoplantar keratoderma (*keratin 1* mutation).

5.1. Histology

There is massive orthohyperkeratosis and acanthosis of the epidermis. The suprabasal keratinocytes reveal vacuolization and distinct hypereosinophilic granules. In the stratum granulosum, the keratohyalin granules are coarse and irregular. The boundaries between keratinocytes are poorly demarcated, and clefts and blisters occur. Minor lymphocytic infiltrates may impose in the dermis (Figure 6) [8].

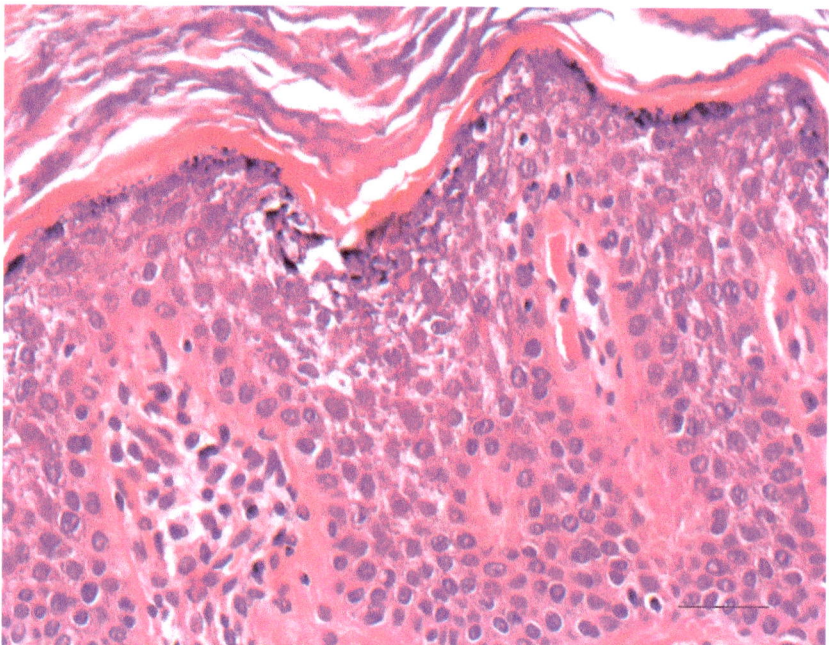

Figure 6. Epidermolytic ichthyosis. Acanthotic epidermis with massive orthohyperkeratosis. Suprabasal keratinocytes vacuolated with distinct hypereosinophilic granules and irregular keratohyalin granules. HE stain, bar = 50 µm.

Electron microscopically, the hypereosinophilic granules correspond to clumps of the keratin skeleton. A collapse of the mutant keratins causes the vacuolar aspect of the cytoplasm and results in mechanical instability.

5.2. Differential Diagnoses

The histologic reaction pattern of epidermolytic hyperkeratosis is also found in superficial epidermolytic ichthyosis with a *keratin 2* mutation (ichthyosis bullosa Siemens), or epidermal nevi in the setting of mosaicism of keratinopathic ichthyoses [15,16]. Very discrete and circumscribed, these changes are also found incidentally in normal skin (preferentially in the vicinity of epithelial or melanocytic tumors), as well as in cysts, scars, or various inflammatory dermatoses.

6. Erythrokeratoderma

Erythrokeratodermas are defined by localized erythematous keratoses on the body and are now classified in the ichthyosis group [5]. They are caused by mutations of connexin 30.3 or 31 (Table 3). These transmembrane protein gap junctions are essential for intercellular communication and, thus, for epidermal differentiation [17].

Autosomal dominantly inherited erythrokeratodermia variabilis (Mendes da Costa syndrome) initially manifests with migratory figured erythema, and later persistent keratoses. The expression varies between intra- and interfamilial, and sometimes only circumscribed keratoses are found on pressure-exposed areas of the sole of the foot. Progressive symmetric erythrokeratodermia (Gottron) is no longer distinguished as a separate entity from erythrokeratodermia variabilis [18].

Histology

The epidermis shows acanthosis and undulating surface with hyperkeratosis, focal parakeratosis, dyskeratotic keratinocytes, and preserved stratum granulosum. Superficial perivascular lymphocytic infiltrate may be present (Figure 7). Overall, the histologic changes mentioned are highly variable and complicate diagnosis. The deficiency of the affected connexin can be easily visualized by immunohistochemistry; at the same time, compensatory connexin 43 expression is increased.

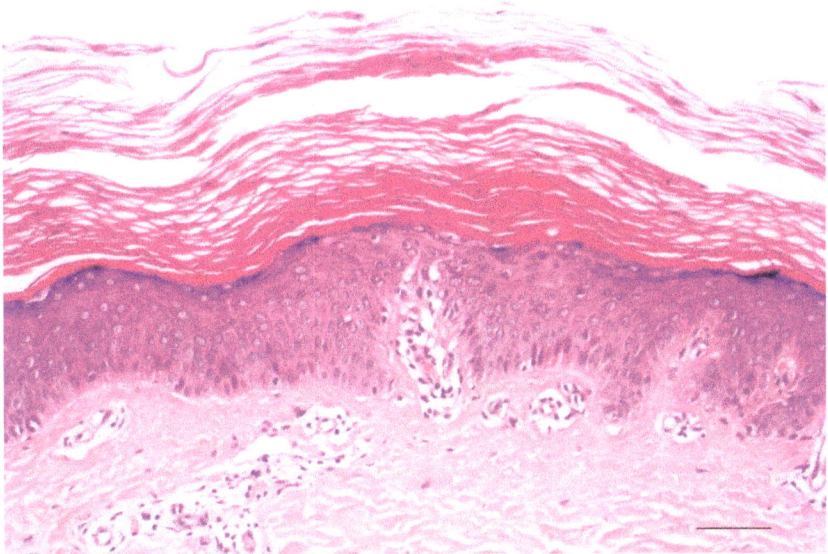

Figure 7. Erythrokeratoderma. Acanthotic epidermis with orthohyperkeratosis, focal parakeratosis, dyskeratotic keratinocytes, and preserved stratum granulosum. Discrete superficial perivascular lymphocytic infiltrate. HE stain, bar = 100 µm.

7. KID Syndrome and HID Syndrome

Keratitis–ichthyosis–deafness (KID) syndrome and hystrix-like–ichthyosis–deafness (HID) syndrome are different forms of an autosomal dominant inherited ichthyosis caused by a mutation of connexin 26 (Table 3) [19]. Because this connexin performs important functions in the inner ear, neurosensory hearing loss also exists. Patients with KID syndrome develop sharply circumscribed wart-like hyperkeratotic plaques on the face and extremities; in HID syndrome, hystrix-like generalized ichthyosis predominates. In the setting of this syndromic ichthyosis, keratitis, alopecia, nail dystrophy, dental abnormalities, or hypohidrosis, and an increased risk of infection and carcinoma occur.

7.1. Histology

The epidermis is acanthotic with a partially verruciform appearance. The hyperkeratotic stratum corneum contains parakeratoses with large round nuclear remnants, and occasionally shadow cells with vacuolated nuclei (Figure 8). Dyskeratotic keratinocytes with perinuclear halo ("bird's eye") appear as a dominant criterion. The stratum granulosum may be absent or strongly pronounced. Subepidermal dense lymphocytic infiltrates occur in some cases. The openings of the hair follicles and sweat glands are highly keratinized.

The sweat glands may be diminished and atrophic. Highly differentiated squamous cell carcinoma may also occur at a young age [8].

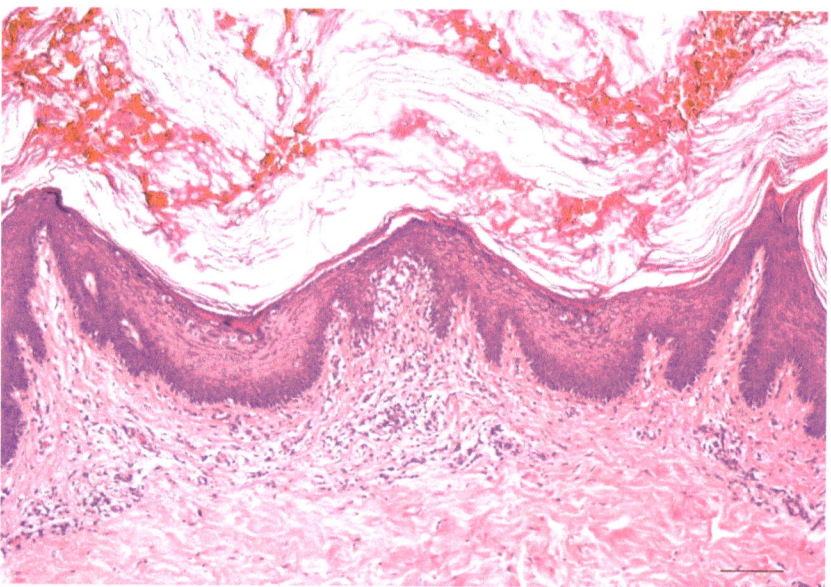

Figure 8. KID syndrome (keratitis–ichthyosis–deafness). Dyskeratotic keratinocytes with perinuclear halo ("bird's eye"). HE stain, bar = 100 µm.

7.2. Differential Diagnoses

Verrucae vulgares also show vacuolated cells, but in KID/HID syndrome these persist in the stratum corneum. Vacuolization is absent in erythrokeratodermia.

8. Ichthyoses with Inflammatory Psoriasiform Pattern

Some hereditary ichthyoses have a histologic pattern that closely resembles psoriasis vulgaris or chronic dermatitis in the setting of atopic eczema, which is why misdiagnosis is common (Table 2). Because of the significant and sometimes lethal complications associated with this group of ichthyoses, prompt dermatohistologic diagnosis is important [20].

9. Netherton Syndrome

In autosomal recessive Netherton syndrome, there is a mutation of the *SPINK5* gene, which encodes LEKTI ("lymphoepithelial Kazal-type related inhibitor"), a major serine protease inhibitor of the epidermis and thymus (Table 3) [21]. Patients are born with marked erythroderma, which later often changes into anular eyrthema with a typical double-edged scale ("ichthyosis linearis circumflexa") (Figure 9). Later, brittle hairs are also noticeable ("bamboo hairs", trichorrhexis invaginata). Type 1 allergies, elevated IgE levels, and hypereosinophilia, as well as immunodeficiency and enteropathy, which can lead to massive failure to thrive, especially in the first year of life, are associated with this cornification disorder. Electrolyte disturbances and sepsis are lethal risks for infants.

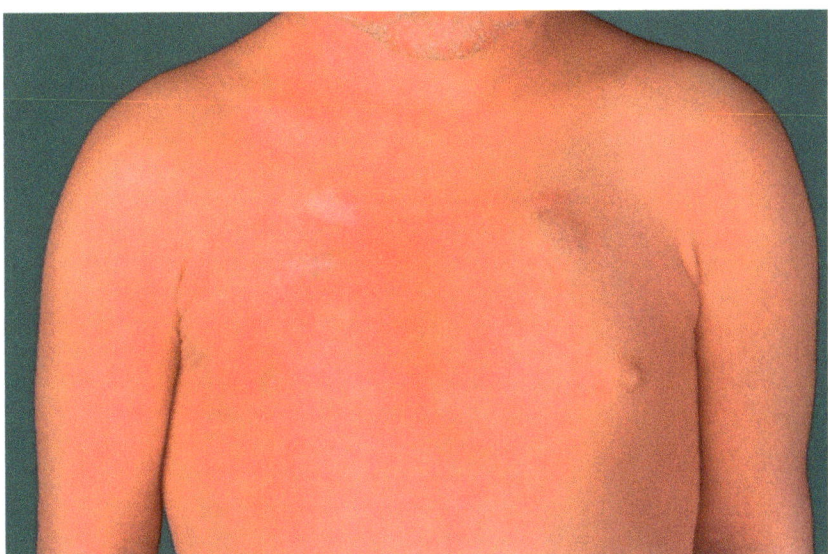

Figure 9. Netherton syndrome. Erythema and scaling of the trunk and face.

9.1. Histology

There is psoriasiform hyperplasia with a moderately widened stratum corneum showing focal parakeratosis and accumulations of neutrophils. The stratum granulosum is absent or severely diminished. The papillary dermis is papillomatously elongated and contains dilated vessels and inflammatory infiltrates with lymphocytes, neutrophils, and eosinophilic granulocytes (Figure 10). Sometimes, however, there are histologic changes, as found in atopic dermatitis. Immunohistochemically, staining for LEKTI is absent in the epidermis and hair follicles (Figure 11) [22].

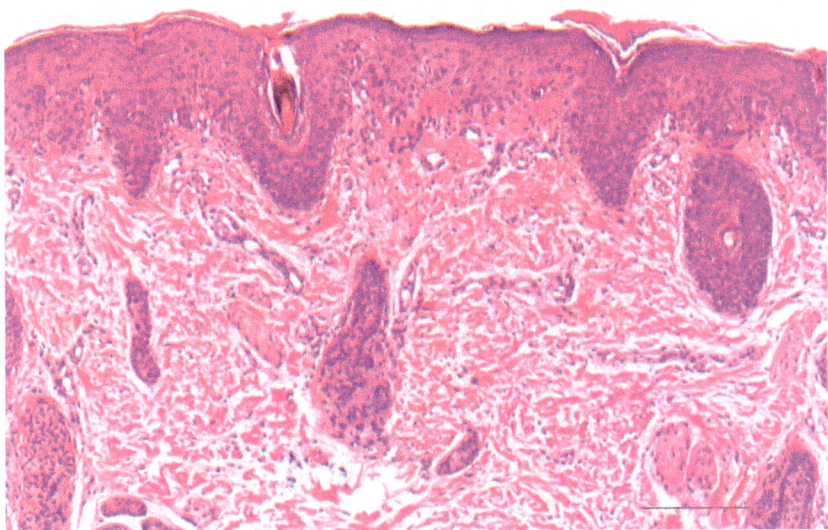

Figure 10. Netherton syndrome. Regular (psoriasiform) hyperplasia with focal parakeratosis and thinned stratum granulosum. Dilated vessels in the papillary dermis and inflammatory infiltrates. HE stain, bar = 100 μm.

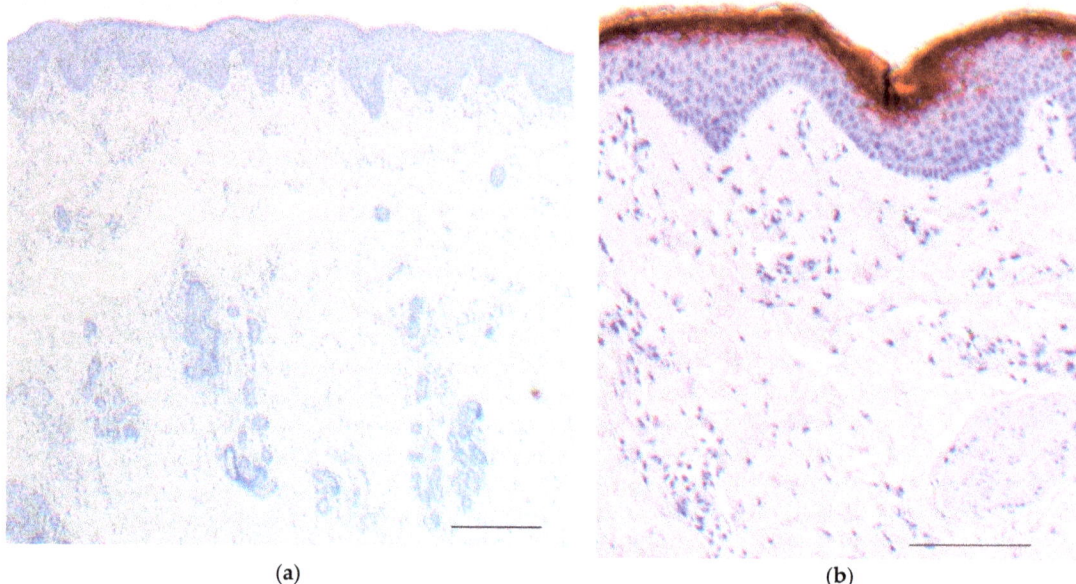

Figure 11. Netherton syndrome, immunohistochemistry, bar = 200 µm (**a**,**b**). Immunohistochemistry shows a lack of staining for LEKTI in the epidermis and hair follicles (**a**); regular expression of LEKTI in the upper layers of the epidermis of healthy skin, bar = 200 µm (**b**). Immunoperoxidase staining.

9.2. Differential Diagnoses

Psoriasis vulgaris or atopic dermatitis cannot always be differentiated histologically. PAS-positive granules in the stratum corneum cannot always be detected and are not specific. The immunohistochemically detectable lack of LEKTI expression is important evidence for Netherton syndrome. Other forms of ichthyosis with psoriasis-like histology are listed in Table 2.

10. Peeling Skin Disease

In peeling skin disease (peeling skin syndrome B), generalized erythema with superficial skin detachment is evident from birth and persists throughout life with seasonal variation (Figure 12). In addition, episodic detachment of the nail plates (onychomadesis) may occur. Hair status is inconspicuous except for a transient slight epilation of fine hairs [23].

There is a mutation of corneodesmosin, an important adhesion protein expressed in the extracellular sections of desmosomes in the stratum corneum of the epidermis, as well as at the inner hair root sheath of hair follicles (Table 3). Ultrastructurally, there is detachment of intact corneocytes from the stratum granulosum (extracellular cleft formation) [20,23]. Autosomal dominant mutations in other domains of corneodesmosin cause hypotrichosis simplex.

Concomitant barrier disruption leads to inflammation with massive pruritus, urticaria, angioedema, food allergy, and asthma with elevated IgE levels and blood eosinophilia.

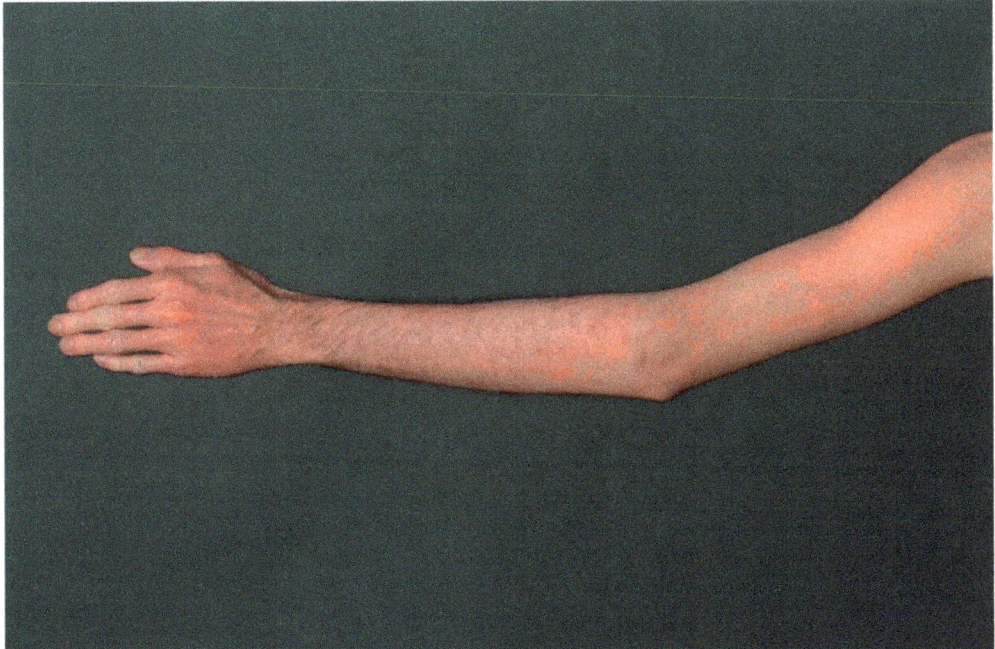

Figure 12. Peeling skin disease. Diffuse erythema with superficial skin detachment is evident from birth and persists throughout life with seasonal variation.

10.1. Histology

The epidermis is hyperplastic with prominent rete ridges. There is mild hyperkeratosis with focal parakeratosis and thinned stratum granulosum. Some biopsies show a focal detachment of the stratum corneum, and in some cases, the stratum corneum is completely absent. However, these changes cannot always be detected on a paraffin section. There are superficial and perivascular lymphocytic infiltrates with single neutrophils, which are also found in the stratum corneum. The papillary body is elongated and edematous, vessels are not dilated [7]. Immunohistochemically, staining for corneodesmosin is absent in the stratum corneum [23].

10.2. Differential Diagnosis

Psoriasis vulgaris, Netherton syndrome, and CHILD syndrome cannot be differentiated without immunohistochemistry.

11. CHILD Syndrome

Congenital Hemidysplasia with Ichthyosiform nevus and Limb Defect (CHILD) syndrome is a very rare X-linked dominant disorder that is usually lethal for male offspring. It is characterized by unilateral inflammatory, often waxy, yellow skin lesions, emphasized in the large flexures and perianogenital region [8,24]. Extracutaneous symptoms range from discrete hypoplasia of the limbs to severe deformities. Monosymptomatic cases are often misdiagnosed as psoriasis or ILVEN [25].

The disorder is caused by nonsense or missense mutations in the so-called *NSDHL* gene, which lead to a disturbance of cholesterol biosynthesis (Table 3) [26,27].

11.1. Histology

Hyperplastic epidermis with elongated rete ridges and marked orthohyperkeratosis with focal parakeratosis are found. The stratum granulosum may be prominent in some areas but can also be absent. A perivascular lymphocytic infiltrate and xanthomatous macrophages that are markedly immunoreactive for adipophilin are apparent in the papillary body [7].

11.2. Differential Diagnoses

Verruciform xanthomas also contain xanthomatous macrophages, which are absent in the other major differential diagnoses as psoriasis inversa and epidermal nevus. The presence of verruciform xanthomas or verruciform xanthoma-like changes in the setting of CHILD syndrome is possible.

12. Severe Dermatitis, Multiple Allergies, Metabolic Wasting Syndrome (SAM Syndrome)

SAM syndrome was identified as a severe life-threatening genodermatosis by Liat Samuelov et al. in 2013 [28]. The acronym stands for severe dermatitis, multiple allergies, metabolic wasting syndrome. It is caused by a mutation of desmoglein−1 (DSG1) (Table 3), a major desmosomal adhesion molecule also involved in pemphigus disease. Later, a *desmoplakin* mutation was also identified [29]. The disease is inherited in an autosomal recessive manner; heterozygous carriers of the *DSG1* mutation develop only striate palmoplantar keratoderma [30].

Clinically, there is ichthyosiform erythroderma in newborns similar to autosomal recessive lamellar ichthyosis, Netherton syndrome, or peeling skin disease. Other symptoms are pruritus, hypotrichosis, food allergies with elevated IgE, dysphagia, decreased growth, and recurrent skin and respiratory infections. In varying degrees, pustular formation, palmoplantar keratoses, onychodystrophy, dental anomalies, cardiac abnormalities, and eosinophilic esophagitis are found. There is marked inter- and intrafamilial variability [30]. The accompanying inflammation can be explained by proinflammatory activity in keratinocytes in the context of impaired barrier function and downregulated blockage of signal transduction pathways [31]. Furthermore, the intracytoplasmic portion of DSG1 blocks the RAS-RAF signaling pathway and, thus, affects epidermal differentiation [32,33]. Similar to Netherton syndrome, anti-inflammatory therapies with biologics improve the clinical picture (Oji V, unpublished).

12.1. Histology

Histologically, there is a superficial lymphocytic dermatitis with hyperplastic epidermis, parakeratosis, and neutrophil granulocytes that strongly resembles psoriasis (psoriasiform dermatitis). However, there are typically dilated intercellular spaces of the epidermis without blistering (Figure 13). Intracellular edema and serum exudate (as in spongiotic dermatitis), and rounding of keratinocytes and pyknosis of nuclei (as in pemphigus disease), hypereosinophilia of cytoplasm (as in M. Darier or Hailey–Hailey), ballooning, and typical viropathic nuclear changes, as in herpes disease, are absent.

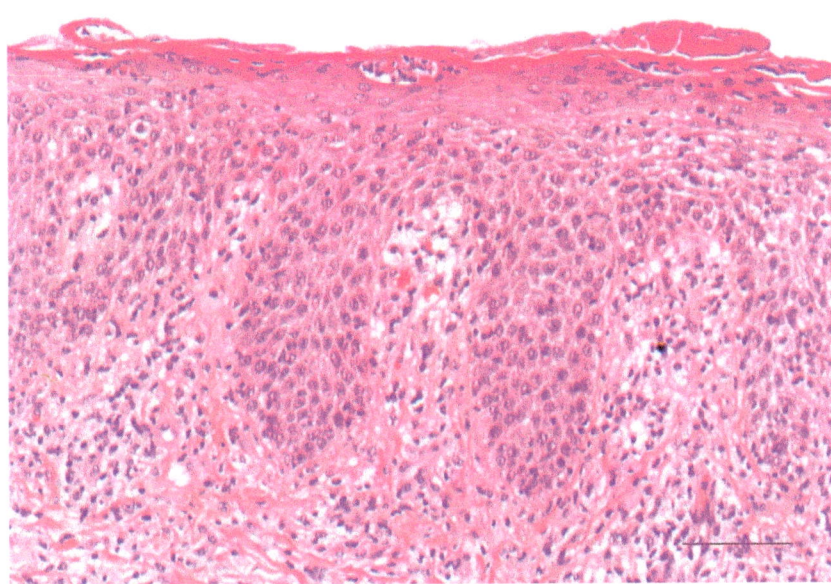

Figure 13. SAM syndrome. Psoriasiform dermatitis with dilated intercellular spaces of the epidermis without blistering ("desmosomal acantholysis"). HE stain, bar = 100 µm.

12.2. Differential Diagnoses

All genodermatoses with mutations of desmosomal proteins leading to the pattern of "desmosomal acantholysis" (Metze, unpublished). These include keratosis palmoplantaris areata et striata (striate palmoplantar keratoderma types 1 and 2), Carvajal-Huerta syndrome, Naxos syndrome, ectodermal dysplasia skin fragility syndrome (McGrath syndrome), or peeling skin disease [34].

Author Contributions: Conceptualization, D.M. and K.S.; methodology, D.M. and K.S.; investigation, D.M., K.S. and H.T.; resources, D.M.; data curation, D.M. and K.S.; writing—original draft preparation, D.M. and K.S.; writing—review and editing, D.M., K.S. and H.T.; visualization, D.M.; supervision, H.T.; project administration, D.M. All authors have read and agreed to the published version of the manuscript.

Funding: This research received no external funding.

Institutional Review Board Statement: Not applicable.

Informed Consent Statement: Not applicable.

Conflicts of Interest: The authors declare no conflict of interest.

Abbreviations

CHILD syndrome	Congenital hemidysplasia with ichthyosiform erythroderma and limb defects syndrome
CRIE	Congenital reticular ichthyosiform erythroderma
EI	Epidermolytic ichthyosis
KID syndrome	Keratitis ichthyosis deafness syndrome
SAM syndrome	Congenital erythroderma–hypotrichosis–recurrent infections–multiple food allergies syndrome
SEI	Superficial epidermolytic ichthyosis

References

1. Krug, M.; Oji, V.; Traupe, H.; Berneburg, M. Ichthyoses-Part 1: Differential diagnosis of vulgar ichthyoses and therapeutic options. *J. Dtsch. Dermatol. Ges.* **2009**, *7*, 511–519. [CrossRef]
2. Krug, M.; Oji, V.; Traupe, H.; Berneburg, M. Ichthyoses-Part 2: Congenital ichthyoses. *J. Dtsch. Dermatol. Ges.* **2009**, *7*, 577–588. [CrossRef] [PubMed]
3. Traupe, H. The Ichthyoses. In *A Guide to Clinical Diagnosis, Genetic Counseling, and Therapy*; Springer: Berlin, Germany, 1989; pp. 103–138.
4. Oji, V.; Traupe, H. Ichthyoses: Differential diagnosis and molecular genetics. *Eur. J. Dermatol.* **2006**, *16*, 349–359. [PubMed]
5. Oji, V.; Tadini, G.; Akiyama, M.; Blanchet Bardon, C.; Bodemer, C.; Bourrat, E.; Coudiere, P.; DiGiovanna, J.J.; Elias, P.; Fischer, J.; et al. Revised nomenclature and classification of inherited ichthyoses: Results of the First Ichthyosis Consensus Conference in Sorèze 2009. *J. Am. Acad. Dermatol.* **2010**, *63*, 607–641. [CrossRef]
6. Metze, D.; Traupe, H. Hereditäre Verhornungsstörungen und epidermale Fehlbildungen. In *Histopathologie der Haut*, 2nd ed.; Cerroni, L., Garbe, C., Metze, D., Kutzner, H., Kerl, H., Eds.; Springer: Berlin, Germany, 2016; Chapter 20; pp. 404–438.
7. Metze, D. Disorders of Keratinization. In *McKee's Pathology of the Skin*, 5th ed.; 2-Volume-Set; Calonje, E., Brenn, T., Lazar, A., McKee, P.H., Eds.; Elsevier: Amsterdam, The Netherlands, 2019; Volume 1, Chapter 3, pp. 53–117.
8. Oji, V.; Metze, D.; Traupe, H. Inherited disorders of cornification. In *Rook's Textbook of Dermatology*, 9th ed.; Burns, T., Breathnach, S., Cox, N., Griffiths, C., Eds.; Wiley-Blackwell: Hoboken, NJ, USA, 2016; Volume 2, Part 6; Chapter 65, pp. 1–75.
9. Majmundar, V.D.; Baxi, K. Hereditary and Acquired Ichthyosis Vulgaris. In *Treasure Island (FL)*; StatPearls Publishing: Treasure Island, FL, USA, 2021.
10. Süßmuth, K.; Gruber, R.; Rodriguez, E.; Traupe, H.; Amler, S.; Sánchez-Guijo, A.; Valentin, F.; Tarinski, T.; Straub, N.; Metze, D.; et al. Increased prevalence of filaggrin deficiency in 51 patients with recessive X-linked ichthyosis presenting for dermatologic examination. *J. Investig. Dermatol.* **2018**, *138*, 709–711. [CrossRef] [PubMed]
11. Kütting, B.; Traupe, H. Der erworbene Ichthyosis-ähnliche Hautzustand. *Hautarztand* **1995**, *46*, 836–840. [CrossRef]
12. Hotz, A.; Kopp, J.; Bourrat, E.; Oji, V.; Komlosi, K.; Giehl, K.; Bouadjar, B.; Bygum, A.; Tantcheva-Poor, I.; Hellström Pigg, M.; et al. Meta-Analysis of Mutations in *ALOX12B* or *ALOXE3* Identified in a Large Cohort of 224 Patients. *Genes* **2021**, *12*, 80. [CrossRef]
13. Raghunath, M.; Hennies, H.C.; Velten, F.; Wiebe, V.; Steinert, P.M.; Reis, A.; Traupe, H. A novel in situ method for the detection of deficient transglutaminase activity in the skin. *Arch. Dermatol. Res.* **1998**, *290*, 621–627. [CrossRef]
14. Rothnagel, J.A.; Dominey, A.M.; Dempsey, L.D.; Longley, M.A.; Greenhalgh, D.A.; Gagne, T.A.; Huber, M.; Frenk, E.; Hohl, D.; Roop, D.R. Mutations in the rod domains of keratins 1 and 10 in epidermolytic hyperkeratosis. *Science* **1992**, *257*, 1128–1130. [CrossRef]
15. Rothnagel, J.A.; Traupe, H.; Wojcik, S.; Huber, M.; Hohl, D.; Pittelkow, M.R.; Saeki, H.; Ishibashi, Y.; Roop, D.R. Mutations in the rod domain of keratin 2e in patients with ichthyosis bullosa of Siemens. *Nat. Genet.* **1994**, *7*, 485–490. [CrossRef]
16. Traupe, H.; Kolde, G.; Hamm, H.; Happle, R. Ichthyosis bullosa of Siemens: A unique type of epidermolytic hyperkeratosis. *J. Am. Acad. Dermatol.* **1986**, *14*, 1000–1005. [CrossRef]
17. Avshalumova, L.; Fabrikant, J.; Koriakos, A. Overview of skin diseases linked to connexin gene mutations. *Int. J. Dermatol.* **2014**, *53*, 192–205. [CrossRef] [PubMed]
18. van Steensel, M.A.M.; Oranje, A.P.; van der Schroeff, J.G.; Wagner, A.; van Geel, M. The missense mutation G12D in connexin30.3 can cause both erythrokeratodermia variabilis of Mendes da Costa and progressive symmetric erythrokeratodermia of Gottron. *Am. J. Med. Genet. A* **2009**, *149A*, 657–661. [CrossRef]
19. van Geel, M.; van Steensel, M.A.; Küster, W.; Hennies, H.C.; Happle, R.; Steijlen, P.M.; König, A. HID and KID syndromes are associated with the same connexin 26 mutation. *Br. J. Dermatol.* **2002**, *146*, 938–942. [CrossRef]
20. Süßmuth, K.; Traupe, H.; Metze, D.; Oji, V. Ichthyoses in everyday practice: Management of a rare group of diseases. *J. Dtsch. Dermatol. Ges.* **2020**, *18*, 225–243. [CrossRef]
21. Chavanas, S.; Bodemer, C.; Rochat, A.; Hamel-Teillac, D.; Ali, M.; Irvine, A.D.; Bonafé, J.L.; Wilkinson, J.; Taïeb, A.; Barrandon, Y.; et al. Mutations in SPINK5, encoding a serine protease inhibitor, cause Netherton syndrome. *Nat. Genet.* **2000**, *25*, 141–142. [CrossRef] [PubMed]
22. Leclerc-Mercier, S.; Bodemer, C.; Furio, L.; Hadj-Rabia, S.; de Peufeilhoux, L.; Weibel, L.; Bursztejn, A.C.; Bourrat, E.; Ortonne, N.; Molina, T.J.; et al. Skin biopsy in Netherton Syndrome: A Histological review of a large series and new findings. *Am. J. Dermatopathol.* **2016**, *38*, 83–91. [CrossRef] [PubMed]
23. Oji, V.; Eckl, K.M.; Aufenvenne, K.; Nätebus, M.; Tarinski, T.; Ackermann, K.; Seller, N.; Metze, D.; Nürnberg, G.; Fölster-Holst, R.; et al. Loss of corneodesmosin leads to severe skin barrier defect, pruritus, and atopy: Unraveling the peeling skin disease. *Am. J. Hum. Genet.* **2010**, *87*, 274–281. [CrossRef] [PubMed]
24. Ramphul, K.; Kota, V.; Mejias, S.G. Child Syndrome. In *Treasure Island (FL)*; StatPearls Publishing: Treasure Island, FL, USA, 2021.
25. Happle, R.; Koch, H.; Lenz, W. The CHILD syndrome. Congenital hemidysplasia with ichthyosiform erythroderma and limb defects. *Eur. J. Pediatr.* **1980**, *134*, 27–33. [CrossRef]
26. Bergqvist, C.; Abdallah, B.; Hasbani, D.J.; Abbas, O.; Kibbi, A.G.; Hamie, L.; Kurban, M.; Rubeiz, N. CHILD syndrome: A modified pathogenesis-targeted therapeutic approach. *Am. J. Med. Genet. A* **2018**, *176*, 733–738. [CrossRef]
27. König, A.; Happle, R.; Bornholdt, D.; Engel, H.; Grzeschik, K.H. Mutations in the NSDHL gene, encoding a 3beta-hydroxysteroid dehydrogenase, cause CHILD syndrome. *Am. J. Med. Genet.* **2000**, *90*, 339–346. [CrossRef]

28. Samuelov, L.; Sarig, O.; Harmon, R.M.; Rapaport, D.; Ishida-Yamamoto, A.; Isakov, O.; Koetsier, J.L.; Gat, A.; Goldberg, I.; Bergman, R.; et al. Desmoglein 1 deficiency results in severe dermatitis, multiple allergies and metabolic wasting. *Nat. Genet.* **2013**, *45*, 1244–1248. [CrossRef]
29. McAleer, M.A.; Pohler, E.; Smith, F.J.D.; Wilson, N.J.; Cole, C.; MacGowan, S.; Koetsier, J.L.; Godsel, L.M.; Harmon, R.M.; Gruber, R.; et al. Severe dermatitis, multiple allergies, and metabolic wasting syndrome caused by a novel mutation in the N-terminal plakin domain of desmoplakin. *J. Allergy. Clin. Immunol.* **2015**, *136*, 1268–1276. [CrossRef]
30. Taiber, S.; Samuelov, L.; Mohamad, J.; Barak, E.C.; Sarig, O.; Shalev, S.A.; Lestringant, G.; Sprecher, E. SAM syndrome is characterized by extensive phenotypic heterogeneity. *Exp. Dermatol.* **2018**, *27*, 787–790. [CrossRef] [PubMed]
31. Polivka, L.; Hadj-Rabia, S.; Bal, E.; Leclerc-Mercier, S.; Madrange, M.; Hamel, Y.; Bonnet, D.; Mallet, S.; Lepidi, H.; Ovaert, C.; et al. Epithelial barrier dysfunction in desmoglein-1 deficiency. *J. Allergy Clin. Immunol.* **2018**, *142*, 702–706.e7. [CrossRef]
32. Hammers, C.M.; Stanley, J.R. Desmoglein-1, differentiation, and disease. *J. Clin. Investig.* **2013**, *123*, 1419–1422. [CrossRef] [PubMed]
33. Ishida-Yamamoto, A.; Igawa, S. Genetic skin diseases related to desmosomes and corneodesmosomes. *J. Dermatol. Sci.* **2014**, *74*, 99–105. [CrossRef] [PubMed]
34. Metze, D.; Oji, V. Palmoplantar Keratodermas. In *Dermatology, Series: Expert Consult*, 4th ed.; Bolognia, J., Schaffer, J., Cerroni, L., Eds.; Elsevier: Philadelphia, PA, USA, 2018; Volume 1, Chapter 58, pp. 924–943.

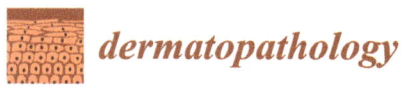

Review

How to Deal with Skin Biopsy in an Infant with Blisters?

Stéphanie Leclerc-Mercier

Reference Center for Genodermatoses (MAGEC Center), Department of Pathology,
Necker-Enfants Malades Hospital, Paris Centre University, 75015 Paris, France; stephanie.leclerc@aphp.fr

Abstract: The onset of blisters in a neonate or an infant is often a source of great concern for both parents and physicians. A blistering rash can reveal a wide range of diseases with various backgrounds (infectious, genetic, autoimmune, drug-related, traumatic, etc.), so the challenge for the dermatologist and the pediatrician is to quickly determine the etiology, between benign causes and life-threatening disorders, for a better management of the patient. Clinical presentation can provide orientation for the diagnosis, but skin biopsy is often necessary in determining the cause of blister formations. In this article, we will provide information on the skin biopsy technique and discuss the clinical orientation in the case of a neonate or infant with a blistering eruption, with a focus on the histology for each etiology.

Keywords: blistering eruption; infant; skin biopsy; genodermatosis; SSSS; hereditary epidermolysis bullosa; keratinopathic ichthyosis; incontinentia pigmenti; mastocytosis; auto-immune blistering diseases

1. Introduction

The onset of blisters in a neonate or an infant (<2 years old) is a source of great concern for both parents and physicians. Therefore, a precise diagnosis, between benign causes and life-threatening disorders, is quickly needed for the best management of the baby.

Several diseases with various backgrounds (infectious, genetic, autoimmune, drug-related, traumatic, etc.) can lead to a blistering eruption.

Skin biopsy is often necessary in determining the cause of the blister formation.

In the present article, only the most frequent etiologies specific to this age group will be described, with a special emphasis on histology in the clinical context (Table 1).

Table 1. Most frequent blistering disorders in neonates and infants.

Infections	Staphylococcal scalded skin syndrome Impetigo Scabies
Genodermatosis	Hereditary epidermolysis bullosa Keratinopathic ichthyosis Incontinentia pigmenti
Cell proliferation	Mastocytosis Langerhans cell histiocytosis
Autoimmune blistering diseases	Bullous pemphigoid and others
Drug reactions	SJS, TEN, etc.

Vesicular and pustular eruptions will not be discussed in this review.

1.1. How Can the Clinical Context Provide Information Concerning the Etiology?

The underlying context of blistering lesions in newborns or infants will sometimes be helpful to provide a clinical orientation. Some elements important to investigate are listed below with examples of etiology:

- distribution of the lesions: localized blisters (traumatic/suction blister, local infection, solitary mastocytosis, etc.)
- general symptoms: fever, systemic disorders (infection, toxic epidermal necrosis, metabolic disorder, etc.)
- tense or flaccid blister/erosion (giving indications on the level of splitting)

1.2. What Is the Appropriate Technique for Skin Biopsy in This Context?

Even if invasive, a skin biopsy is often necessary in this situation for a quick diagnosis and a better management of the patient.

The physician should give the pathologist a precise report with the clinical data, the precise topography of the biopsy, the anesthetic procedure, and a description of the lesion collected. The injection of an anesthetic product will be performed, but an anesthetic cream containing lidocaine prilocaine should not be applied prior to the biopsy since it can be responsible for histopathologic changes and lead to misdiagnosis, and also prevent ultrastructural analysis (vacuolization of keratinocytes) [1].

A skin biopsy will be taken for routine examination, and another will be frozen for immunohistochemistry techniques (split skin is not usually performed in this acute situation). A biopsy for electron microscopy is usually not routinely available but could be useful for genodermatosis diagnosis.

The biopsy should be taken on the most recent lesion within 24 h (and within 12 h when possible):

- for routine histology, it must be performed between the normal skin and the edge of the blister so that the epidermis does not detach as in Figure 1, fixed in formalin, and processed routinely (paraffin embedded, haematoxylin and eosin (HE) staining) in order to determine the anatomic level of the blister
- for immunohistochemistry, it will be frozen or can be put in Michel media
    - if an autoimmune blistering disease (AIBD) is suspected, the biopsy will be performed on healthy perilesional skin and processed for direct immunofluorescence (DIF)
    - if a genodermatosis is suspected, the biopsy will also be taken between the normal skin and the edge of the blister and processed for immunomapping with specialized antibodies (DIF or immunoperoxidase)

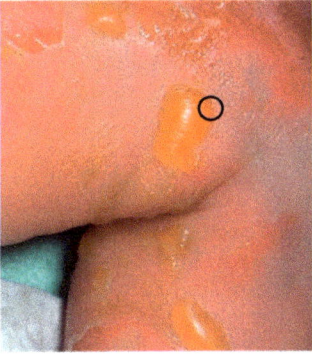

Figure 1. Skin biopsy for EBH, between normal skin and the edge of the blister.

2. Etiologies

2.1. Infections

Infections are the first cause of blistering eruption in neonates and infants.

2.1.1. Staphylococcal Scalded Skin Syndrome (SSSS)

SSSS is an exfoliative, toxin-mediated eruption caused by certain strains of *Staphylococcus aureus* producing an epidermolytic toxin (formerly named exfoliatin). The disease affects mostly neonates and children under 5 years of age but can also affect adults. In neonates, omphalitis is often the origin of the infection [2].

SSSS usually presents with prodromes (irritability, malaise, and fever) followed by a painful erythema, blistering with large areas of epidermal detachment, beginning on the face, neck, axillae, and groin. SSSS is associated with a positive Nikolsky sign (Figure 2a). Mucosae are not affected.

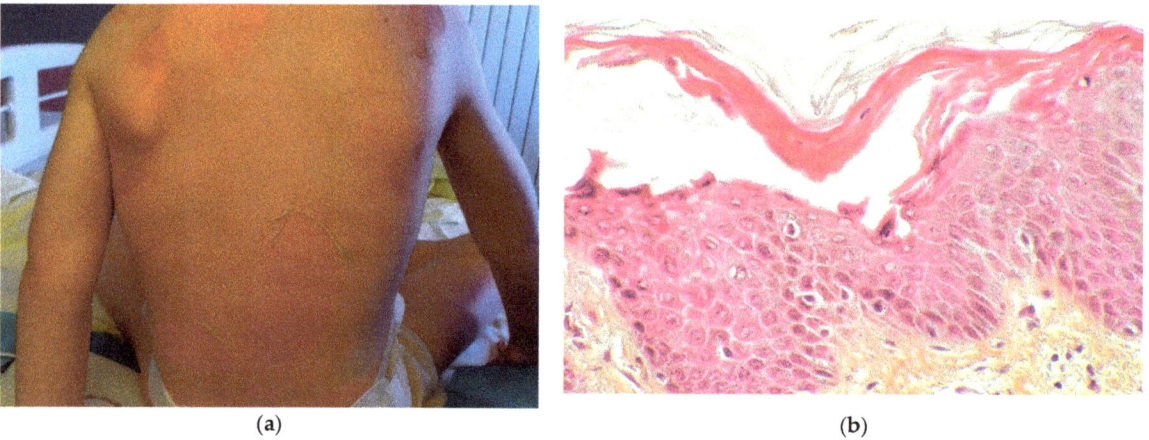

Figure 2. SSSS. (**a**) Clinical appearance of SSSS with Nikolsky sign. (**b**) Hematein eosin ×40: subcorneal blister with acantholysis.

The toxin in SSSS (and also bullous impetigo) causes a cleavage in the granular layer. Skin biopsy is not always performed except in case of toxic epidermal necrosis (TEN) suspicion.

2.1.2. Histology

A subcorneal blister is observed along the granular layer and accompanied by a mild inflammatory infiltrate in the epidermis or dermis. Acantholysis is often present, as shown in Figure 2b, and except in the situation of an old blister, no necrosis is observed. Dermal edema and blood vessel dilatation can be observed in the superficial dermis.

In TEN, the blister is subepidermal and epidermal necrosis is present; a frozen section can be performed for quick results [3].

2.1.3. Impetigo

Bullous impetigo usually affects children between 2 and 5 years of age but can be observed in infants. The disease is usually transmitted through direct contact and cutaneous trauma is often found. Bullous impetigo is considered as a localized form of SSSS and caused by the same strains of *S. aureus* producing an epidermolytic toxin. Superficial vesicles progress to a flaccid blister replaced with yellow crusting after rupture with a peripheral peeling, which is helpful for the diagnosis (Figure 3a). Bullous impetigo is often located in infants in moist areas, such as the perineum, axillae, and neck folds, sparing the mucosae [4].

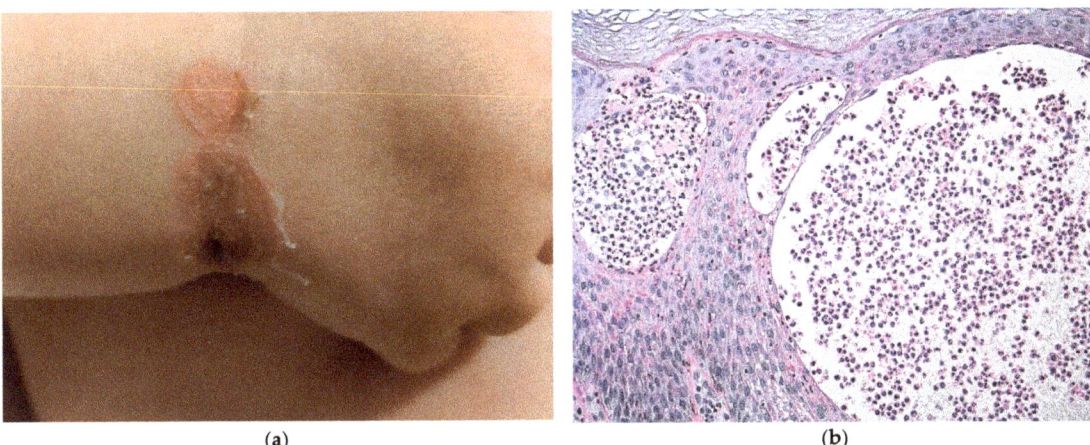

Figure 3. Impetigo. (**a**) Post-bullous lesion of impetigo. (**b**) PAS staining × 20: Impetigo, vesicles filled with neutrophils.

2.1.4. Histology

Skin biopsy is rarely necessary. As in SSSS, the cleavage is subcorneal and the blister usually contains neutrophils (Figure 3b), acantholytic cells, and sometimes Gram-positive germs.

Superficial dermis is inflammatory (lymphocytes and neutrophils).

The main differential diagnosis of impetigo is superficial pemphigus in cases with acantholytic cells [5].

2.1.5. Scabies

Scabies is a contagious disorder caused by the infestation of the skin with *Sarcoptes scabiei* var. *hominis*. It can occasionally have a blistering presentation, as in Figure 4a.

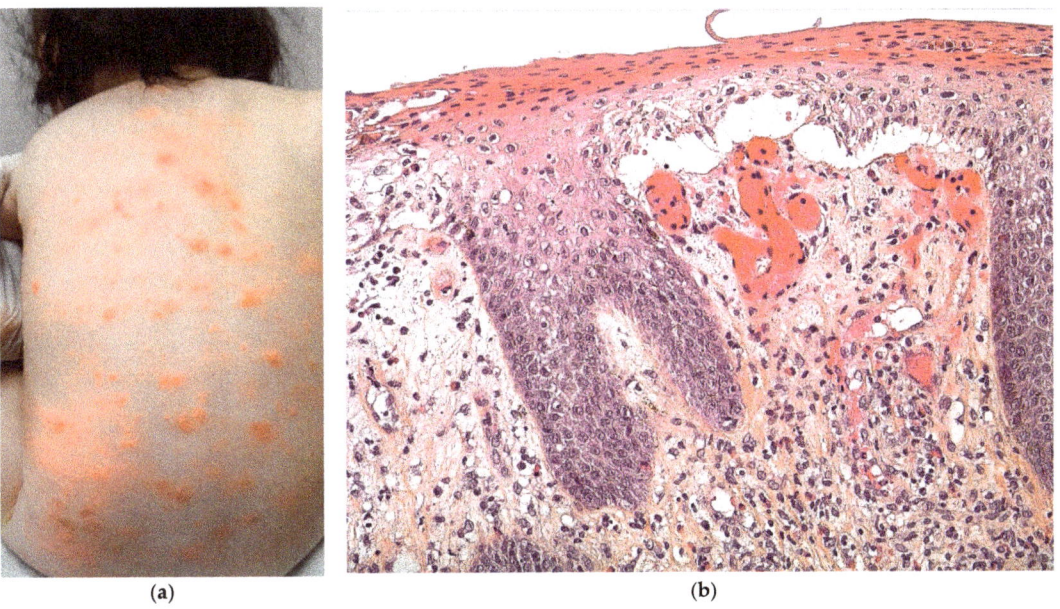

Figure 4. Scabies. (**a**) Blistering scabies. (**b**) Hematein eosin ×20: dermo-epidermal blister and inflammatory infiltrate with eosinophils in the dermis.

In infants, palms and soles are often involved as well as the sides of the feet.

The presence of an individual or familial pruritus, often during night, provides clinical orientation [5].

2.1.6. Histology

A skin biopsy is not performed to confirm the diagnosis of scabies but usually because of the suspicion of another diagnosis, such as an autoimmune blistering disease.

The epidermis is acanthotic with an important spongiosis resulting in vesiculation and blistering (Figure 4b), with exocytosis of eosinophils and neutrophils. Serial cuts can reveal the female mite and her eggs in the stratum corneum. An important inflammatory cell infiltrate is present in the dermis, along the vessels and adnexae, made of lymphocytes, histiocytes, and eosinophils. Langerhans cells may be numerous and sometimes, if an immunohistochemistry with anti-CD1a antibody is performedit can be misleading and result in a Langerhans cell histiocytosis diagnosis. Flame figures are often present in infants.

2.2. Genodermatosis

2.2.1. Hereditary Epidermolysis Bullosa

Inherited epidermolysis bullosa (EB) comprises a highly heterogeneous group of rare diseases characterized by fragility and/or blistering of the skin and mucosae. EB type and subtype classification is presently defined by "onion skin", terminology based on the combination of level of skin cleavage corresponding to the major EB type, the clinical severity, the inheritance pattern, and the molecular defect, including the relative protein expression and the disease-causing sequence variant (Table 2) [6].

Table 2. Classical types of EB (adapted from Ref. [6]).

Level of Skin Cleavage	EB Type	Inheritance	Mutated Gene (s)	Targeted Protein (s)
Intraepidermal	EB simplex	Autosomal dominant	KRT5, KRT14	Keratin 5, keratin 14
			PLEC	Plectin
			KLHL24	Kelch-like member 24
		Autosomal recessive	KRT5, KRT14	Keratin 5, keratin 14
			DST	Bullous pemphigoid antigen 230 (BP230) (syn. BPAG1e, dystonin)
			EXPH5 (syn. SLAC2B)	Exophilin-5 (syn. synaptotagmin-like protein homolog lacking C2 domains b, Slac2-b)
			PLEC	Plectin
			CD151(syn. TSPAN24)	CD151 antigen (syn. tetraspanin 24)
Junctional	Junctional EB	Autosomal recessive	LAMA3, LAMB3, LAMC2	Laminin 332
			COL17A1	Type XVII collagen
			ITGA6, ITGB4	Integrin a6b4
			ITGA3	Integrin a3 subunit
Dermal	Dystrophic EB	Autosomal dominant	COL7A1	Type VII collagen
		Autosomal recessive	COL7A1	Type VII collagen
Mixed	Kindler EB	Autosomal recessive	FERMT1 (syn. KIND1)	Fermitin family homolog 1 (syn. kindlin-1)

There are four main subtypes: EB simplex (EBS), junctional EB (JEB), dystrophic EB (DEB), and Kindler syndrome [7].

In these four subtypes, mucocutaneous fragility is the result of abnormalities of the cutaneous basement membrane zone (BMZ) (hemidesmosomes, focal adhesions, anchoring filaments, and anchoring fibrils) [8].

The clinical appearance depends on the level of skin cleavage: superficial blisters or erosions will occur with EBS, and blisters will be more profound with JEB, DEB, and KS, and lead to ulcerations. Blisters may be generalized or localized to the extremities, as shown in Figure 5a,b.

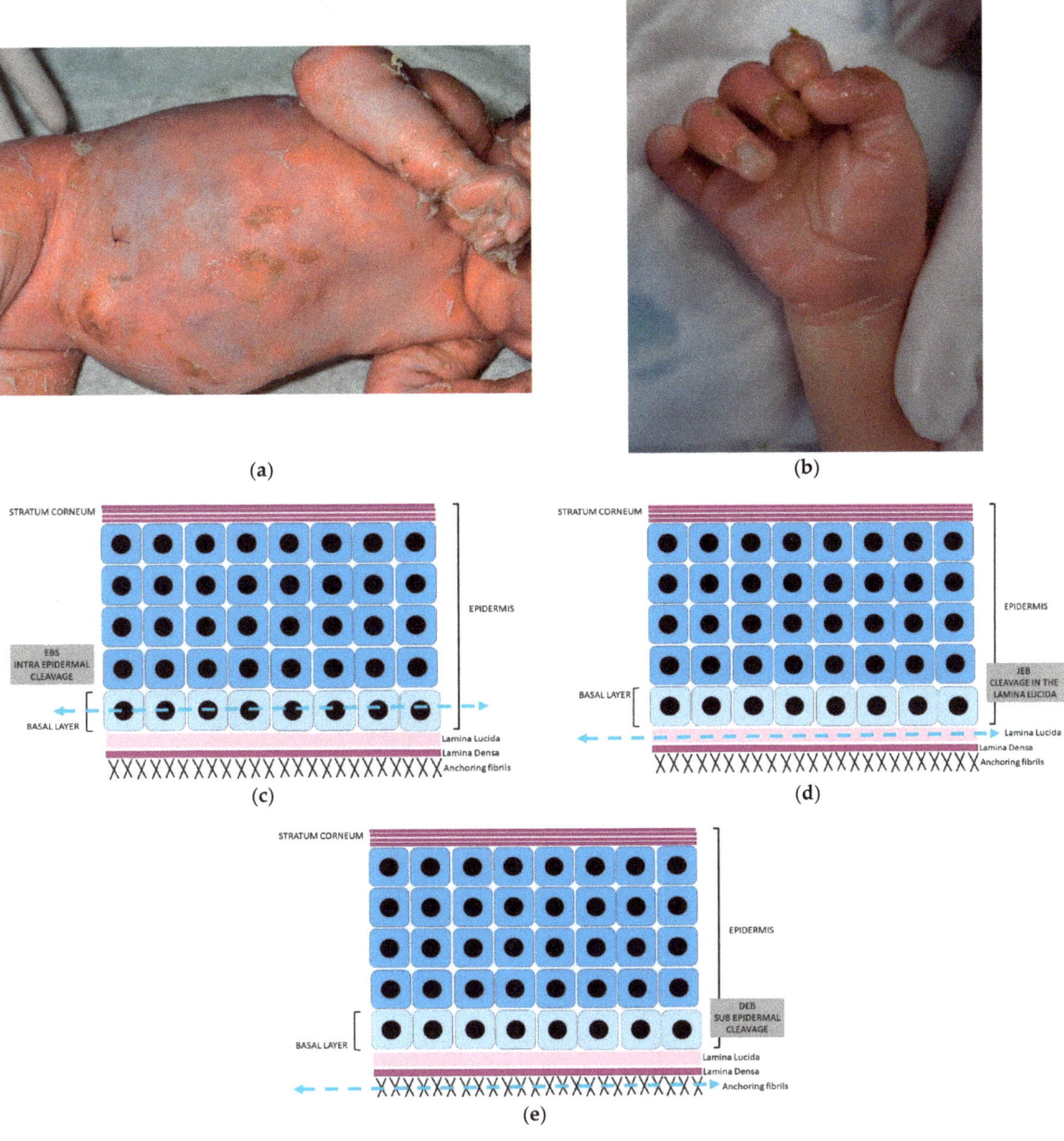

Figure 5. Cont.

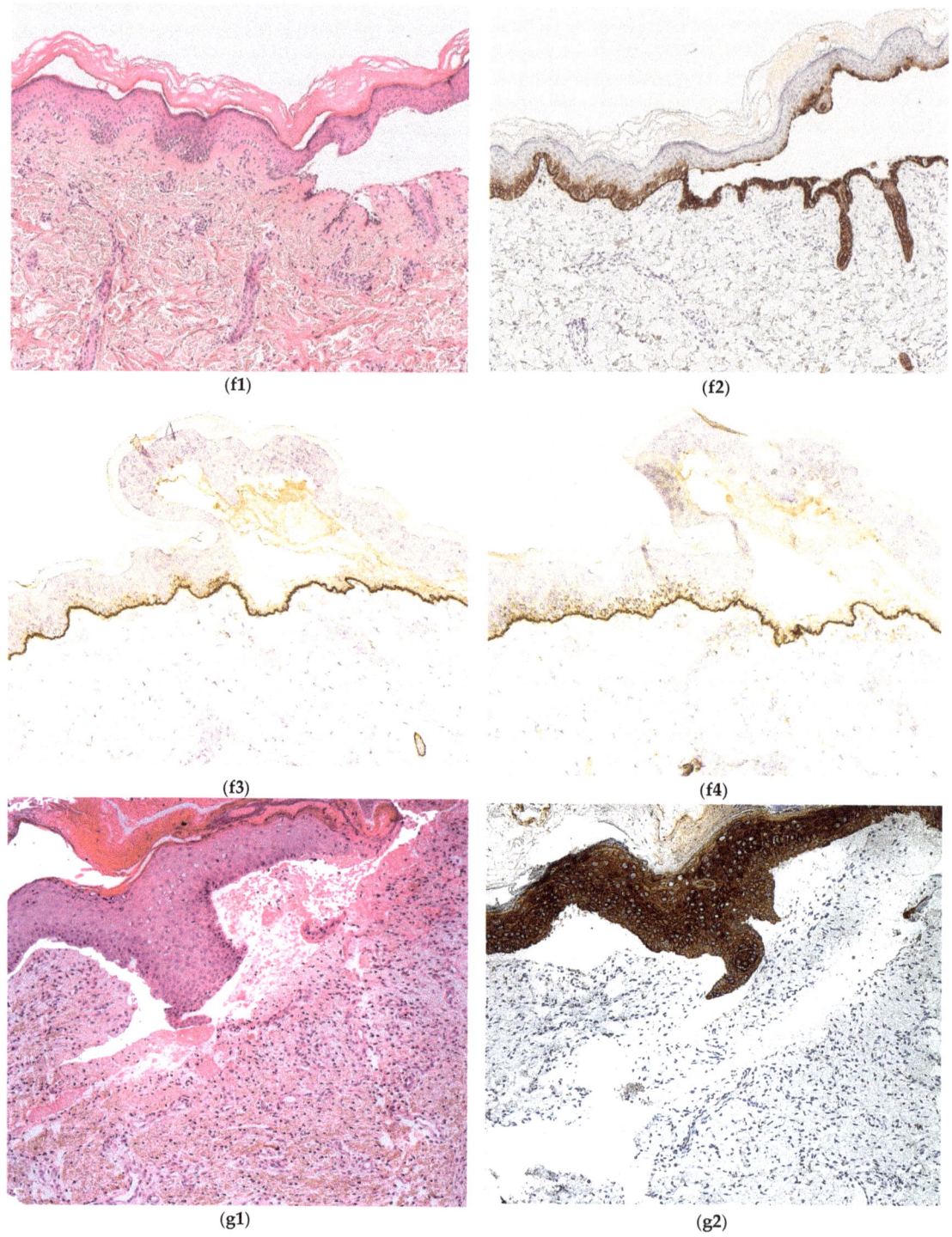

Figure 5. Cont.

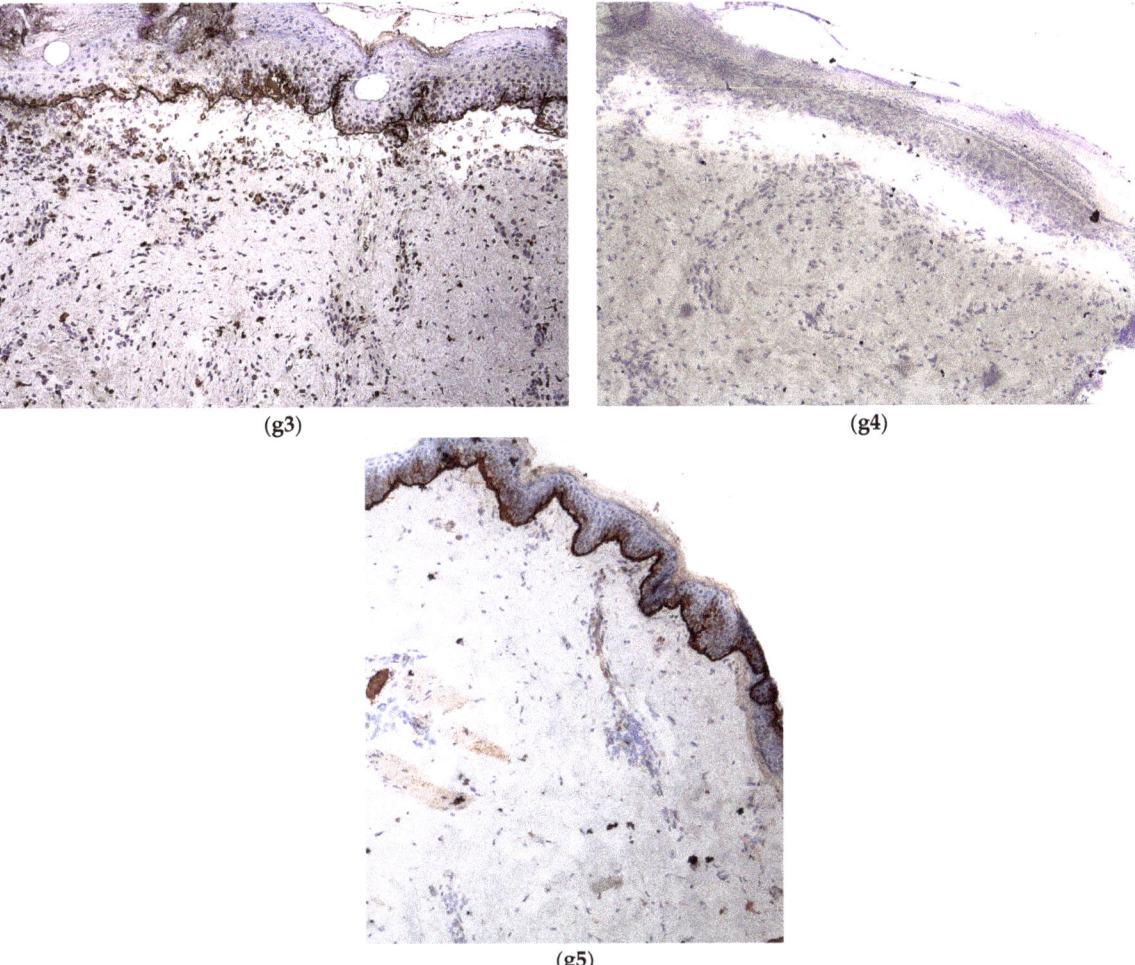

Figure 5. Hereditary epidermolysis bullosa. (**a**) Generalised blisters in EBS. (**b**) Cutaneous aplasia in EBJ. (**c**) EBS: intraepidermal cleavage. (**d**) EBJ: cleavage in lamina lucida. (**e**) EBD: cleavage in anchoring fibrils. EB simplex: (**f1**) Hematein eosin ×10: blister at the DEJ with vacuolization of basal keratinocytes (arrows) and remnants of basal keratinocytes (asterisk) on the floor of the blister; (**f2**) immunohistochemistry with anti-pan cytokeratin antibody showing positivity on the roof and the floor of the blister; (**f3,f4**) immunohistochemistry with anti-laminin and anti-collagen VII antibodies showing positivity on the floor of the blister. Dystrophic EB: (**g1**) Hematein eosin X10 blister at the DEJ; (**g2**) immunohistochemistry with anti-pan cytokeratin antibody showing positivity on the roof of the blister; (**g3**) immunohistochemistry with anti-laminin showing positivity on the roof of the blister; and (**g4**) anti-collagen VII antibodies showing absence of expression compared to a control (**g5**).

The skin defects heal with dyschromia, atrophy, and scarring. Mucosae and skin adnexa (nails, hair) are also affected.

A correct and rapid diagnosis of EB type is mandatory for an optimal management of the baby, for parent information about prognosis, for therapeutic options, and also for genetic counseling.

Immunomapping is the first diagnostic step as it can deliver rapid results in less than 48 h [8].

2.2.2. Histology

The biopsy (see technique above) must be taken in a fresh lesion because, after a short delay, re-epithelialization occurs, and the real level of the blister will be difficult to assess.

Standard histology will usually show a subepidermal blister in all subtypes; the epidermis is usually intact, except in an old biopsy in which necrosis of the epidermis can be observed. In EBS, eosinophilic granules corresponding to tonofilaments clumping may be present, as well as modifications of basal keratinocytes (vacuolisation) and occasionally keratinocyte remnants are present on the floor (Figure 5(f1)).

The blister is usually empty without inflammatory cells when recent, but inflammation can occasionally be observed. The floor of the blister is made of dermis with conservation of the papillary relief and no or little inflammation, except in the case of generalized EBS.

Immunomapping will be performed on the fixed and frozen biopsies to assess the level of cleavage of the blister (Figure 6).

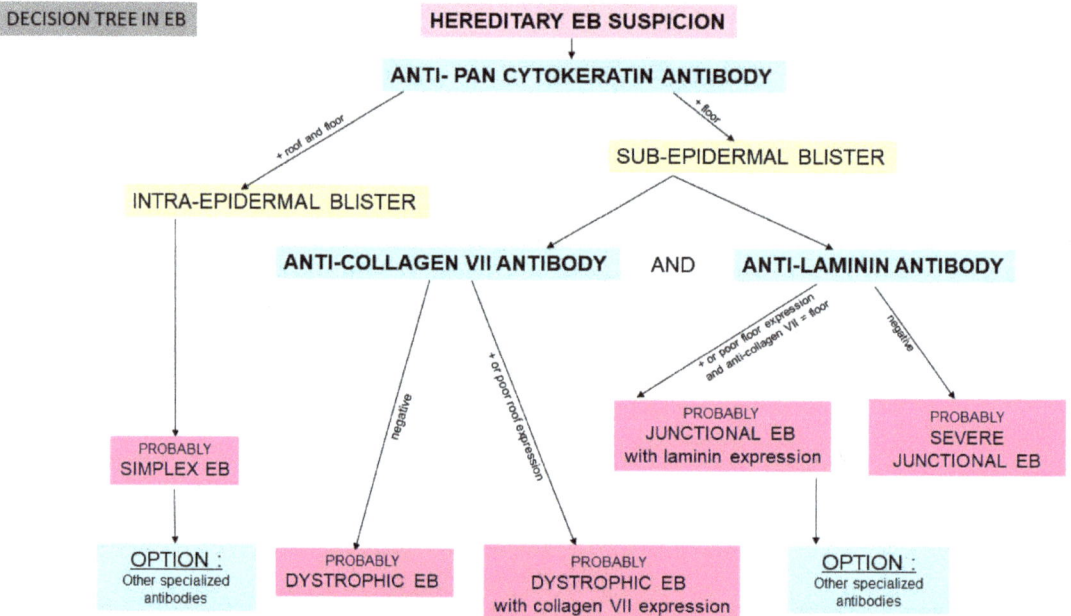

Figure 6. Decision tree.

The location of the cleavage is detailed in Figure 5c–e.

In general pathology laboratories, immunohistochemistry with anti-pan cytokeratin and anti-collagen 4 antibodies can be used to provide rapid results.

In specialized centers, three main antibodies can be introduced as a first step for immunomapping because they are necessary for diagnosis of the three main EB subtypes (EBS, JEB, DEB):

- anti-pan cytokeratin AE1/AE3
- anti-laminin antibody
- anti-collagen VII antibody

If necessary, other specialized antibodies are introduced to study the other proteins of the DEJ (anti-integrin, anti-plectin, anti-BP180).

Figure 5(f1–g5) show examples of immunomapping in two different subtypes of EB.

2.2.3. Keratinopathic Ichthyosis (KI)

KI is a new umbrella term defined by the First Ichthyosis Consensus Conference in Sorèze in 2009, which revised the nomenclature and classification of inherited ichthyoses [9].

KI encompasses ichthyoses caused by keratin mutations, namely epidermolytic ichthyosis (EI), superficial epidermolytic ichthyosis (SEI), and other non-blistering variants.

Newborns may show widespread blistering resembling epidermolysis bullosa (Figure 7a), or have severe erythroderma requiring a specific management, so an early diagnosis is therefore necessary.

A correct diagnosis of ichthyosis is essential for genetic counseling but also for patient information about prognosis and therapeutic options.

These rare keratinization disorders are due to pathogenic variants in the genes encoding keratins 1, 2, or 10. Mutations result in keratin clumping and collapse of the cytoskeleton in the suprabasal keratinocytes (keratin 1 or 10) or upper layers (keratin 2).

The presence of palmoplantar keratoderma (Figure 7b) provides clinical orientation for keratin 1 mutations as keratin 10 is absent in palms and soles.

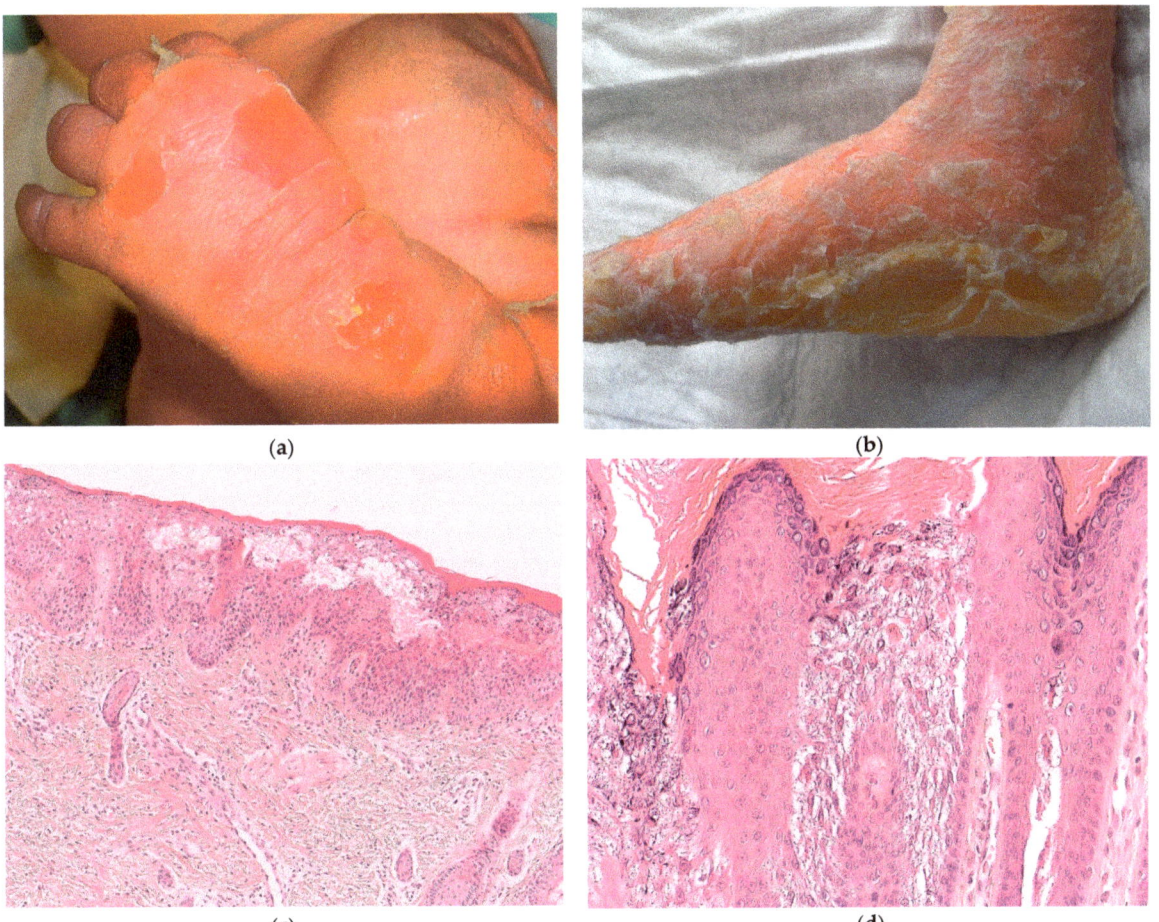

Figure 7. Cont.

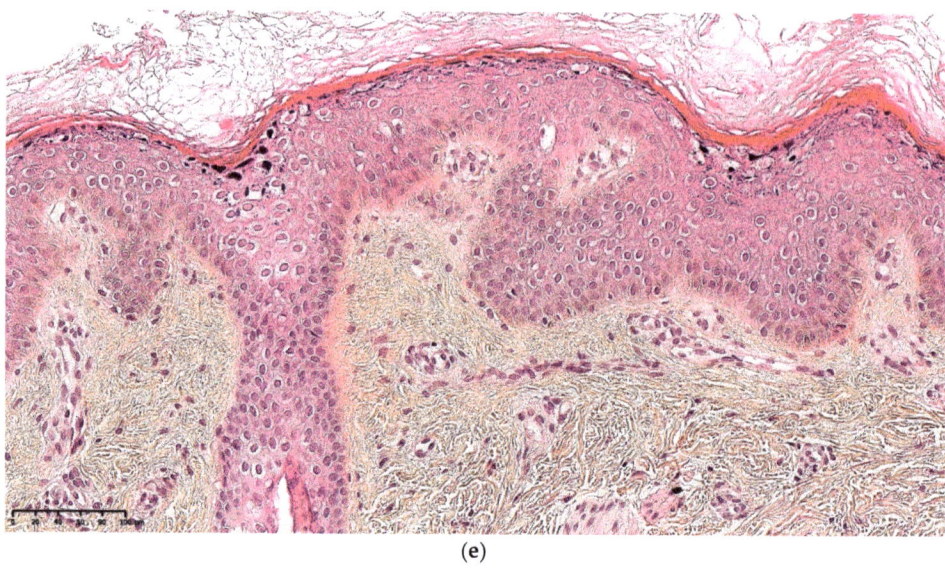

(e)

Figure 7. Epidermolytic ichthyosis. (**a**) Newborn with superficial blisters and erythroderma. (**b**) Palmoplantar keratoderma in *CK1 mutation*. (**c**) Hematein eosin ×10: confluent epidermolysis leading to blister. (**d**) Hematein eosin ×20: epidermolysis with basophilic and eosinophilic granules. (**e**) Hematein eosin ×20: SEI, epidermolysis is located in the granular layer.

2.2.4. Histology

The histological diagnosis of EI will easily and quickly help the physician, since the appearance of epidermolysis is visible at a low magnification with the typical appearance of epidermolytic hyperkeratosis [10–12], with vacuolated suprabasal keratinocytes, affecting the upper part or the entire epidermis with or without a blister formation (Figure 7c). The stratum corneum can become very thick following the first days of life, sometimes compact or more basket-weave like. The granular layer is also affected, containing basophilic granules and the keratinocytes containing eosinophilic granules, corresponding to clumps of tonofilaments in electron microscopy (Figure 7d).

Interestingly, the diagnosis of KI can be performed very early in life and the diagnosis can be very fast in a newborn just by the examination of a frozen section, therefore eliminating the other differential diagnosis of extensive skin blisters, such as infection or hereditary epidermolysis bullosa. In our experience, the clinical appearance does not correlate with the intensity of histologic abnormalities.

Recently, Galler et al. [13] reported the opportunity of a quick diagnosis with minimal trauma to the patient by performing the "jelly-roll" technique. The observation of the roof of a blister shows characteristic findings of epidermolytic hyperkeratosis, which included hyperkeratosis with granular layer degeneration, vacuolization, and eosinophilic globules. The authors suggest that this technique can be used for the diagnosis of EI.

The histology of SEI shares the appearance of classical EI but is restricted to the more superficial spinous and granular cell layers (Figure 7e) with possible intracorneal blister formation [14]. The distribution of granular degeneration is consistent with the expression site of keratin 2.

2.2.5. Incontinentia Pigmenti (IP)

IP is a rare X-linked dominant genodermatosis caused by mutations in the inhibitor of the kappa B kinase gamma (IKBKG) (previously known as NEMO or nuclear factor kappa B essential modulator) gene. IP affects mostly female patients and is usually lethal in utero for males, but cases in boys are reported [15,16]. The phenotype in females is variable, manifestations being dependent on the effects of mosaicism resulting from X-chromosome lyonization.

IP is a multisystem disorder of ectodermal origin and skin lesions may be associated with dental, ocular, and neurologic abnormalities. The skin is almost always involved in neonates. The lesions are classically vesiculobullous, following the Blaschko lines, and represent the first stage of cutaneous involvement. They are usually located on the limbs, trunk, and scalp (Figure 8a). Later stages are characterized by verrucous papules (stage 2), whorled hyperpigmentation (stage 3), and pallor and scarring (stage 4); different stages may overlap and only stages 1, 2, and 3 can be seen in infants. Skin histology is helpful for all 4 stages [17].

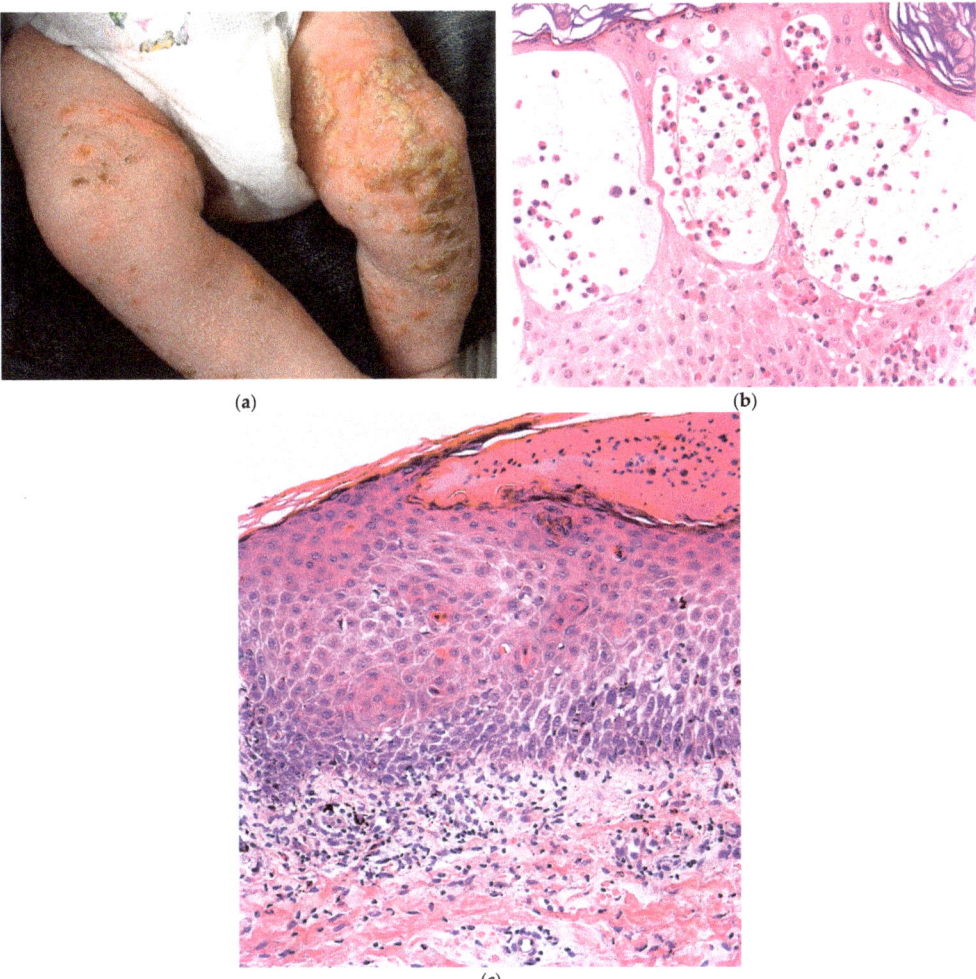

Figure 8. Incontinentia pigmenti. (**a**) Newborn with blistering Blaschko-linear eruption. (**b**) Hematein eosin ×40: spongiosis with eosinophils leading to vesicles. (**c**) Hematein eosin ×20: numerous apoptotic keratinocytes.

The differential diagnosis of IP lesions in newborns are herpes simplex infection, congenital varicella, and autoimmune blistering diseases, but the Blaschko-linear disposition of the lesion is helpful. Genodermatosis, including Conradi–Hunermann–Happle syndrome or Goltz syndrome, needs to be ruled out with histology.

The skin biopsy is therefore always performed and of great help.

2.2.6. Histology

At stage 1, eosinophilic spongiosis is observed, and its confluence leads to vesiculation and blisters (Figure 8b). Dyskeratotic/apoptotic keratinocytes (isolates or aggregates) are an important clue for diagnosis and can be assessed with serial cuts when necessary (Figure 8c). An inflammatory dermal infiltrate with eosinophils may be present. Free melanin can be observed in the dermis even at stage 1. In cases with an overlap between stages 1 and 2, hyperkeratosis, papillomatosis, and acanthosis can be present, as well as numerous apoptotic cells.

2.3. Cell Proliferation

2.3.1. Mastocytosis

Mastocytosis is caused by a clonal mast cell proliferation associated with somatic activating mutations in *c-kit*. All forms of cutaneous mastocytosis may be associated with blistering in infancy, but the most frequent form associated with blisters is solitary mastocytoma. Clinical assessment will find a history of infiltrated red/purple lesions associated with the occurrence of blisters. Another very rare presentation is diffuse cutaneous mastocytosis (DCM) in a neonate having erythroderma and generalized blisters, and may be so serious that it mimics staphylococcal scalded skin syndrome (Figure 9a). The episodes of skin blisters are accompanied by pruritus and redness all over the body. The tendency to blister usually improves over 3–4 years [18–20].

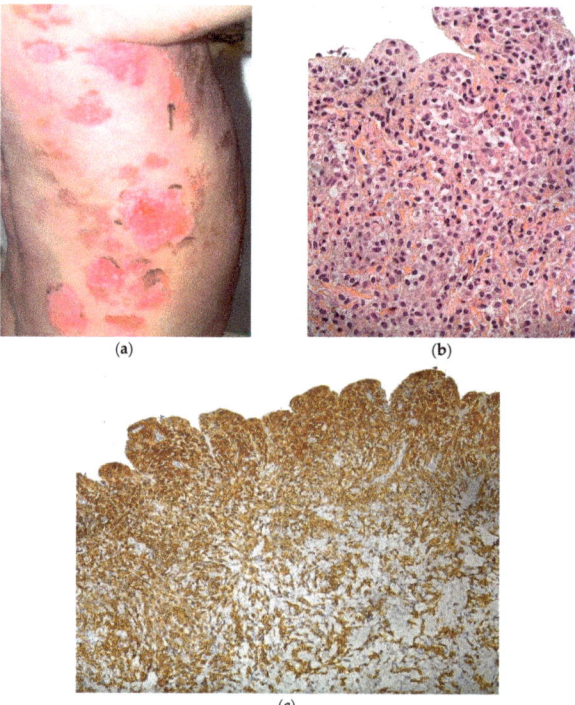

Figure 9. Mastocytosis. (**a**) Generalized blisters. (**b**) Hematein eosin ×40: floor of the blister, conservation of papillary relief, and dense mastocytes infiltrate. (**c**) Immunohistochemistry with anti-CD117 antibody ×10: positivity of the dermal infiltrate.

2.3.2. Histology

Skin biopsy shows a subepidermal blister surrounding a dense dermal mast cell infiltrate (Figure 9b). Immunohistochemistry is positive for the *c-kit* (anti-CD117) antibody(Figure 9c).

2.3.3. Langerhans Cell Histiocytosis (LCH)

LCH is a rare disease characterized by the aberrant clonal proliferation of Langerhans cells. Blistering presentation in cutaneous Langerhans cell histiocytosis, even if infrequent, may happen in the self-healing form (Figure 10a) [21–24].

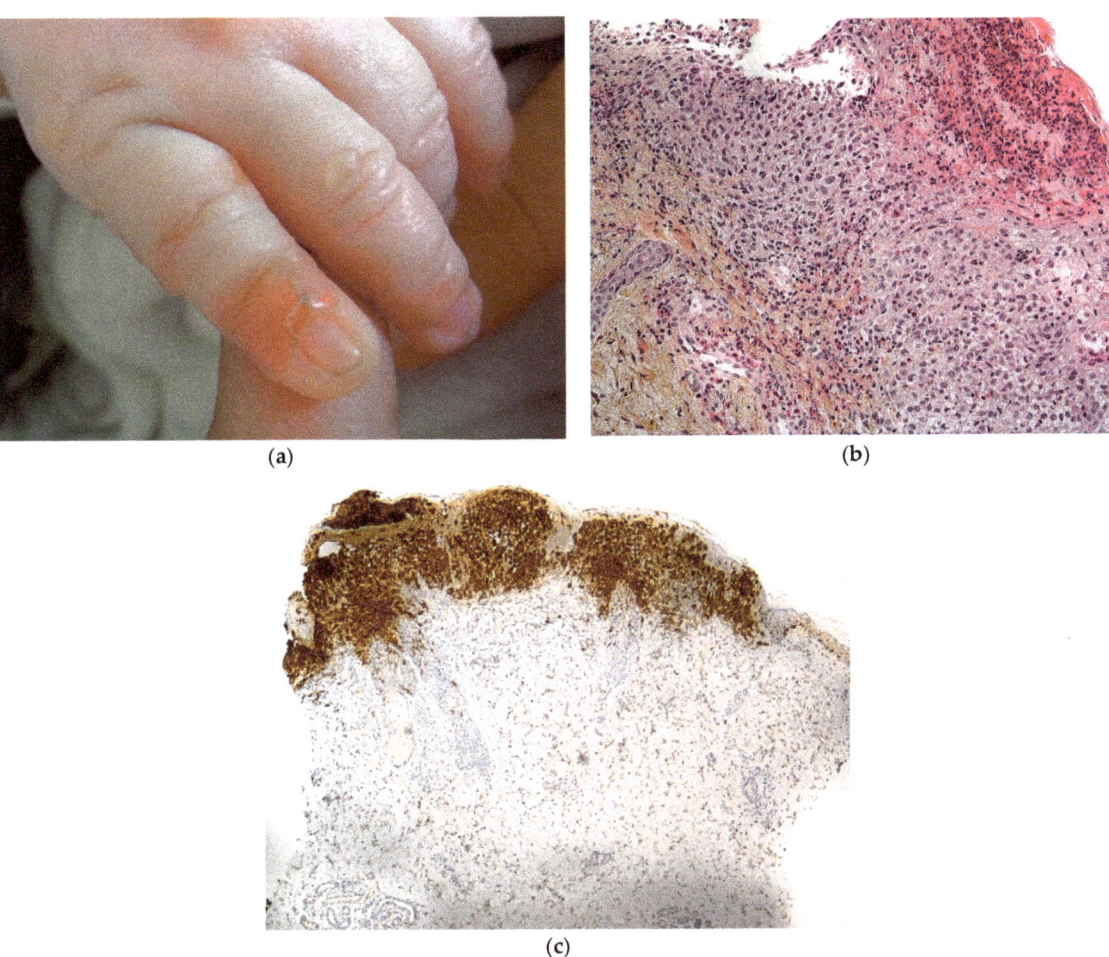

Figure 10. Langerhans cell histiocytosis. (**a**) Blister in a neonate. (**b**) Hematein eosin ×40: papillary infiltration with Langerhans cell, exocytosis resulting in blister and crusts, eosinophilic infiltrate in the dermis. (**c**) Immunohistochemistry with anti-CD1a antibody ×5: positivity of the dermal infiltrate.

2.3.4. Histology

Langerhans cells (LC) have coffee-bean or kidney-shaped nuclei. The histiocytic infiltrate is epidermotropic and also situated in the papillary dermis, sometimes extending to the reticular dermis. The blister is situated at the dermo-epidermal junction. In the dermis, the infiltration is often associated with eosinophils and lymphocytes (Figure 10b).

Detection of LC markers (CD1a and CD207 on formalin-fixed sample) is mandatory to confirm the diagnosis (Figure 10c).

2.3.5. Auto-Immune Blistering Diseases

Bullous Pemphigoid (BP)

Bullous pemphigoid (BP), usually seen in elderly populations, is a rare condition in children. Like in adults, tense serous fluid-filled or hemorrhagic bullae occur on an inflammatory base or urticated plaques. The eruption is widespread and mucous membranes are not affected. Acral involvement (palms, soles, and head) is more common in infantile BP, sometimes with a bunch of grapes appearance (Figure 11) [25–27].

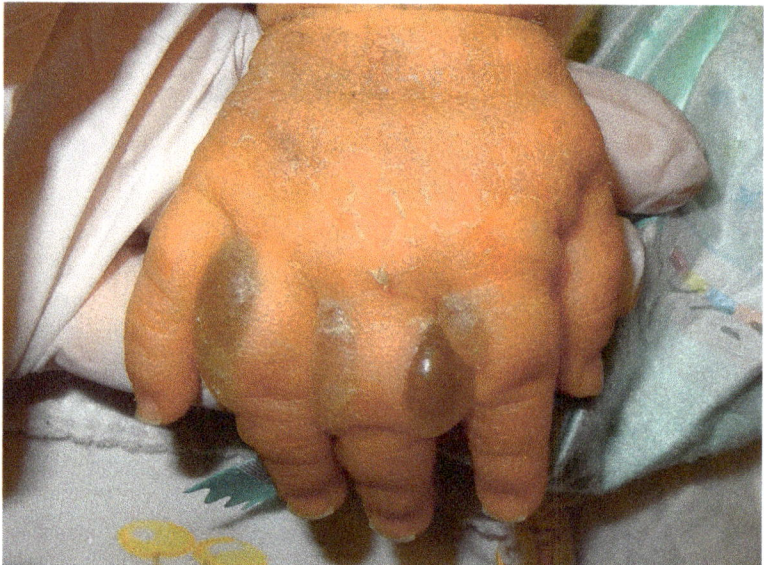

Figure 11. Bullous pemphigoid with typical appearance of bunch of grapes on the hand of an infant.

2.3.6. Histology

Skin histology is not different from BP in adults: subepidermal blistering is observed associated with an inflammatory infiltrate made of eosinophils and often neutrophils.

Histopathology shows eosinophilic spongiosis with clefting. DIF reveals linear deposition of IgG and/or C3 along the basement membrane. IgA deposition is also often seen.

2.3.7. Other AIBDs

The other AIBDs are less frequent in this age group, since only about 50 cases of neonatal AIBDs were identified in a systematic review of the literature [28].

Pemphigus vulgaris, pemphigus foliaceus, bullous pemphigoid, pemphigoid gestationis, IgA-linear dermatosis, and epidermolysis bullosa acquisita have been reported in babies of affected mothers (antibodies are passively transferred from the mother to the neonate). Pemphigoid diseases are more likely to present after birth and were more predominant in males [25–27].

Skin histology does not differ from adult AIBDs.

2.3.8. Drug Reactions

Exposure to different medications can occur for the first time during infancy. Adverse drug reactions can have a blistering presentation, mostly in erythema multiforme (EM), Stevens–Johnson syndrome (SJS), and toxic epidermal necrolysis.

In children, EM and SJS cases are often due to infections of herpes simplex virus (HSV) or *Mycoplasma*, while TEN is often associated with drugs [4].

As discussed above, TEN and SSSS can have a close clinical presentation and skin biopsy is useful to differentiate SSSS and TEN.

However, skin histology does not differ from adults for EM, SJS, and TEN.

3. Conclusions

The onset of blisters in a neonate or an infant is most often a diagnostic challenge for physicians, and the underlying cause has to be determined quickly between several etiologies.

The clinical context must be discussed with the clinician as well as the best technique for the biopsy.

Skin biopsy, often necessary, is particularly helpful for a rapid and precise diagnosis, leading to an appropriate management of the baby.

Funding: This research received no external funding.

Institutional Review Board Statement: Not applicable.

Informed Consent Statement: Not applicable.

Conflicts of Interest: The author declares no conflict of interest.

References

1. Cazes, A.; Prost-Squarcioni, C.; Bodemer, C.; Heller, M.; Brousse, N.; Fraitag, S. Histologic cutaneous modifications after the use of EMLA cream, a diagnostic pitfall: Review of 13 cases. *Arch. Dermatol.* **2007**, *143*, 1073–1087. [CrossRef] [PubMed]
2. Liy-Wong, C.; Pope, E.; Weinstein, M.; Lara-Corrales, I. Staphylococcal scalded skin syndrome: An epidemiological and clinical review of 84 cases. *Pediatr. Dermatol.* **2021**, *38*, 149–153. [CrossRef]
3. Amon, R.B.; Dimond, R.L. Toxic epidermal necrolysis. Rapid differentiation between staphylococcal and drug induced disease. *Arch. Dermatol.* **1975**, *111*, 1433–1437. [CrossRef] [PubMed]
4. Mahon, C.; Martinez, A.E. Vesiculopustular, bullous and erosive diseases of the neonate. In *Harper's Textbook of Pediatric Dermatology*; Hoeger, P., Kinsler, V., Yan, A., Harper, J., Oranje, A., Bodemer, C., Larralde, M., Luk, D., Mendiratta, V., Purvis, D., Eds.; Wiley Global Research: Hoboken, NJ, USA, 2019; Volume 1, pp. 134–153.
5. Grayson, W.; Calonje, E. Infectious diseases of the skin. In *McKee's Pathology of the Skin*, 5th ed.; Calonje, J.E., Brenn, T., Lazar, A., Billings, S., Eds.; Elsevier: Amsterdam, The Netherlands, 2019; Volume 1, pp. 858–862.
6. Has, C.; Bauer, J.; Bodemer, C.; Bolling, M.; Bruckner-Tuderman, L.; Diem, A.; Fine, J.-D.; Heagerty, A.; Hovnanian, A.; Marinkovich, M.; et al. Consensus reclassification of inherited epidermolysis bullosa and other disorders with skin fragility. *Br. J. Dermatol.* **2020**, *183*, 614–627. [CrossRef]
7. Fine, J.-D.; Bruckner-Tuderman, L.; Eady, R.A.; Bauer, E.A.; Bauer, J.W.; Has, C.; Heagerty, A.; Hintner, H.; Hovnanian, A.; Jonkman, M.F.; et al. Inherited epidermolysis bullosa: Updated recommendations on diagnosis and classification. *J. Am. Acad. Dermatol.* **2014**, *70*, 1103–1126. [CrossRef] [PubMed]
8. Has, C.; Liu, L.; Bolling, M.; Charlesworth, A.; El Hachem, M.; Escámez, M.J.; Fuentes, I.; Büchel, S.; Hiremagalore, R.; Pohla-Gubo, G.; et al. Clinical practice guidelines for laboratory diagnosis of epidermolysis bullosa. *Br. J. Dermatol.* **2019**, *182*, 574–592. [CrossRef]
9. Oji, V.; Tadini, G.; Akiyama, M.; Bardon, C.B.; Bodemer, C.; Bourrat, E.; Coudiere, P.; DiGiovanna, J.J.; Elias, P.; Fischer, J.; et al. Revised nomenclature and classification of inherited ichthyoses: Results of the First Ichthyosis Consensus Conference in Sorèze 2009. *J. Am. Acad. Dermatol.* **2010**, *63*, 607–641. [CrossRef]
10. Ross, R.; DiGiovanna, J.J.; Capaldi, L.; Argenyi, Z.; Fleckman, P.; Robinson-Bostom, L. Histopathologic characterization of epidermolytic hyperkeratosis: A systematic review of histology from the National Registry for Ichthyosis and Related Skin Disorders. *J. Am. Acad. Dermatol.* **2008**, *59*, 86–90. [CrossRef]
11. Metze, D.; Oji, V. Disorders of keratinization. In *McKee's Pathology of the Skin*, 5th ed.; Calonje, J.E., Brenn, T., Lazar, A., Billings, S., Eds.; Elsevier: Amsterdam, The Netherlands, 2019; Volume 1, pp. 63–66.
12. Bergman, R.; Khamaysi, Z.; Sprecher, E. A unique pattern of dyskeratosis characterizes epidermolytic hyperkeratosis and epidermolytic palmoplantar keratoderma. *Am. J. Dermatopathol.* **2008**, *30*, 101–105. [CrossRef]
13. Galler, B.; Bowen, C.; Arnold, J.; Kobayashi, T.; Dalton, S.R. Use of the frozen section 'jelly-roll' technique to aid in the diagnosis of bullous congenital ichthyosiform erythroderma (epidermolytic hyperkeratosis). *J. Cutan. Pathol.* **2016**, *43*, 434–437. [CrossRef]
14. McLean, W.H.I.; Morley, S.M.; Lane, E.B.; Eady, R.A.J.; Griffiths, W.A.D.; Paige, D.G.; Harper, J.I.; Higgins, C.; Leigh, I.M. Ichthyosis bullosa of Siemens–A disease involving keratin 2e. *J. Investig. Dermatol.* **1994**, *103*, 277–281. [CrossRef]

15. Hadj-Rabia, S.; Froidevaux, D.; Bodak, N.; Hamel-Teillac, D.; Smahi, A.; Touil, Y.; Fraitag, S.; De Prost, Y.; Bodemer, C. Clinical study of 40 cases of incontinentia pigmenti. *Arch. Dermatol.* **2003**, *139*, 1163–1170. [CrossRef]
16. Bodemer, C.; Diociaiuti, A.; Hadj-Rabia, S.; Robert, M.P.; Desguerre, I.; Manière, M.C.; de la Dure-Molla, M.; De Liso, P.; Federici, A.; Galeotti, A.; et al. Multidisciplinary consensus recommendations from a European network for the diagnosis and practical management of patients with incontinentia pigmenti. *J. Eur. Acad. Dermatol. Venereol.* **2020**, *34*, 1415–1424. [CrossRef] [PubMed]
17. Fraitag, S.; Rimella, A.; de Prost, Y.; Brousse, N.; Hadj-Rabia, S.; Bodemer, C. Skin biopsy is helpful for the diagnosis of incontinentia pigmenti at late stage (IV): A series of 26 cutaneous biopsies. *J. Cutan. Pathol.* **2009**, *36*, 966–971. [CrossRef] [PubMed]
18. Polivka, L.; Bodemer, C. Paediatric mastocytosis. In *Harper's Textbook of Pediatric Dermatology*; Hoeger, P., Kinsler, V., Yan, A., Harper, J., Oranje, A., Bodemer, C., Larralde, M., Luk, D., Mendiratta, V., Purvis, D., Eds.; Wiley Global Research: Hoboken, NJ, USA, 2019; Volume 1, pp. 1097–1108.
19. Goodlad, J.; Calonje, E. Cutaneous lymphoproliferative diseases and related disorders (mastocytosis). In *McKee's Pathology of the Skin*, 5th ed.; Calonje, J.E., Brenn, T., Lazar, A., Billings, S., Eds.; Elsevier: Amsterdam, The Netherlands, 2019; Volume 2, pp. 1515–1519.
20. Kamat, D.; Chatterjee, D.; Vinay, K. Recurrent blistering in an infant. *JAMA Dermatol.* **2020**, *156*, 212. [CrossRef] [PubMed]
21. Morren, M.A.; Broecke, K.V.; Vangeebergen, L.; Sillevis-Smitt, J.H.; Van Den Berghe, P.; Hauben, E.; Jacobs, S.; Van Gool, S.W. Diverse cutaneous presentations of langerhans cell histiocytosis in children: A retrospective cohort study. *Pediatr. Blood Cancer* **2016**, *63*, 486–492. [CrossRef]
22. Chan, M.M.H.; Tan, D.J.A.; Koh, M.J.-A.; Tan, L.S. Blistering Langerhans cell histiocytosis. *Lancet Oncol.* **2018**, *19*, e500. [CrossRef]
23. Emile, J.-F.; Abla, O.; Fraitag, S.; Horne, A.; Haroche, J.; Donadieu, J.; Requena-Caballero, L.; Jordan, M.B.; Abdel-Wahab, O.; Allen, C.E.; et al. Revised classification of histiocytoses and neoplasms of the macrophage-dendritic cell lineages. *Blood* **2016**, *127*, 2672–2681. [CrossRef]
24. Fraitag, S.; Donadieu, J. Langerhans Cell Histiocytosis. In *Harper's Textbook of Pediatric Dermatology*; Hoeger, P., Kinsler, V., Yan, A., Harper, J., Oranje, A., Bodemer, C., Larralde, M., Luk, D., Mendiratta, V., Purvis, D., Eds.; Wiley Global Research: Hoboken, NJ, USA, 2019; Volume 1, pp. 1071–1077.
25. Hill, S.F.; Murrell, D.F. Differential diagnosis of vesiculobullous lesions. In *Harper's Textbook of Pediatric Dermatology*; Hoeger, P., Kinsler, V., Yan, A., Harper, J., Oranje, A., Bodemer, C., Larralde, M., Luk, D., Mendiratta, V., Purvis, D., Eds.; Wiley Global Research: Hoboken, NJ, USA, 2019; Volume 1, pp. 868–897.
26. Welfringer-Morin, A.; Bekel, L.; Bellon, N.; Gantzer, A.; Boccara, O.; Hadj-Rabia, S.; Leclerc-Mercier, S.; Frassati-Biaggi, A.; Fraitag, S.; Bodemer, C. Long-term evolving profile of childhood autoimmune blistering diseases: Retrospective study on 38 children. *J. Eur. Acad. Dermatol. Venereol.* **2019**, *33*, 1158–1163. [CrossRef]
27. Marathe, K.; Lu, J.; Morel, K.D. Bullous diseases: Kids are not just little people. *Clin. Dermatol.* **2015**, *33*, 644–656. [CrossRef]
28. Zhao, C.Y.; Chiang, Y.Z.; Murrell, D.F. Neonatal autoimmune blistering disease: A systematic review. *Pediatr. Dermatol.* **2016**, *33*, 367–374. [CrossRef] [PubMed]

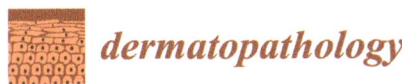

Review

Histologic Patterns and Clues to Autoinflammatory Diseases in Children: What a Cutaneous Biopsy Can Tell Us

Athanassios Kolivras [1,*], Isabelle Meiers [1,2], Ursula Sass [1] and Curtis T. Thompson [3,4,5]

[1] Department of Dermatology and Dermatopathology, Saint-Pierre, Brugmann and Queen Fabiola Children's University Hospitals, Université Libre de Bruxelles, 1000 Brussels, Belgium; isabelle.meiers@stpierre-bru.be (I.M.); ursula.sass@stpierre-bru.be (U.S.)
[2] Department of Pathology, Laboratoire Luc Olivier, 5380 Fernelmont, Belgium
[3] Department of Dermatology, Oregon Health and Sciences University, Portland, OR 97239, USA; curtisinportland@gmail.com
[4] Department of Pathology, Oregon Health and Sciences University, Portland, OR 97239, USA
[5] CTA Pathology, Portland, OR 97223, USA
* Correspondence: athanassios.kolivras@stpierre-bru.be

Abstract: Autoinflammation is defined by aberrant, antigen-independent activation of the innate immune signaling pathways. This leads to increased, pro-inflammatory cytokine expression and subsequent inflammation. In contrast, autoimmune and allergic diseases are antigen-directed immune responses from activation of the adaptive immune system. The innate and adaptive immune signaling pathways are closely interconnected. The group of 'complex multigenic diseases' are a result of mutual dysregulation of both the autoinflammatory and autoimmune physiologic components. In contrast, monogenic autoinflammatory syndromes (MAIS) result from single mutations and are exclusively autoinflammatory in their pathogenesis. Studying the clinical and histopathological findings for the various MAIS explains the phenotypical correlates of their specific mutations. This review aims to group the histopathologic clues for autoinflammation into three recognizable patterns. The presence of these histologic patterns in a pediatric patient with recurrent fevers and systemic inflammation should raise suspicion of an autoinflammatory component in MAIS, or, more frequently, in a complex multigenic disease. The three major histopathological patterns seen in autoinflammation are as follows: (i) the 'neutrophilic' pattern, seen in urticarial neutrophilic dermatosis, pustular psoriasis, aseptic neutrophilic folliculitis, and Sweet's syndrome; (ii) the 'vasculitic' pattern seen in small vessel-vasculitis (including hypersensitivity/leukocytoclastic vasculitis, thrombosing microangiopathy and lymphocytic vasculitis), and intermediate-sized vessel vasculitis, mimicking polyarteritis nodosa; and (iii) the 'granulomatous' pattern. Beyond these three patterns, there are additional histopathologic clues, which are detailed below. It is important for a dermatopathologist to recognize the patterns of autoinflammation, so that a diagnosis of MAIS or complex multigenic diseases may be obtained. Finally, careful histopathologic analyses could contribute to a better understanding of the various clinical manifestations of autoinflammation.

Keywords: autoinflammation; cryopyrin; inflammasome; interferonopathies; pustular psoriasis; lupus erythematosus; neutrophilic urticarial dermatitis; pyoderma gangrenosum; suppurative hidradenitis

Citation: Kolivras, A.; Meiers, I.; Sass, U.; Thompson, C.T. Histologic Patterns and Clues to Autoinflammatory Diseases in Children: What a Cutaneous Biopsy Can Tell Us. *Dermatopathology* **2021**, *8*, 202–220. https://doi.org/10.3390/dermatopathology8020026

Academic Editors: Sylvie Fraitag and Gürkan Kaya

Received: 22 April 2021
Accepted: 31 May 2021
Published: 8 June 2021

Publisher's Note: MDPI stays neutral with regard to jurisdictional claims in published maps and institutional affiliations.

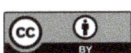

Copyright: © 2021 by the authors. Licensee MDPI, Basel, Switzerland. This article is an open access article distributed under the terms and conditions of the Creative Commons Attribution (CC BY) license (https://creativecommons.org/licenses/by/4.0/).

1. Introduction

1.1. Innate versus Adaptive Immunity: Autoinflammatory Versus Autoimmune Disease—What the Dermatopathologist Needs to Know

Innate immunity is our first line of defense and rapidly recognizes molecules unique to pathogens via pattern recognition receptors, such as the toll-like receptors. However, there is no memory after repeated exposure. Innate immunity employs macrophages, neutrophils and mast cells, and at a molecular level, complement and antimicrobial peptides. In contrast, adaptive immunity is a second line of defense, utilizing T- and B-lymphocytes.

Adaptive immunity is highly specific since highly diverse lymphocytes can target specific antigens. Adaptive immunity remembers these specific antigens upon subsequent exposure to the antigen, with the ability to be reactivated. Adaptive immunity is also self-tolerant as it distinguishes self-antigens from foreign antigens [1].

Dysfunction of innate immunity is rare and results from an antigen-independent hyperactivation of molecular pro-inflammatory pathways, leading to 'autoinflammatory' diseases. Dysfunction of adaptive immunity is frequent and results from non-pathogen activation of inflammation. The non-pathogen is a self-antigen in autoimmune diseases and an environmental antigen in allergic diseases. The inherited diseases that cause autoinflammation, called 'monogenic autoinflammatory syndromes' (MAIS), are characterized by recurrent fever, increased cytokine expression, and episodic inflammation, resulting in potential end-organ damage. In contrast to autoimmune diseases, the increased, chronically active cytokine expression does not require auto-reactive lymphocytes or immunoglobulins to self-antigens. Although MAIS may be triggered by an infectious pathogen, their hallmark is the persistence of inflammation in the absence of a recognizable infection [2–6].

Despite these differences, autoinflammation and autoimmunity are interlinked. Complex multigenic diseases have different amounts of both autoinflammatory and autoimmune components within their pathogenesis. Complex multigenic diseases include common diseases such as lupus erythematosus (LE), Crohn's disease, spondyloarthropathies, and type-1 diabetes mellitus, among others. In contrast to complex multigenic diseases, the rarely-encountered group of monogenic syndromes are either entirely autoimmune or autoinflammatory [7].

The MAIS encountered in pediatric dermatology may arise due to four major modes of activation of the innate immunity as follows: (1) interleukin (IL)-1 activation; (2) type-I-interferon (IFN) activation; (3) nuclear-factor-kappa B (NF-κB) activation; and (4) M1 macrophage activation: [1,5,6,8–10].

1. IL-1 activation. The binding of an antigen to a pattern recognition receptor activates a pro-inflammatory cascade of intracellular, multimeric protein complexes called 'inflammasomes.' Inflammasomes are defined by their sensor proteins, which oligomerize to activate caspase-1, also called IL-1–converting enzyme, leading to proteolytic activation of IL-1b. Multiple inflammasomes are well-understood, including pyrin and cryopyrin. Cryopyrin is also called NLR family pyrin domain containing 3 (NLRP3). MAIS resulting from mutations within inflammasomes are also called 'inflammasomopathies'. Unleashed IL1-induced inflammation can also result from deficiency of IL1 and IL36 receptor antagonists. Phospholipase C gamma 2 (PLCγ2) is a cytoplasmic signaling enzyme, which, when recruited to the membrane upon receptor activation, induces the release of endoplasmic reticulum calcium stores, thereby leading to increased intracellular calcium levels and activation of the NLRP3 inflammasome.

2. Type I interferon (IFN) activation (Type I interferonopathies). Autoinflammatory diseases related to IFN activation, also called interferonopathies, reflect aberrant activation of type I IFN pathways (IFN-α and IFN-β), which are involved in antiviral defense. Type I IFN production is triggered by viral RNA or DNA, and interferonopathies may arise through disorders of intracytoplasmic accumulation of endogenous nucleic acid due to their decreased degradation, through inherent, increased intracytoplasmic nucleic acid sensing or through a proteasome dysfunction.

3. NF-κB activation (NFkBopathies). The NF-κB complex is a central signaling hub within the cytoplasm, integrating signals from multiple cell-surface receptors, including TNF receptors and intracellular pattern recognition receptors, like the nucleotide-binding oligomerization domain 2 (NOD2) receptor. NF-κB allows the freeing of several transcription factors, which move to the nucleus and trigger expression of proinflammatory genes. Activation of caspase-activating recruitment domain, member 14 (CARD14) also leads to enhanced NF-κB activity. A20 is a negative regulator of NF-κB and A20 insufficiency also results in an NFkBopathy.

4. M1 macrophage activation. Adenosine deaminase 2 deficiency results in increased proinflammatory M1 macrophages (as opposed to anti-inflammatory M2 macrophages).

Figure 1 summarizes the major activated pathways with their corresponding MAIS and mutated genes. Dysregulation of innate immunity is far more complex than this illustration, which has been simplified for didactic purposes. Of note, this dysregulation of innate immunity is interdependent with adaptive immunity.

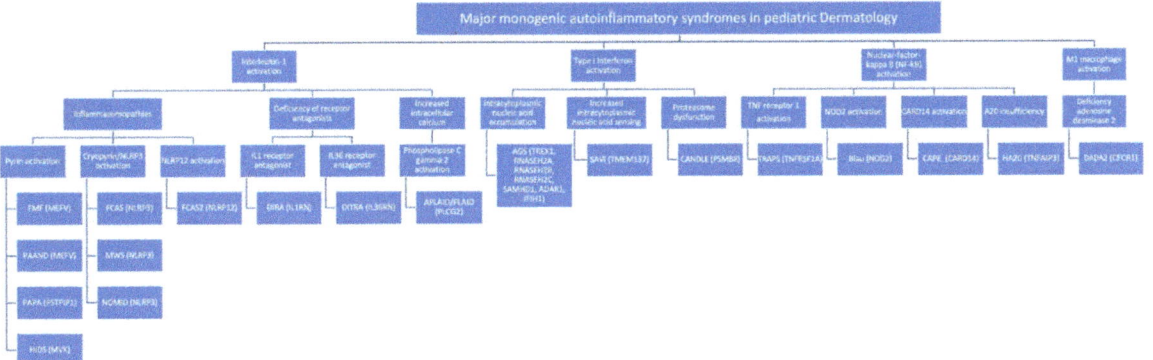

Figure 1. The major monogenic autoinflammatory syndromes in pediatric dermatology based on the major pathogenesis pathways. Mutated genes in parenthesis next to their corresponding syndrome; AGS, Aicardi Goutières Syndrome; APLAID, autoinflammation and phospholipase C gamma 2 associated antibody deficiency and immune dysregulation; CANDLE, Chronic atypical neutrophilic dermatosis with lipodystrophy and elevated temperature; CAPE, Caspase-activating recruitment domain, member 14 associated papulosquamous eruption; DADA2, Deficiency of adenosine deaminase 2; DIRA, Deficiency of IL-1 receptor antagonist syndrome; DITRA, Deficiency of IL-36 receptor antagonist; FCAS, Familial cold autoinflammatory syndrome; FMF, Familial Mediterranean fever syndrome; HA20, Haploinsufficiency of A20; HIDS, Hyperimmunoglobulinemia D syndrome; MWS, Muckle–Wells syndrome; NOMID, Neonatal-onset multisystem inflammatory disease; PAAND, Pyrin-associated autoinflammation with neutrophilic dermatosis; PAPA, Pyogenic Arthritis, pyoderma gangrenosum and acne; PLAID, Phospholipase C gamma 2 associated antibody deficiency and immune dysregulation; SAVI, Stimulator of interferon genes (STING) associated vasculopathy of infancy; TRAPS, TNF receptor-associated periodic syndrome.

1.2. Histopathological Clues to the Diagnosis of Autoinflammation

Autoinflammation is devoid of any specific histopathological clue. In fact, different mutations in the same molecular pathway can produce different clinical and histopathological findings. MAIS, which result from single mutations in a pathway, demonstrate close, phenotypic correlations with specific mutations. This information has led to a better understanding of the aberrant activation of the same pathways in the group of complex multigenic diseases [9]. With this knowledge, the dermatopathologist can better recognize histologic patterns associated with autoinflammation and integrate them into a patient's particular clinical presentation. Beyond recognition, this understanding also provides an opportunity for the use of more targeted treatments. Finally, the identification of histologic patterns associated with MAIS allows for a better understanding and classification of inflammatory diseases in general.

This review will focus on the identification of the three main histopathological patterns, followed by the identification of more subtle histopathological clues. These patterns will then be correlated with clinical findings, which are usually from pediatric patients. The three main histopathologic groups are: (1) neutrophilic; (2) vasculitic; and (3) granulomatous. Identification of any pattern may lead to a diagnosis of either a MAIS or a complex multigenic disease. Figure 2 delineates the histopathological patterns of autoinflammation in both major MAIS and complex multigenic diseases and Table 1 classifies the main monogenic autoinflammatory syndromes based on their mechanism of pathogenesis and relevant histopathological findings.

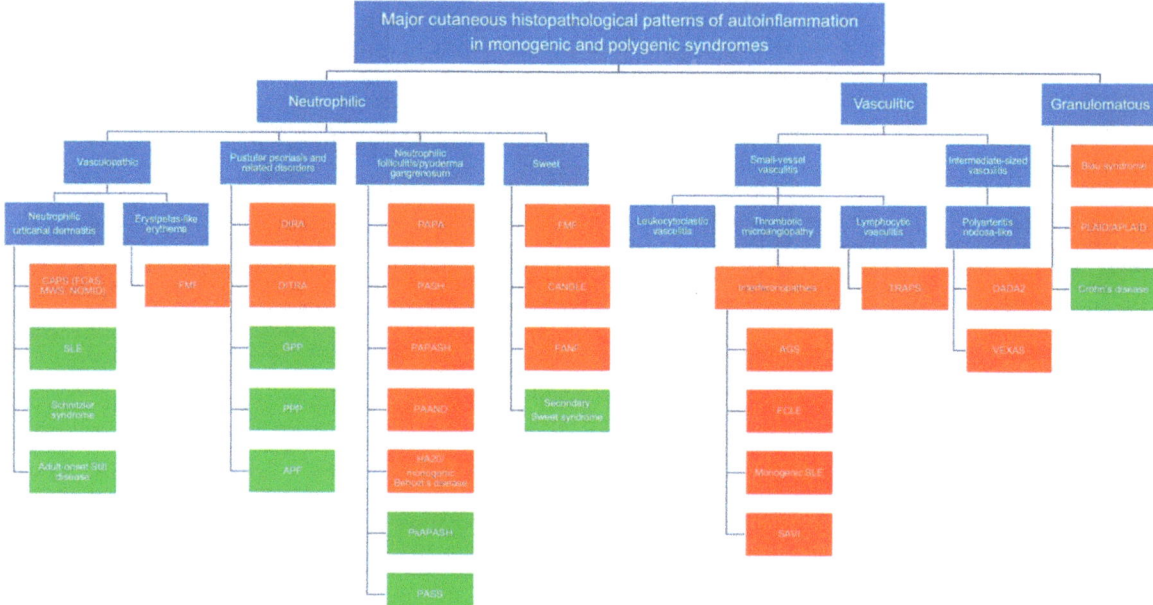

Figure 2. Major cutaneous histopathological patterns (neutrophilic, vasculitic and granulomatous) seen in autoinflammation in both monogenic autoinflammatory syndromes (Red) and complex multigenic diseases (Green); AGS, Aicardi Goutières syndrome; APF, Amicrobial pustulosis of the folds; APLAID, Autoinflammation and phospholipase C gamma 2 associated antibody deficiency and immune dysregulation; CANDLE, Chronic atypical neutrophilic dermatosis with lipodystrophy and elevated temperature; CAPS, Cryopyrin-associated periodic syndromes; DADA2, Deficiency of adenosine deaminase 2; DIRA, Deficiency of IL-1 receptor antagonist syndrome; DITRA, Deficiency of IL-36 receptor antagonist; FCAS, Familial cold autoinflammatory syndrome; FCLE, Familial chilblain lupus erythematosus; FANF, Familial autoinflammatory necrotising fasciitis; FMF, Familial Mediterranean fever syndrome; GPP, Generalized pustular psoriasis; HA20, Haploinsufficiency of A20; MWS, Muckle–Wells syndrome; NOMID, Neonatal-onset multisystem inflammatory disease; PAAND, Pyrin-associated autoinflammation with neutrophilic dermatosis; PAPA, Pyogenic arthritis, pyoderma gangrenosum and acne; PAPASH, Pyogenic Arthritis, pyoderma gangrenosum, acne, suppurative hidradenitis; PASH, Pyoderma gangrenosum, acne, suppurative Hidradenitis; PASS, Pyoderma gangrenosum, acne, suppurative hidradenitis and ankylosing spondylitis; PLAID, Phospholipase C gamma 2 associated antibody deficiency and immune dysregulation; PPP, Palmoplantar pustulosis; PsAPASH, Psoriatic arthritis, pyoderma gangrenosum, acne, suppurative hidradenitis; SAVI, Stimulator of interferon genes (STING) associated vasculopathy of infancy; SLE, Systemic lupus erythematosus; TRAPS, TNF receptor-associated periodic syndrome; VEXAS, vacuoles, E1 enzyme, X-linked, autoinflammatory, somatic syndrome.

Table 1. Main histopathological findings for the major monogenic autoinflammatory syndromes with their mechanism of pathogenesis and identified mutated genes (in parenthesis): AGS, Aicardi Goutières Syndrome; APLAID, autoinflammation and phospholipase C gamma 2 associated antibody deficiency and immune dysregulation; CANDLE, Chronic atypical neutrophilic dermatosis with lipodystrophy and elevated temperature; CAPE, caspase-activating recruitment domain member 14 associated papulosquamous eruption, DADA2, deficiency of adenosine deaminase 2; DIRA, Deficiency of IL-1 receptor antagonist syndrome; DITRA, Deficiency of IL-36 receptor antagonist; FCLE, Familial chilblain lupus erythematosus; FMF, Familial Mediterranean fever syndrome; HA20, Haploinsufficiency of A20; MWS, Muckle–Wells syndrome; NAID, NOD-2 associated autoinflammatory syndrome; NOMID, Neonatal-onset multisystem inflammatory disease; PAAND, pyrin-associated autoinflammation with neutrophilic dermatosis; PAPA, Pyogenic Arthritis, pyoderma gangrenosum and acne; PLAID, Phospholipase C gamma 2 associated antibody deficiency and immune dysregulation; SAVI, Stimulator of interferon genes (STING) associated vasculopathy of infancy; TRAPS, TNF receptor-associated periodic syndrome.

Inflammasomopathies	Pyrin activation	FMF (MEFV)	Erysipelas-like erythema in the only pathognomonic cutaneous marker of FMF and is characterized by mild papillary dermal edema, dilated vessels, sparse perivascular mononuclear cell infiltrate admixed with neutrophils and nuclear dust
		PAAND (MEFV) and PAPA (PSTPIP1)	Neutrophilic dermatosis comprising the phenotypical spectrum of pyoderma gangrenosum, neutrophilic folliculitis, abscess and acne, PAAND also shows small vessel leukocytoclastic vasculitis
	Cryopyrin/NLRP3 activation	Cryopyrinopathies: FCAS, MWS, NOMID	Neutrophilic urticarial dermatitis: perivascular and interstitial neutrophilic infiltrate with variable leukocytoclasia, linear interstitial arrangement of neutrophils as 'Indian file', neutrophilic epitheliotropism including intraepidermal and peri-eccrine involvement, absence of fibrin in vessel walls, no significant dermal edema
Interleukin-1 activation	IL1 receptor antagonist	DIRA (IL1RN)	Pustular psoriasis (psoriasiform epidermal hyperplasia, subcorneal spongiform pustulation, neutrophilic aggregates within parakeratotic stratum corneum), dense intradermal neutrophilic infiltrate with peri-eccrine involvement
	IL36 receptor antagonist	DITRA (IL36RN)	
	Phospholipase C gamma 2 activation	APLAID (PLCG2)	Dense perivascular and interstitial granulomatous infiltrate, palisading granulomas around necrobiotic collagen, dense neutrophilic infiltrate, intense papillary dermal oedema leading to subepidermal blistering
		PLAID (PLCG2)	Neutrophilic urticarial dermatitis (cold-induced urticaria) and non-caseating sarcoidal granulomas
Type I Interferon activation	Intracytoplasmic nucleic acid accumulation	AGS (TREX1, RNASEH2A, RNASEH2B, RNASEH2C, SAMHD1, ADAR1, IFIH1) and FCLE (TREX1, SAMHD1)	Thrombotic microangiopathy associated with findings of chilblain lupus erythematosus (vacuolar interface dermatitis, lymphocytic vasculitis, peri-eccrine lymphocytic infiltrate)
	Increased intracytoplasmic nucleic acid sensing	SAVI (TMEM137)	Thrombotic microangiopathy
	Proteasome dysfunction	CANDLE (PSMB8)	Histiocytoid Sweet syndrome: dense perivascular and interstitial mononuclear cell infiltrate composed of immature myeloid cells admixed with mature neutrophils, eosinophils and leukocytoclasia

NF-κB activation	TNF receptor 1 activation	TRAPS (TNFRSF1A)	Lymphocytic vasculitis: perivascular lymphocytic infiltrate showing tight cuffing within both superficial and deep dermis, absence of fibrin within vessel walls
	NOD2 activation	Blau (NOD2)	Non-caseating sarcoidal granulomas with lymphocytic coronas
	NOD2 activation	NAID (NOD2)	Subacute spongiotic dermatitis, irregular epidermal acanthosis with overlying parakeratotic hyperkeratosis
	CARD14 activation	CAPE (CARD14)	Pityriasis rubra pilaris (psoriasiform epidermal hyperplasia, irregular hyperkeratosis, alternating vertical and horizontal orthokeratosis and parakeratosis, follicular plugging), absence of acantholysis
	A20 insufficiency	HA20 (TNFAIP3)	Non-specific (oral aphtous erosions or ulcerations similarly to Behcet's disease)
M1 macrophage activation	Deficiency adenosine deaminase 2	DADA2 (CECR1)	Polyarteritis nodosa: neutrophilic infiltrate around and within muscular arteriole walls (intermediate-sized vessels at the dermo-hypodermal junction), disruption of the internal elastic lamina, fibrin deposition and intraluminal thrombosis

2. Autoinflammatory Diseases: Correlating Histologic Patterns with Specific Diseases

2.1. The Neutrophilic Pattern

The neutrophilic pattern can be further subdivided into 4 groups as follows: (a) vasculopathic; (b) pustular psoriasis; (c) aseptic neutrophilic folliculitis, including pyoderma gangrenosum (PG); and (d) Sweet's syndrome.

2.1.1. The Vasculopathic Pattern

The vasculopathic reaction pattern includes a group of diseases in which inflammation produces erythematous and slightly infiltrated plaques, resulting from vasodilatation, increased vessel wall permeability with resulting slight dermal edema. In contrast to the 'vasculitic' pattern, there is no vessel wall damage and the lesions resolve rapidly. The vasculopathic pattern contains the spectrum of diseases in neutrophilic urticarial dermatitis (NUD), and the erysipelas-like erythema of the familial Mediterranean fever (FMF) syndrome. The NUD group contains the spectrum of cryopyrin-associated periodic syndromes (CAPS) or 'cryopyrinopathies'. CAPS includes three main diseases: (1) familial cold autoinflammatory syndrome (FCAS); (2) Muckle–Wells syndrome (MWS); and (3) neonatal onset multisystem inflammatory disorder (NOMID). The remaining diseases associated with NUD are systemic LE, Schnitzler syndrome and adult-onset Still-disease in adults. The two latter diagnoses are only seen in adults and will only be briefly mentioned.

NUD is characterized by chronic, recurrent urticarial wheals lasting 24–48 h. Unlike usual urticaria, the lesions may last more than 24 h and are not responsive to antihistamine treatment. Of note, the eruption has a diurnal variation, being absent or discrete in the morning but gradually increasing in severity into the evenings. Histopathological examination of NUD shows no epidermal change or subjacent edema. There is a dense, perivascular and interstitial neutrophilic infiltrate with leukocytoclasia. The neutrophils may show a linear interstitial arrangement between collagen bundles. Neutrophils may show epitheliotropism and a peri-eccrine accentuation ('neutrophilic hidradenitis') [11,12]. Dilated vessels often contain neutrophils. No true leukocytoclastic vasculitis is present with fibrin in venule walls. A few eosinophils may be present [13,14].

CAPS are due to mutations leading to cryopyrin activation. There exists a spectrum of different disease-severity syndromes, from mild disease in the FCAS; intermediate disease in MWS; and severe disease in NOMID [15,16]. FCAS starts in the first year of life with an urticarial eruption and flu-like symptoms induced by cold stimuli, including ingestion of cold liquid [17]. A less common variant, termed 'FCAS2' (NLRP12-related disease), has a later onset in childhood with symptoms lasting 2–10 days [18]. MWS is intermediate in terms of disease severity and characterized by fever, a chronic evanescent urticarial eruption, arthralgia, conjunctivitis and systemic AA amyloidosis, often leading to renal impairment. Fever may be absent. Symptoms usually appear within the first 6 months of life but may also develop later in adolescence. In contrast to FCAS, attacks in MWS are not cold-induced, and the episodes tend also to last longer, usually 1 to 2 days. Similar to FCAS, patients with MWS describe a pattern of worsening symptoms in the evening. The course of the disease varies among individuals, ranging from recurrent attacks to near-continuous symptoms [16]. NOMID, is also called chronic infantile neurologic cutaneous and articular syndrome (CINCA). NOMID is the most severe form of CAPS and is characterized by an urticarial eruption associated with arthralgia and neurologic manifestations. The onset is within 6 months of age with two thirds of patients being affected at birth, or even in utero. The duration of attacks is usually less than 24 h. The initial presentation is similar to other CAPS disease with variable degrees of articular and neurologic involvement [19,20]. A histologic finding of NUD with a peri-eccrine neutrophilic hidradenitis in the correct clinical setting should raise suspicion of NOMID (Figure 3) [12,21].

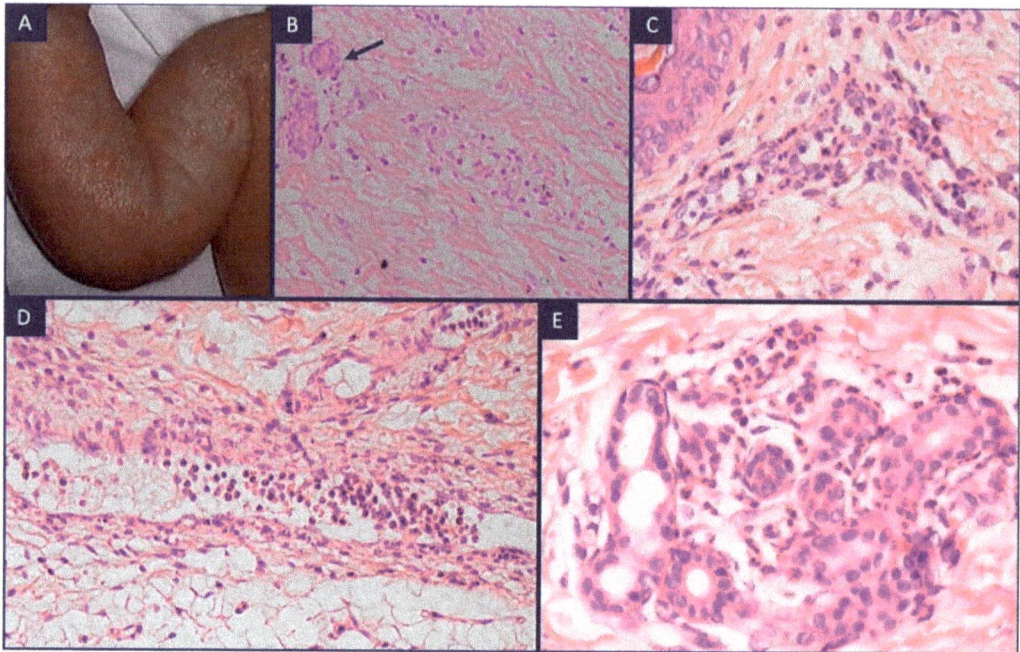

Figure 3. Neutrophilic urticarial dermatitis (NUD) in neonatal-onset multisystem inflammatory disease (NOMID). (**A**) Female newborn with an urticarial eruption associated with recurrent fever, increased serologic inflammatory markers, and aseptic purulent meningitis; (**B**) H&E, ×10. A perivascular, interstitial and peri-eccrine (arrow) mononuclear cell infiltrate admixed with neutrophils and rare eosinophils; (**C**) H&E, ×20. A perivascular neutrophilic infiltrate with leukocytoclasia but no fibrinoid necrosis in vessel walls; (**D**) H&E, ×10. Dilated lymphatics containing numerous neutrophils; (**E**) H&E, ×20. Peri-eccrine neutrophilic hidradenitis.

Non-bullous neutrophilic LE, a variant of systemic LE which clinically and histopathologically resembles NUD, is a cutaneous marker suggesting progression to systemic disease. On histology, there is a vacuolar interface dermatitis with apoptotic keratinocytes in addition to typical NUD. Direct immunofluorescence studies show granular IgG deposition along the dermal-epidermal junction. Neutrophil-rich lupus panniculitis can also be seen in the context of progression to systemic LE, in contrast to the usual lymphocytic panniculitis seen in chronic cutaneous LE [22].

NUD is also seen in Schnitzler syndrome and adult-onset disease, which are only briefly mentioned because they appear in adulthood. Schnitzler syndrome is characterized by chronic urticaria associated with recurrent fever, lymphadenopathy, increased erythrocyte sedimentation rate, leukocytosis and a monoclonal gammopathy, which is usually IgM, or rarely, IgG in the 'Schnitzler variant'. The disease may progress to a blood dyscrasia, especially 'Waldenstrom' macroglobulinemia. Histopathology in Schnitzler syndrome shows typical NUD or mononuclear-cell infiltrate with a perivascular accentuation. Eosinophils are sparse or absent [23]. Adult-onset Still's disease has a 'typical' and an 'atypical' clinical presentation. The typical presentation has an evanescent urticarial eruption of NUD. The atypical presentation has more persistent lesions, often in a photo-distributed pattern with a reticular or rippled-like pattern and associated with a more aggressive disease course and associated malignancy (lymphoma, breast cancer). In addition to histologic features of NUD, the 'atypical' eruption also shows psoriasiform hyperplasia with focal parakeratosis, dyskeratotic keratinocytes in the superficial epidermis, and small intraepidermal clusters of neutrophils. The dermis has superficial perivascular lymphocytes with or without interstitial neutrophils [24].

The final disease in the vasculopathic group is erysipelas-like erythema (ELE), which is a minor diagnostic criterion for the diagnosis of the familial Mediterranean fever (FMF) syndrome. Clinically, FMF has recurrent, self-limited attacks of fever for ~3 days with polyserositis involving the peritoneum, pleura and synovium [25–27]. There is a favorable response to colchicine and progression to amyloidosis if untreated. ELE is the only pathognomonic cutaneous marker of FMF and is seen in a minority of cases of FMF (7–46% of all patients and 15–20% of children). ELE typically occurs on the lower extremities with well-demarcated plaques, no larger than 15 cm in diameter, and it may be triggered by physical exercise. The lesions subside with rest over 48–72 h [28]. Histopathological findings for ELE are subtle with no epidermal change, mild papillary dermal edema, dilated blood and lymphatic vessels and a perivascular infiltrate of lymphocytes and neutrophils with variable amounts of leukocytoclasia. Eosinophils are absent (Figure 4) [29]. Endothelial cells may appear swollen. Although blurring of some vessel walls may be observed, no fibrin deposition occurs and leukocytoclastic vasculitis is not observed. This may be due to the short duration of the attacks, which is insufficient to provoke vessel wall damage [29,30]. However, direct immunofluorescence shows deposits of IgM, C3, and fibrinogen in the small-sized vessel walls within the papillary dermis [28,30]. A recurrent subepidermal bullous eruption has been reported with ELE with negative direct immunofluorescence study findings [31].

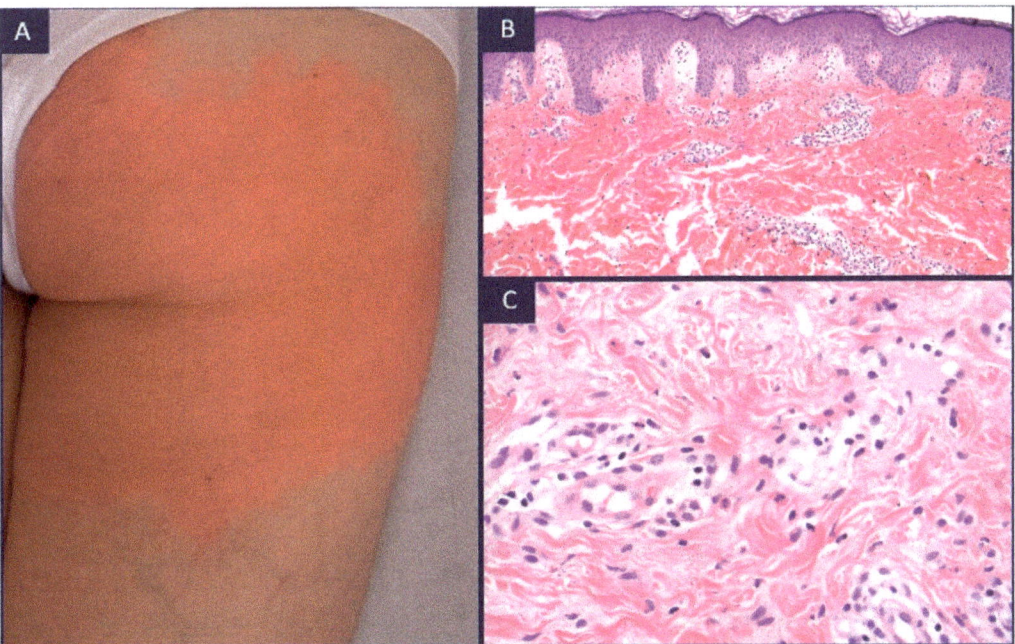

Figure 4. Erysipelas-like erythema in familial Mediterranean fever syndrome (FMF): (**A**) 34-year-old female with a recurrent, well-demarcated erythematous plaque on the right buttock, spontaneously resolving within 2–3 days; (**B**) H&E, ×4. Mild papillary dermal edema, dilated blood and lymphatic vessels surrounded by a mild inflammatory cell infiltrate; (**C**) H&E, ×20. Perivascular infiltrate of lymphocytes and neutrophils with slightly thickened vessel walls, but devoid of fibrin deposition.

2.1.2. The Pustular Psoriasis Pattern

Pustular psoriasis with its related disorders is the second type of neutrophilic pattern. This pattern occurs in the deficiency of IL-1 receptor antagonist syndrome (DIRA), deficiency of IL-36 receptor antagonist syndrome (DITRA), pustular psoriasis (including generalized pustular psoriasis and palmoplantar pustulosis), and amicrobial pustulosis of the skin folds.

DIRA is a recessive loss-of-function mutation of the IL-1RN gene, which encodes the IL-1 receptor antagonist. The result is neonatal generalized pustular psoriasis, fever with elevated inflammatory markers, joint swelling, multifocal osteolytic lesions, hepatosplenomegaly and interstitial lung disease. The outcome is poor, leading to death with multi-organ failure. The rash mostly involves the face including oral and conjunctival involvement, and there is also diffuse pustular psoriasis with erythematous, scaly plaques. Nails may be involved. Pathergy may also be present. Histopathologically, the changes are identical to pustular psoriasis with psoriasiform epidermal hyperplasia, neutrophils in parakeratotic foci, and spongiform subcorneal pustules. In contrast to usual pustular psoriasis, neutrophils may densely infiltrate the dermis and show peri-eccrine accentuation. Leukocytoclastic vasculitis has also been reported, with vasculitis being present even in the deeper subcutaneous adipose tissue adjacent to bone [32,33].

IL-36RN is a negative regulator of IL-36 receptor signaling, and loss of function is present in the monogenic syndrome called DITRA and in complex multigenic diseases such as generalized pustular psoriasis, palmoplantar pustular psoriasis, and acrodermatitis continua of Hallopeau. DITRA is characterized by recurrent episodes of generalized pustular psoriasis, fever, systemic inflammation and leukocytosis. Histopathological findings, like DIRA, are identical to pustular psoriasis though the density of the neutrophilic infiltrate in the papillary dermis appears to be denser than in pustular psoriasis (Figure 5) [34,35].

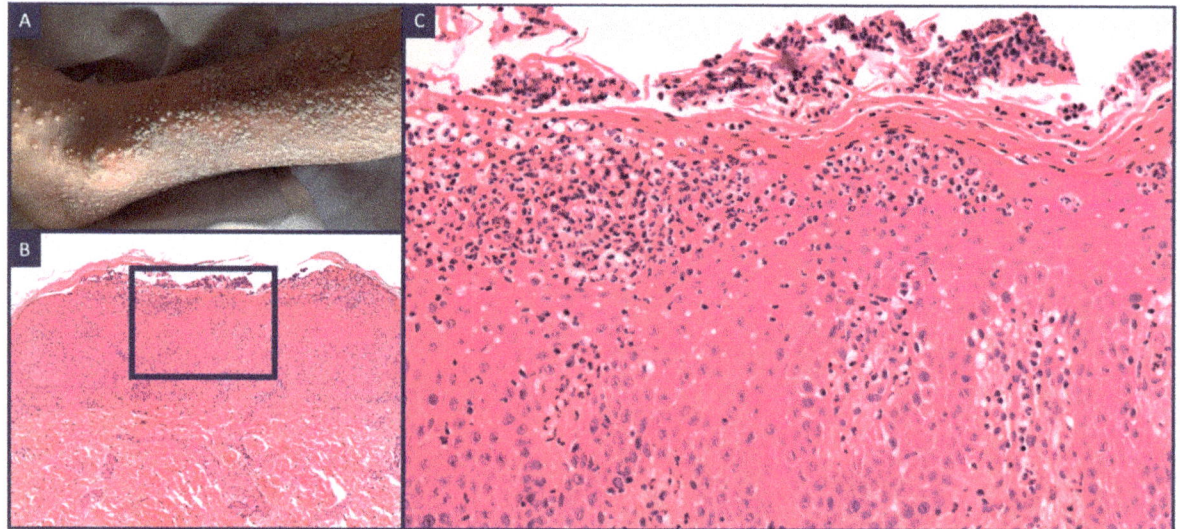

Figure 5. Pustular-psoriasis in deficiency of IL-36 receptor antagonist syndrome (DITRA): (**A**) 5-year-old boy with an erythrodermic eruption showing confluent, non-follicular, aseptic pustules on an erythematous background; (**B**) H&E, ×4. Psoriasiform epidermal hyperplasia with aggregates of subcorneal and intra-epidermal neutrophils; (**C**) H&E, ×10. Spongiform pustules, neutrophils in a parakeratotic stratum corneum, and a neutrophilic infiltrate in the papillary dermis. Courtesy of Deborah Salik.

CARD14 gain-of-function mutations result in a monogenic syndrome called CARD-14-associated-papulosquamous eruption (CAPE) and the complex multigenic diseases of generalized pustular psoriasis and palmoplantar pustular psoriasis [35–37]. CAPE is identical to pityriasis rubra pilaris (PRP) type V, which causes a hereditary, pediatric form of PRP. There is early onset in life with prominent facial involvement, typically sparing the lower lip, and associated arthritis. The patients have features of psoriasis, PRP, or a combination of both with erythroderma [38,39]. The histopathological findings for CAPE are identical to PRP, showing psoriasiform hyperplasia with irregular hyperkeratosis, alternating vertical and horizontal orthokeratosis and parakeratosis and follicular plugging. In contrast to typical PRP, both psoriasis and CAPE lack acantholysis [40].

Amicrobial pustulosis of the folds and the scalp, rather than occurring in monogenic diseases, occurs in a few complex multigenic inflammatory diseases, most frequently systemic LE, mixed connective tissue disease, Sjögren syndrome and Crohn's disease. Age ranges from 12 to 63-years-old (mean 30 years). Clinically, there are non-follicular-based pustules on an erythematous ground. Histopathology shows spongiform pustulation identical to pustular psoriasis [41].

2.1.3. The Aseptic Neutrophilic Folliculitis Pattern

Aseptic neutrophilic folliculitis is the third type of neutrophilic pattern. Aseptic neutrophilic folliculitis is the primary lesion seen in PG, hidradenitis suppurativa (HS) and acne.

The folliculitis may occur in a variety of overlapping syndromes that show neutrophilic folliculitis, pyogenic arthritis and seronegative spondyloarthropathies including ankylosing spondylitis and psoriatic arthritis. The syndromes have been grouped in a set of so-called 'P' syndromes as follows: PAPASH (pyogenic arthritis, pyoderma gangrenosum, acne, suppurative hidradenitis); PsAPASH (psoriatic arthritis, pyoderma gangrenosum, acne, suppurative hidradenitis); PASS (pyoderma gangrenosum, acne, suppurative hidradenitis and ankylosing spondylitis); PASH (pyoderma gangrenosum, acne, suppurative hidradenitis); and PAPA (pyogenic arthritis, pyoderma gangrenosum, acne) [42]. PAPASH, PASH and PAPA syndromes are all MAIS [43,44]. PAPA syndrome is variably expressed with onset of joint disease between 1 and 16 years of age and acne beginning in puberty, associated with mild physical trauma. Severe, cystic, disfiguring acne appears after the joint disease [45,46].

Some consider erosive pustular dermatosis of the scalp to be a neutrophilic folliculitis similar to PG, especially because it may start after mechanical trauma (younger patients) or treatment of actinic keratoses (older patients). It is possible, however, that the disease in younger patients is an aseptic neutrophilic folliculitis, while the disease in older patients is the result of an inability to maintain epithelialization in severely actinic-damaged skin. Reports of histopathologic findings, though, do propose that the primary lesion may be, similarly to PG, a neutrophilic folliculitis [47].

Pyrin-associated auto-inflammation with neutrophilic dermatosis (PAAND) is due to mutations in the MEFV gene. Features of FMF such as amyloidosis and serositis are absent. PAAND is characterized by childhood-onset of recurrent episodes of PG, acne, fever (which last for weeks as opposed to days in FMF), elevated acute-phase reactants, arthralgia, and myalgia/myositis and pyogenic arthritis. Leukocytoclastic vasculitis, reported as 'neutrophilic small-vessel vasculitis', has also been described (see below) [48].

Haploinsufficiency of A20 (HA20) causes recurrent oral and genital ulcers mimicking the bipolar aphthosis of Behçet's disease. Although the histopathological findings for this syndrome have not yet been elucidated, this syndrome can be included in this group since mucosal ulceration, acne and folliculitis have been described [49]. Monogenic Behçet's disease can be also caused by rare, identified mutations in genes of the NF-κB pathway [50].

2.1.4. Sweet's Syndrome

Sweet's syndrome is the last group of neutrophilic patterns. Various MAIS produce the neutrophilic, histiocytoid and necrotizing variants. FMF can produce the neutrophilic variant [51]. Chronic atypical neutrophilic dermatosis with lipodystrophy and elevated temperature (CANDLE) syndrome is similar to the histiocytoid variant of Sweet's syndrome. CANDLE causes annular violaceous plaques, persistent eyelid swelling and lipodystrophy. Histopathological findings for CANDLE show a superficial and deep dermal interstitial infiltrate of CD68+, CD163+, myeloperoxidase+, CD45+ mononuclear myeloid cells, admixed with leukocytoclasia [52]. Necrotizing Sweet syndrome, often misdiagnosed as infectious necrotizing fasciitis, is a diagnostic pitfall, and occurrence after a surgical procedure or a trauma is an important clinical clue. A careful clinical correlation can help exclude a hematologic disorder, particularly myelodysplastic syndrome, a connective tissue disease, an endocrine disorder, or a drug eruption (granulocyte colony-stimulating factor) [53]. Familial autoinflammatory necrotizing fasciitis is a recently described NFkBopathy [50,54]. Recurrent sterile necrotizing fasciitis should lead one to suspect this disease, since an aggressive surgical therapeutic approach after a misdiagnosis of a bacterial infection can cause rapid disease progression and death.

2.2. The Vasculitic Pattern

The second histopathological pattern leading to suspicion of autoinflammation is vasculitis and it can be seen in either small-sized vessels (capillaries and post-capillary venules), or intermediate-sized vessels that have muscular walls (arterioles).

2.2.1. Small Sized-Vessel Vasculitis

The MAIS that produce small-sized vessel vasculitis include leukocytoclastic vasculitis, the thrombotic microangiopathy seen in the interferonopathies, and the lymphocytic vasculitis seen in tumor necrosis factor receptor-associated periodic syndrome (TRAPS).

Leukocytoclastic vasculitis is a non-specific cutaneous marker of auto-inflammation and has been described in various MAIS, including FMF, PAAND, NOMID, PAPA and hyperimmunoglobulinemia D syndrome (HIDS) [55]. HIDS, also called mevalonate kinase deficiency, is characterized by recurrent fever lasting from 5 to 7 days, cervical lymphadenopathy and splenomegaly, joint disease, and gastrointestinal symptoms. Cutaneous lesions have been reported as morbilliform, urticarial and purpuric. More frequently, however, the lesions lack a morphological description and are reported simply as a 'rash' [56–58]. Histopathology shows small vessel vasculitis, including Henoch–Schonlein purpura and erythema elevatum diutinum [58–60].

Thrombotic microangiopathy is the histopathological hallmark of the interferonopathies, all characterized by mutations that lead to the aberrant release of type I IFN and inflammation simulating viral infection or systemic LE. The thrombotic microangiopathy in the interferonopathies causes severe necrotic chilblains, leading to digital amputations and ear-tissue loss. The patients also present with features of systemic lupus erythematosus (i.e., antinuclear antibodies specific for SLE) [61]. Monogenic systemic LE with cytopenia, glomerulonephritis, arthritis and oral ulcers also belongs to this group of MAIS [1,62]. Aicardi–Goutières syndrome and familial chilblain lupus are allelic phenotypes of the same disease [63,64]. Patients with Aicardi–Goutières syndrome also develop severe neurological disease with intracranial basal ganglia calcifications [65,66]. Stimulator of interferon genes (STING)-associated vasculopathy with onset in infancy (SAVI) has interstitial lung disease and may be misdiagnosed as granulomatosis with polyangiitis [67–70]. Finally, spondyloenchondrodysplasia is characterized by skeletal dysplasia, and neurological developmental delay with intracranial calcification [61]. Histopathological findings for Aicardi–Goutières syndrome and familial chilblain lupus are identical to chilblain LE. There is vacuolar interface dermatitis, absent or mild papillary dermal edema and a superficial and deep lymphocytic infiltrate, often with a peri-eccrine accentuation. There may also be a lymphocytic vasculitis, with thick vessel walls, red cell extravasation and formation of intraluminal thrombi (Figure 6) [61,65].

TRAPS, another of the MAIS, is characterized by prolonged episodes of fever and systemic inflammation (myalgia, arthralgia, fasciitis, pericarditis, periorbital edema and conjunctivitis). Abdominal pain is the most prominent finding. Eighty percent of cases occur in childhood, with the episodes lasting 2–4 weeks, with intervals from months to years. Periorbital edema and cellulitis-like subcutaneous inflammation of the upper limbs is a characteristic feature. The cutaneous lesions start as erythematous macules and patches, which are variable in size. They may migrate proximal-to-distal on the extremity [71–73]. Histopathology shows a superficial and deep lymphocytic infiltrate with tight venule cuffing but no fibrin within vessel walls [73,74].

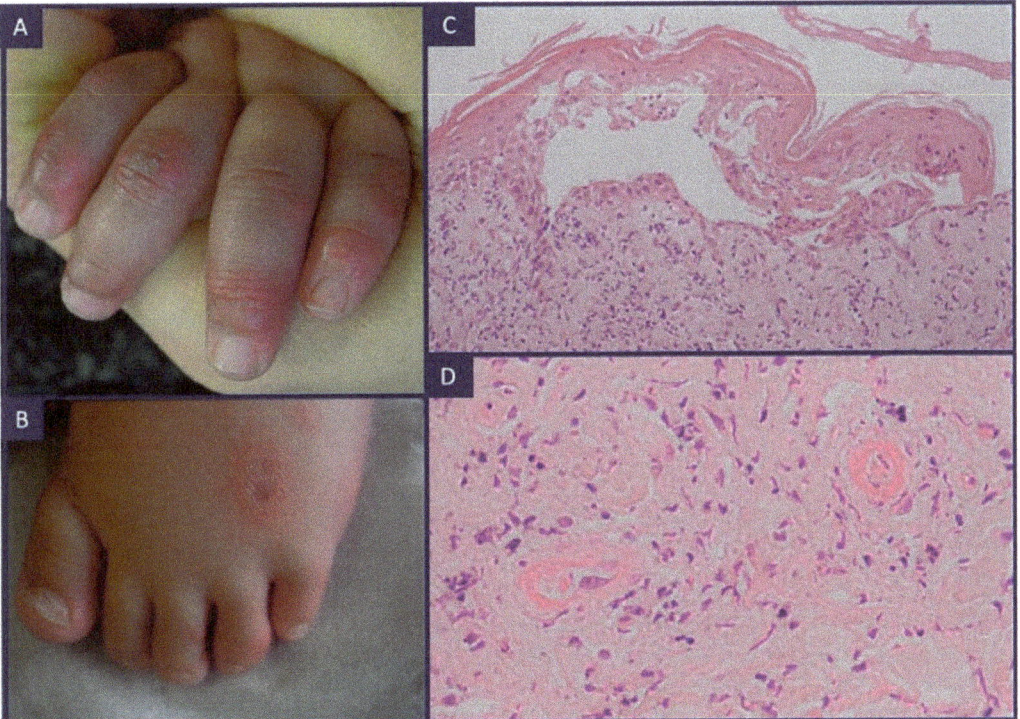

Figure 6. Thrombotic microangiopathy in Aicardi–Goutières syndrome: (**A**,**B**) 1-year-old female with acral necrotic bullous chilblains (**C**) H&E, ×4. Vacuolar interface dermatitis associated with numerous apoptotic keratinocytes, epidermal necrosis and subepidermal bulla. similar to necrotic chilblain lupus erythematosus; (**D**) H&E, ×20. Fibrin deposition in small-sized vessel walls associated with intraluminal thrombi.

2.2.2. Intermediate-Sized Vessel Vasculitis

The MAIS that cause intermediate-sized vessel vasculitis are deficiency in adenosine deaminase 2 (DADA2) and VEXAS (vacuoles, E1 enzyme, X-linked, autoinflammatory, somatic) syndrome. Histopathology shows features identical to cutaneous polyarteritis nodosa (PAN).

DADA2 or monogenic polyarteritis is an autosomal recessive vasculopathy due to CECR1 (cat eye syndrome chromosome region, candidate 1) mutation. The disease is characterized by PAN, lymphopenia and pancytopenia, and a B-cell immunodeficiency [75,76]. The vasculitis starts early in life and is characterized by the triad of livedo racemosa, recurrent fever and strokes [77–79]. DADA2 also has microangiopathic involvement, with clinical findings similar to the interferonopathies with necrotic chilblains [77,80]. Importantly, any diagnosis of PAN in a child should always exclude DADA2, since early implementation of anti-TNF therapy may prevent a stroke. Histopathological findings for DADA2 show a neutrophilic infiltrate with the neutrophils being present in and around and muscular arteriole walls where there is fibrinoid necrosis. The internal elastic lamina is disrupted, and there are hyalin fibrin rings with intraluminal thrombi [79,81]. We have also been confronted by a case of DADA2 in a child with extensive livedo, whose skin biopsy revealed a mononuclear cell infiltrate surrounding thrombosed intermediate-sized vessels simulating lymphocytic thrombophilic arteritis (Figure 7).

The VEXAS syndrome is caused by mutations of the UBA1 gene. No pediatric cases have been reported. VEXAS syndrome is characterized by fever, cytopenias, characteristic vacuoles in myeloid and erythroid precursor cells, dysplastic bone marrow (myelodysplastic syndrome or multiple myeloma), relapsing polychondritis, Sweet's syndrome, polyarteritis nodosa, and giant-cell arteritis [82].

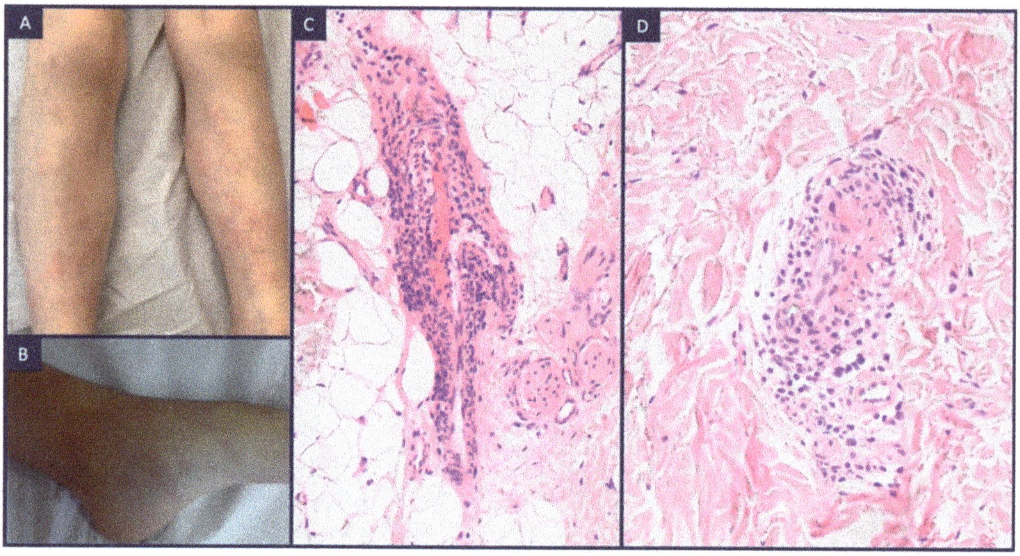

Figure 7. Deficiency of adenosine deaminase 2 syndrome (DADA2): (**A,B**) 6-year-old boy with livedo racemosa on the lower limbs; (**C,D**) H&E, ×10 (**C**), ×20 (**D**). Intraluminal thrombi within intermediate-sized vessels at the dermal-subcutaneous junction and a surrounding mononuclear cell infiltrate simulating lymphocytic thrombophilic arteritis.

2.3. The Granulomatous Pattern

The granulomatous pattern is the third pattern seen in autoinflammation. This pattern is seen with NOD2 mutations in Blau syndrome and with PLCγ2 mutations in 'autoinflammation and phospholipase C gamma 2 associated antibody deficiency and immune dysregulation' (APLAID) and 'phospholipase C gamma 2 associated antibody deficiency and immune dysregulation' (PLAID). Both NOD2 and PLCγ2 mutations are associated with Crohn's disease [83,84].

Blau syndrome (early-onset sarcoidosis) is characterized by the triad of articular, cutaneous and ocular non-caseating granulomatous inflammation. The disease begins very early in life. The cutaneous lesions initially are monomorphic, non-confluent papules, and late lesions are heterogenous with confluent papules, plaques, nodules and panniculitis. Histopathological findings are consistently sarcoidal granulomas in both early and late lesions [85–87]. Granulomas in Blau syndrome and granulomas in NOD2-associated Crohn's disease show distinct morphologic features with granulomas with large lymphocytic coronas, emperipolesis of lymphocytes within multinucleated giant cells and giant cell apoptosis seen only in Blau syndrome [88]. In contrast to Blau syndrome, NOD2-associated autoinflammatory syndrome (NAID) occurs in adults. NAID has gastro-intestinal symptoms instead of uveitis with cutaneous erythematous patches and plaques. Histopathological findings in NAID show a non-specific spongiotic dermatitis [89]. Patients may show phenotypical overlap between Blau syndrome, NAID, and Crohn's disease [84,86,90,91].

PLAID and APLAID are allelic diseases that are both caused by PLCγ2 mutations, which produce a B-cell immunodeficiency. Mutations responsible for PLAID are deletions that result in enhanced PLCγ2 signaling and mutations responsible for APLAID are missense mutations that decrease the threshold required for PLCγ2 activation. PLAID is associated with autoimmune diseases (thyroiditis, vitiligo, positive antinuclear antibodies) and cold-induced urticaria. The histopathological findings for cold-induced urticaria are similar to the NUD already discussed in the cryopyrinopathy section. Neonates with

PLAID also have blistering ulcerations, especially on the nose, ears and fingers. Ulceration usually spontaneously resolves, but, in a few cases, it may progress, thereby leading to destruction of ear and nose cartilage. In neonates with self-resolving ulceration, isolated granulomatous patches may develop later in life. The histopathology of these patches shows non-caseating granulomatous inflammation. APLAID is associated with a neonatal-onset vesicular-bullous eruption and recurrent acral hemorrhagic blisters. Histopathology in APLAID shows a dense perivascular and interstitial granulomatous infiltrate, palisading granulomas around areas of collagen necrobiosis, and a dense neutrophilic infiltrate. Leukocytoclastic vasculitis is also observed. Bulla formation can result from intense papillary dermal edema [92–95].

3. Conclusions

Autoinflammation can be suspected upon cutaneous histopathological examination and based on recognition of three main histopathological patterns: the neutrophilic, the vasculitic and the granulomatous patterns. In this review we have described the journey of the dermatopathologist, beginning with the identification of these histopathological patterns, followed by the identification of additional histopathological clues and the correlation of these findings with the clinical manifestations in the pediatric patient. This would lead to the identification of an activated regulatory pathway and the diagnosis of a MAIS or a complex multigenic disease.

Author Contributions: Writing—original draft preparation, A.K.; writing—review and editing, A.K., I.M., U.S. and C.T.T.; visualization, A.K., I.M., U.S. and C.T.T. All authors have read and agreed to the published version of the manuscript.

Funding: This review received no external funding.

Institutional Review Board Statement: Not applicable.

Informed Consent Statement: Not applicable.

Acknowledgments: We gratefully acknowledge Josette André, Chantal Dangoisse, Aline Ferster, Florence Goffin, Olivia Paduart, Philippe Provost, Deborah Salik, Anne Theunis for their contribution.

Conflicts of Interest: The authors declare no conflict of interest.

Abbreviations

APLAID	autoinflammation and phospholipase C gamma 2 associated antibody deficiency and immune dysregulation
CANDLE	Chronic Atypical Neutrophilic Dermatosis with Lipodystrophy and Elevated temperature
CAPE	caspase-activating recruitment domain, member 14 associated papulosquamous eruption
CAPS	cryopyrin-associated periodic syndromes
DADA2	deficiency of adenosine deaminase 2
DIRA	Deficiency of IL-1 Receptor Antagonist syndrome
DITRA	Deficiency of IL-36 Receptor Antagonist
FCAS	Familial Cold Autoinflammatory syndrome
FMF	Familial Mediterranean Fever syndrome
HA20	Haploinsufficiency of A20
HIDS	Hyperimmunoglobulinemia D syndrome
IFN	interferon
IL	interleukin
LE	lupus erythematosus
MAIS	monogenic autoinflammatory syndromes
MWS	Muckle–Wells syndrome
NOMID	neonatal-onset multisystem inflammatory disease
PAAND	pyrin-associated autoinflammation with neutrophilic dermatosis

PAPA	Pyogenic Arthritis, Pyoderma gangrenosum and Acne
PAPASH	Pyogenic Arthritis, Pyoderma gangrenosum, Acne, Suppurative Hidradenitis
PASH	Pyoderma gangrenosum, Acne, Suppurative Hidradenitis
PASS	Pyoderma gangrenosum, Acne, Suppurative hidradenitis and ankylosing Spondylitis
PLAID	Phospholipase C gamma 2 associated antibody deficiency and immune dysregulation
PLCγ2	Phospholipase C gamma 2
PsAPASH	Psoriatic Arthritis, Pyoderma gangrenosum, Acne, Suppurative Hidradenitis
SAVI	Stimulator of interferon genes (STING) associated vasculopathy of infancy
TRAPS	TNF receptor-associated periodic syndrome
VEXAS	Vacuoles, E1 enzyme, X-linked, Autoinflammatory, Somatic syndrome

References

1. Nigrovic, P.A.; Lee, P.Y.; Hoffman, H.M. Monogenic autoinflammatory disorders: Conceptual overview, phenotype, and clinical approach. *J. Allergy Clin. Immun.* **2020**, *146*, 925–937. [CrossRef] [PubMed]
2. Stojanov, S.; Kastner, D.L. Familial autoinflammatory diseases: Genetics, pathogenesis and treatment. *Curr. Opin. Rheumatol.* **2005**, *17*, 586–599. [CrossRef] [PubMed]
3. Chitkara, P.; Stojanov, S.; Kastner, D.L. The hereditary autoinflammatory syndromes. *Pediatr. Infect. Dis. J.* **2007**, *26*, 353–354. [CrossRef]
4. McDermott, M.F.; Aksentijevich, I. The autoinflammatory syndromes. *Curr. Opin. Allergy Clin. Immunol.* **2002**, *2*, 511–516. [CrossRef] [PubMed]
5. Figueras-Nart, I.; Mascaró, J.M.; Solanich, X.; Hernández-Rodríguez, J. Dermatologic and Dermatopathologic Features of Monogenic Autoinflammatory Diseases. *Front. Immunol.* **2019**, *10*, 2448. [CrossRef]
6. Shwin, K.W.; Lee, C.R.; Goldbach-Mansky, R. Dermatologic Manifestations of Monogenic Autoinflammatory Diseases. *Derm. Clin.* **2017**, *35*, 21–38. [CrossRef] [PubMed]
7. Lipsker, D.; Saurat, J.-H. Neutrophilic cutaneous lupus erythematosus. At the edge between innate and acquired immunity? *Dermatology* **2008**, *216*, 283–286. [CrossRef]
8. Stankovic, K.; Grateau, G. What's new in autoinflammatory diseases? *Rev. Med. Interne* **2008**, *29*, 994–999. [CrossRef]
9. Nguyen, T.V.; Cowen, E.W.; Leslie, K.S. Autoinflammation: From monogenic syndromes to common skin diseases. *J. Am. Dermatol.* **2013**, *68*, 1–20. [CrossRef]
10. Kelley, N.; Jeltema, D.; Duan, Y.; He, Y. The NLRP3 Inflammasome: An Overview of Mechanisms of Activation and Regulation. *Int. J. Mol. Sci.* **2019**, *20*, 3328. [CrossRef] [PubMed]
11. Broekaert, S.M.C.; Böer-Auer, A.; Kerl, K.; Herrgott, I.; Schulz, X.; Bonsmann, G.; Brehler, R.; Metze, D. Neutrophilic Epitheliotropism Is a Histopathological Clue to Neutrophilic Urticarial Dermatosis. *Am. J. Dermatopathol.* **2016**, *38*, 39–49. [CrossRef] [PubMed]
12. Kolivras, A.; Theunis, A.; Ferster, A.; Lipsker, D.; Sass, U.; Dussart, A.; André, J. Cryopyrin-associated periodic syndrome: An autoinflammatory disease manifested as neutrophilic urticarial dermatosis with additional perieccrine involvement. *J. Cutan. Pathol.* **2011**, *38*, 202–208. [CrossRef] [PubMed]
13. Gusdorf, L.; Lipsker, D. Neutrophilic urticarial dermatosis. An entity bridging monogenic and polygenic autoinflammatory disorders, and beyond. *J. Eur. Acad. Dermatol. Venereol.* **2020**, *34*, 685–690. [CrossRef] [PubMed]
14. Gusdorf, L.; Lipsker, D. Neutrophilic urticarial dermatosis: A review. *Ann. Dermatol. Vénéréologie* **2018**, *145*, 735–740. [CrossRef]
15. Aksentijevich, I.; Putnam, C.D.; Remmers, E.F.; Mueller, J.L.; Le, J.; Kolodner, R.D. The clinical continuum of cryopyrinopathies: Novel CIAS1 mutations in North American patients and a new cryopyrin model. *Arthritis Rheumatism.* **2007**, *56*, 1273–1285. [CrossRef]
16. Neven, B.; Prieur, A.-M.; Maire, P.Q.D. Cryopyrinopathies: Update on pathogenesis and treatment. *Nat. Clin. Pract. Rheumatol.* **2008**, *4*, 481–489. [CrossRef] [PubMed]
17. Hoffman, H.M.; Wanderer, A.A.; Broide, D.H. Familial cold autoinflammatory syndrome: Phenotype and genotype of an autosomal dominant periodic fever. *J. Allergy Clin. Immunol.* **2001**, *108*, 615–620. [CrossRef]
18. Jeru, I.; Duquesnoy, P.; Fernandes-Alnemri, T.; Cochet, E.; Yu, J.-W.; Lackmy-Port-Lis, M.; Grimprel, E.; Landman-Parker, J.; Hentgen, V.; Marlin, S.; et al. Mutations in NALP12 cause hereditary periodic fever syndromes. *Proc. Natl. Acad. Sci. USA* **2008**, *105*, 1614–1619. [CrossRef]
19. Kilcline, C.; Shinkai, K.; Bree, A.; Modica, R.; Scheven, E.V.; Frieden, I.J. Neonatal-Onset multisystem inflammatory disorder: The emerging role of pyrin genes in autoinflammatory diseases. *Arch. Dermatol.* **2005**, *141*, 248–253. [CrossRef]
20. Goldbach-Mansky, R.; Dailey, N.J.; Canna, S.W.; Gelabert, A.; Jones, J.; Rubin, B.I.; Kastner, D.L. Neonatal-Onset multisystem inflammatory disease responsive to interleukin-1beta inhibition. *N. Engl. J. Med.* **2006**, *355*, 581–592. [CrossRef]
21. Shinkai, K.; McCalmont, T.H.; Leslie, K.S. Cryopyrin-associated periodic syndromes and autoinflammation. *Clin. Exp. Dermatol.* **2008**, *33*, 1–9. [CrossRef]
22. Brinster, N.K.; Nunley, J.; Pariser, R.; Horvath, B. Nonbullous neutrophilic lupus erythematosus: A newly recognized variant of cutaneous lupus erythematosus. *J. Am. Acad. Dermatol.* **2012**, *66*, 92–97. [CrossRef]

23. Sokumbi, O.; Drage, L.A.; Peters, M.S. Clinical and histopathologic review of Schnitzler syndrome: The Mayo Clinic experience (1972–2011). *J. Am. Dermatol.* **2012**, *67*, 1289–1295. [CrossRef]
24. Santa, E.; McFalls, J.M.; Sahu, J.; Lee, J.B. Clinical and histopathological features of cutaneous manifestations of adult-onset Still disease. *J. Cutan. Pathol.* **2017**, *44*, 591–595. [CrossRef]
25. Livneh, A.; Langevitz, P.; Zemer, D.; Zaks, N.; Kees, S.; Lidar, T.; Migdal, A.; Padeh, S.; Pras, M. Criteria for the diagnosis of familial mediterranean fever. *Arthritis Rheum.* **1997**, *40*, 1879–1885. [CrossRef] [PubMed]
26. Tamir, N.; Langevitz, P.; Zemer, D.; Pras, E.; Shinar, Y.; Padeh, S. Late-Onset familial Mediterranean fever (FMF): A subset with distinct clinical, demographic, and molecular genetic characteristics. *Am. J. Med. Genet.* **1999**, *87*, 30–35. [CrossRef]
27. Padeh, S.; Livneh, A.; Pras, E.; Shinar, Y.; Lidar, M.; Feld, O.; Berkun, Y. Familial Mediterranean Fever in the First Two Years of Life: A Unique Phenotype of Disease in Evolution. *J. Pediatr.* **2010**, *156*, 985–989. [CrossRef]
28. Lidar, M.; Doron, A.; Barzilai, A.; Feld, O.; Zaks, N.; Livneh, A.; Langevitz, P. Erysipelas-like erythema as the presenting feature of familial Mediterranean fever. *J. Eur. Acad. Dermatol. Venereol.* **2012**, *27*, 912–915. [CrossRef]
29. Kolivras, A.; Provost, P.; Thompson, C.T. Erysipelas-like erythema of familial Mediterranean fever syndrome: A case report with emphasis on histopathologic diagnostic clues. *J. Cutan. Pathol.* **2013**, *40*, 585–590. [CrossRef]
30. Barzilai, A.; Langevitz, P.; Goldberg, I.; Kopolovic, J.; Livneh, A.; Pras, M.; Trau, H. Erysipelas-like erythema of familial Mediterranean fever: Clinicopathologic correlation. *J. Am. Acad. Dermatol.* **2000**, *42*, 791–795. [CrossRef] [PubMed]
31. Akman, A.; Cakcak, D.S.; Çoban, E.; Ozbudak, H.I.; Ciftcioglu, M.A.; Alpsoy, E.; Yilmaz, E. Recurrent bullous lesions associated with familial Mediterranean fever: A case report. *Clin. Exp. Dermatol.* **2009**, *34*, 216–218. [CrossRef] [PubMed]
32. Aksentijevich, I.; Masters, S.L.; Ferguson, P.J.; Dancey, P.; Frenkel, J.; Van Royen-Kerkhoff, A.; Laxer, R.; Tedgård, U.; Cowen, E.W.; Pham, T.-H.; et al. An Autoinflammatory Disease with Deficiency of the Interleukin-1–Receptor Antagonist. *N. Engl. J. Med.* **2009**, *360*, 2426–2437. [CrossRef] [PubMed]
33. Minkis, K.; Aksentijevich, I.; Goldbach-Mansky, R.; Magro, C.; Scott, R.; Davis, J.G.; Sardana, N.; Herzog, R. Interleukin 1 Receptor Antagonist Deficiency Presenting as Infantile Pustulosis Mimicking Infantile Pustular Psoriasis. *Arch. Dermatol.* **2012**, *148*, 747–752. [CrossRef]
34. Marrakchi, S.; Guigue, P.; Renshaw, B.R.; Puel, A.; Pei, X.-Y.; Fraitag, S.; Zribi, J.; Bal, E.; Cluzeau, C.; Chrabieh, M.; et al. Interleukin-36–Receptor Antagonist Deficiency and Generalized Pustular Psoriasis. *N. Engl. J. Med.* **2011**, *365*, 620–628. [CrossRef]
35. Bachelez, H. Pustular psoriasis and related pustular skin diseases. *Br. J. Dermatol.* **2018**, *178*, 614–618. [CrossRef]
36. Spoerri, I.; Herms, S.; Eytan, O.; Sarig, O.; Heinimann, K.; Sprecher, E.; Itin, P.; Burger, B. Immune-regulatory genes as possible modifiers of familial pityriasis rubra pilaris—Lessons from a family with PRP and psoriasis. *J. Eur. Acad. Dermatol. Venereol.* **2018**, *32*, e389–e392. [CrossRef]
37. Sugiura, K. Autoinflammatory diseases in dermatology: DITRA and CAMPS. *Nihon Rinsho Men'eki Gakkai Kaishi Jpn. J. Clin. Immunol.* **2017**, *40*, 169–173. [CrossRef] [PubMed]
38. Craiglow, B.G.; Boyden, L.M.; Hu, R.; Virtanen, M.; Su, J.; Rodriguez, G.; McCarthy, C.; Luna, P.; Larralde, M.; Humphrey, S.; et al. CARD14-associated papulosquamous eruption: A spectrum including features of psoriasis and pityriasis rubra pilaris. *J. Am. Acad. Dermatol.* **2018**, *79*, 487–494. [CrossRef]
39. Takeichi, T.; Sugiura, K.; Nomura, T.; Sakamoto, T.; Ogawa, Y.; Oiso, N.; Akiyama, M. Pityriasis Rubra Pilaris Type V as an Autoinflammatory Disease by CARD14 Mutations. *JAMA Dermatol.* **2017**, *153*, 66–70. [CrossRef]
40. Ring, N.G.; Craiglow, B.G.; Panse, G.; Antaya, R.J.; Ashack, K.; Ashack, R.; Faith, E.F.; Paller, A.S.; McNiff, J.M.; Choate, K.A.; et al. Histopathologic findings characteristic of CARD14-associated papulosquamous eruption. *J. Cutan. Pathol.* **2020**, *47*, 425–430. [CrossRef]
41. Schissler, C.; Velter, C.; Lipsker, D. Amicrobial pustulosis of the folds: Where have we gone 25 years after its original description? *Ann. Dermatol. Vénéréol.* **2017**, *144*, 169–175. [CrossRef] [PubMed]
42. Gottlieb, J.; Madrange, M.; Gardair, C.; Sbidian, E.; Frazier, A.; Wolkenstein, P.; Bachelez, H. PAPASH, Ps APASHand PASSautoinflammatory syndromes: Phenotypic heterogeneity, common biological signature and response to immunosuppressive regimens. *Br. J. Dermatol.* **2019**, *181*, 866–869. [CrossRef]
43. Zhang, X.; He, Y.; Xu, H.; Wang, B. First PSENEN mutation in PASH syndrome. *J. Dermatol.* **2020**, *47*, 1335–1337. [CrossRef]
44. Marzano, A.V.; Trevisan, V.; Gattorno, M.; Ceccherini, I.; de Simone, C.; Crosti, C. Pyogenic Arthritis, Pyoderma Gangrenosum, Acne, and Hidradenitis Suppurativa (PAPASH): A New Autoinflammatory Syndrome Associated with a Novel Mutation of the PSTPIP1 Gene. *JAMA Dermatol.* **2013**, *149*, 762–764. [CrossRef]
45. Tallon, B.; Corkill, M. Peculiarities of PAPA syndrome. *Rheumatology* **2006**, *45*, 1140–1143. [CrossRef] [PubMed]
46. Smith, E.J.; Allantaz, F.; Bennett, L.; Zhang, N.; Gao, X.; Wood, G.; Kastner, D.L.; Punaro, M.; Aksentijevich, I.; Pascual, V.; et al. Clinical, Molecular, and Genetic Characteristics of PAPA Syndrome: A Review. *Curr. Genom.* **2010**, *11*, 519–527. [CrossRef] [PubMed]
47. Tomasini, C.; Michelerio, A. Erosive pustular dermatosis of the scalp: A neutrophilic folliculitis within the spectrum of neutrophilic dermatoses: A clinicopathologic study of 30 cases. *J. Am. Acad. Dermatol.* **2018**, *81*, 527–533. [CrossRef]
48. Masters, S.L.; Lagou, V.; Jéru, I.; Baker, P.J.; Van Eyck, L.; Parry, D.A.; Lawless, D.; De Nardo, D.; Garcia-Perez, J.E.; Dagley, L.F.; et al. Familial autoinflammation with neutrophilic dermatosis reveals a regulatory mechanism of pyrin activation. *Sci. Transl. Med.* **2016**, *8*, 332ra45. [CrossRef] [PubMed]

49. Aeschlimann, F.A.; Batu, E.D.; Canna, S.W.; Go, E.; Gül, A.; Hoffmann, P.; Laxer, R.M. A20 haploinsufficiency (HA20): Clinical phenotypes and disease course of patients with a newly recognised NF-κB-mediated autoinflammatory disease. *Ann. Rheum. Dis.* **2018**, *77*, 728. [CrossRef] [PubMed]
50. Kaustio, M.; Haapaniemi, E.; Göös, H.; Hautala, T.; Park, G.; Syrjänen, J.; Einarsdottir, E.; Sahu, B.; Kilpinen, S.; Rounioja, S.; et al. Damaging heterozygous mutations in NFKB1 lead to diverse immunologic phenotypes. *J. Allergy Clin. Immunol.* **2017**, *140*, 782–796. [CrossRef]
51. Oskay, T.; Anadolu, R. Sweet's syndrome in familial Mediterranean fever: Possible continuum of the neutrophilic reaction as a new cutaneous feature of FMF. *J. Cutan. Pathol.* **2009**, *36*, 901–905. [CrossRef]
52. Torrelo, A.; Patel, S.; Colmenero, I.; Gurbindo, D.; Lendinez, F.; Hernandez, A.; Paller, A.S. Chronic atypical neutrophilic dermatosis with lipodystrophy and elevated temperature (CANDLE) syndrome. *J. Am. Acad. Dermatol.* **2010**, *62*, 489–495. [CrossRef]
53. Sanchez, I.M.; Lowenstein, S.; Johnson, K.A.; Babik, J.; Haag, C.; Keller, J.J.; Shinkai, K. Clinical Features of Neutrophilic Dermatosis Variants Resembling Necrotizing Fasciitis. *JAMA Dermatol.* **2019**, *155*, 79–82. [CrossRef]
54. Kaustio, M.; Hautala, T.; Seppänen, M.R.J. Primary Immunodeficiency, a Possible Cause of Neutrophilic Necrotizing Dermatosis. *JAMA Dermatol.* **2019**, *155*, 863–864. [CrossRef]
55. Jain, A.; Misra, D.P.; Sharma, A.; Wakhlu, A.; Agarwal, V.; Negi, V.S. Vasculitis and vasculitis-like manifestations in monogenic autoinflammatory syndromes. *Rheumatol. Int.* **2018**, *38*, 13–24. [CrossRef] [PubMed]
56. Durel, C.-A.; Aouba, A.; Bienvenu, B.; Deshayes, S.; Coppéré, B.; Gombert, B.; Hot, A. Observational Study of a French and Belgian Multicenter Cohort of 23 Patients Diagnosed in Adulthood with Mevalonate Kinase Deficiency. *Medicine* **2016**, *95*, e3027. [CrossRef]
57. Korppi, M.; Van Gijn, M.E.; Antila, K. Hyperimmunoglobulinemia D and periodic fever syndrome in children. Review on therapy with biological drugs and case report. *Acta Paediatr.* **2011**, *100*, 21–25. [CrossRef]
58. Drenth, J.P.; Boom, B.W.; Toonstra, J.; van der Meer, J.W. Cutaneous manifestations and histologic findings in the hyperimmunoglobulinemia D syndrome. International Hyper IgD Study Group. *Arch. Dermatol.* **1994**, *130*, 59–65. [CrossRef] [PubMed]
59. Miyagawa, S.; Kitamura, W.; Morita, K.; Saishin, M.; Shirai, T. Association of hyperimmunoglobulinaemia D syndrome with erythema elevatum diutinum. *Br. J. Dermatol.* **1993**, *128*, 572–574. [CrossRef] [PubMed]
60. Boom, B.W.; Daha, M.R.; Vermeer, B.J.; van der Meer, J.W. IgD immune complex vasculitis in a patient with hyperimmunoglobulinemia D and periodic fever. *Arch. Dermatol.* **1990**, *126*, 1621–1624. [CrossRef]
61. Munoz, J.; Marque, M.; Dandurand, M.; Meunier, L.; Crow, Y.J.; Bessis, D. Interféronopathies de type I. *Ann. Dermatol. Vénéréol.* **2015**, *142*, 653–663. [CrossRef] [PubMed]
62. Omarjee, O.; Picard, C.; Frachette, C.; Moreews, M.; Laucat, F.R.; Sprauel, P.; Belot, A. Monogenic lupus: Dissecting heterobeneity. *Autoimmun. Rev.* **2019**, *18*, 102361. [CrossRef] [PubMed]
63. Günther, C.; Berndt, N.; Wolf, C.; Lee-Kirsch, M.A. Familial Chilblain Lupus Due to a Novel Mutation in the Exonuclease III Domain of 3' Repair Exonuclease 1 (TREX1). *JAMA Dermatol.* **2015**, *151*, 426–431. [CrossRef]
64. Beltoise, A.S.; Audouin-Pajot, C.; Lucas, P.; Tournier, E.; Rice, G.I.; Crow, Y.J.; Mazereeuw-Hautier, J. Lupus-engelures familial: Quatre cas sur trois générations. *Ann. Dermatol. Vénéréol.* **2018**, *145*, 683–689. [CrossRef] [PubMed]
65. Kolivras, A.; Aeby, A.; Crow, Y.J.; Rice, G.I.; Sass, U.; André, J. Cutaneous histopathological findings of Aicardi-Goutières syndrome, overlap with chilblain lupus. *J. Cutan. Pathol.* **2008**, *35*, 774–778. [CrossRef]
66. Lee-Kirsch, M.A.; Wolf, C.; Günther, C. Aicardi-Goutières syndrome: A model disease for systemic autoimmunity. *Clin. Exp. Immunol.* **2014**, *175*, 17–24. [CrossRef]
67. Liu, Y.; Jesus, A.A.; Marrero, B.; Yang, D.; Ramsey, S.E.; Montealegre Sanchez, G.A.; Tenbrock, K.; Wittkowski, H.; Jones, O.Y.; Kuehn, H.S.; et al. Activated STING in a Vascular and Pulmonary Syndrome. *N. Engl. J. Med.* **2014**, *371*, 507–518. [CrossRef]
68. Munoz, J.; Rodière, M.; Jeremiah, N.; Rieux-Laucat, F.; Oojageer, A.; Rice, G.I.; Rozenberg, F.; Crow, Y.J.; Bessis, D. Stimulator of Interferon Genes–Associated Vasculopathy With Onset in Infancy. *JAMA Dermatol.* **2015**, *151*, 872–877. [CrossRef]
69. Crow, Y.J.; Casanova, J.-L. STING-Associated Vasculopathy with Onset in Infancy—A New Interferonopathy. *N. Engl. J. Med.* **2014**, *371*, 568–571. [CrossRef] [PubMed]
70. Chia, J.; Eroglu, F.K.; Özen, S.; Orhan, D.; Montealegre-Sanchez, G.; De Jesus, A.A.; Goldbach-Mansky, R.; Cowen, E.W. Failure to thrive, interstitial lung disease, and progressive digital necrosis with onset in infancy. *J. Am. Acad. Dermatol.* **2016**, *74*, 186–189. [CrossRef] [PubMed]
71. Stojanov, S.; McDermott, M.F. the tumour necrosis factor receptor-associated periodic syndrome: Current concepts. *Expert Rev. Mol. Med.* **2005**, *7*, 1–18. [CrossRef]
72. Masson, C.; Simon, V.; Hoppe, E.; Insalaco, P.; Cissé, I.; Audran, M. Tumor necrosis factor receptor-associated periodic syndrome (TRAPS): Definition, semiology, prognosis, pathogenesis, treatment, and place relative to other periodic joint diseases. *Jt. Bone Spine* **2004**, *71*, 284–290. [CrossRef] [PubMed]
73. Toro, J.R.; Aksentijevich, I.; Hull, K.; Dean, J.; Kastner, D.L. Tumor necrosis factor receptor-associated periodic syndrome: A novel syndrome with cutaneous manifestations. *Arch. Dermatol.* **2000**, *136*, 1487–1494. [CrossRef]
74. Farasat, S.; Aksentijevich, I.; Toro, J.R. Autoinflammatory Diseases: Clinical and Genetic Advances. *Arch. Dermatol.* **2008**, *144*, 392–402. [CrossRef]

75. Elkan, P.N.; Pierce, S.B.; Segel, R.; Walsh, T.; Barash, J.; Padeh, S.; Zlotogorski, A.; Berkun, Y.; Press, J.J.; Mukamel, M.; et al. Mutant Adenosine Deaminase 2 in a Polyarteritis Nodosa Vasculopathy. *N. Engl. J. Med.* **2014**, *370*, 921–931. [CrossRef] [PubMed]
76. Fayand, A.; Sarrabay, G.; Belot, A.; Hentgen, V.; Kone-Paut, I.; Grateau, G.; Georgin-Lavialle, S. Les multiples facettes du déficit en ADA2, vascularite, maladie auto-inflammatoire et immunodéficit: Mise au point à partir des 135 cas de la littérature. *Rev. Méd. Interne* **2018**, *39*, 297–306. [CrossRef] [PubMed]
77. Zhou, Q.; Yang, D.; Ombrello, A.K.; Zavialov, A.; Toro, C.; Zavialov, A.V.; Stone, D.L.; Chae, J.J.; Rosenzweig, S.D.; Bishop, K.; et al. Early-Onset Stroke and Vasculopathy Associated with Mutations in ADA2. *N. Engl. J. Med.* **2014**, *370*, 911–920. [CrossRef]
78. Caorsi, R.; Penco, F.; Grossi, A.; Insalaco, A.; Omenetti, A.; Alessio, M.; Conti, G.; Marchetti, F.; Picco, P.; Tommasini, A.; et al. ADA2 deficiency (DADA2) as an unrecognised cause of early onset polyarteritis nodosa and stroke: A multicentre national study. *Ann. Rheum. Dis.* **2017**, *76*, 1648–1656. [CrossRef]
79. Pichard, D.C.; Ombrello, A.K.; Hoffmann, P.; Stone, D.L.; Cowen, E.W. Early-onset stroke, polyarteritis nodosa (PAN), and livedo racemosa. *J. Am. Acad. Dermatol.* **2016**, *75*, 449–453. [CrossRef]
80. Santiago, T.M.G.; Zavialov, A.; Saarela, J.; Seppanen, M.; Reed, A.M.; Abraham, R.S.; Gibson, L.E. Dermatologic Features of ADA2 Deficiency in Cutaneous Polyarteritis Nodosa. *JAMA Dermatol.* **2015**, *151*, 1230–1234. [CrossRef]
81. Caorsi, R.; Penco, F.; Schena, F.; Gattorno, M. Monogenic polyarteritis: The lesson of ADA2 deficiency. *Pediatr. Rheumatol.* **2016**, *14*, 51. [CrossRef]
82. Beck, D.B.; Ferrada, M.A.; Sikora, K.A.; Ombrello, A.K.; Collins, J.C.; Pei, W.; Balanda, N.; Ross, D.L.; Cardona, D.O.; Wu, Z.; et al. Somatic Mutations in UBA1 and Severe Adult-Onset Autoinflammatory Disease. *N. Engl. J. Med.* **2020**, *383*, 2628–2638. [CrossRef] [PubMed]
83. Szymanski, A.M.; Ombrello, M.J. Using genes to triangulate the pathophysiology of granulomatous autoinflammatory disease: NOD2, PLCG2 and LACC1. *Int. Immunol.* **2018**, *30*, 205–213. [CrossRef] [PubMed]
84. Yao, Q.; Li, E.; Shen, B. Autoinflammatory disease with focus on NOD2-associated disease in the era of genomic medicine. *Autoimmunity* **2019**, *52*, 48–56. [CrossRef]
85. Wlodek, C.; Clinch, J.; Planas, S.; Shaw, L. Widespread papular eruption in an infant. *Clin. Exp. Dermatol.* **2018**, *43*, 212–215. [CrossRef]
86. Caso, F.; Galozzi, P.; Costa, L.; Sfriso, P.; Cantarini, L.; Punzi, L. Autoinflammatory granulomatous diseases: From Blau syndrome and early-onset sarcoidosis to NOD2-mediated disease and Crohn's disease. *RMD Open* **2015**, *1*, e000097. [CrossRef] [PubMed]
87. Poline, J.; Fogel, O.; Pajot, C.; Miceli-Richard, C.; Rybojad, M.; Galeotti, C. Early onset granulomatous arthritis, uveitis and skin rash: Characterisation of skin involvement in Blau syndrome. *J. Eur. Acad. Dermatol. Venereol.* **2019**, *34*, 340–348. [CrossRef]
88. Janssen, C.E.I.; Rosé, C.D.; Hertogh, G.D.; Martin, T.M.; Bader-Meunier, B.; Cimaz, R.; Wouters, C.H. Morphologic and immunohistochemical characterization of granulomas in the nucleotide oligomerization domain 2-related disorders Blau syndrome and Crohn disease. *J. Allergy Clin. Immunol.* **2012**, *129*, 1076–1084. [CrossRef] [PubMed]
89. Yao, Q.; Su, L.-C.; Tomecki, K.J.; Zhou, L.; Jayakar, B.; Shen, B. Dermatitis as a characteristic phenotype of a new autoinflammatory disease associated with NOD2 mutations. *J. Am. Acad. Dermatol.* **2013**, *68*, 624–631. [CrossRef]
90. Shen, M.; Moran, R.; Tomecki, K.J.; Yao, Q. Granulomatous disease associated with NOD2 sequence variants and familial camptodactyly: An intermediate form of NOD2-associated diseases? *Semin. Arthritis Rheu.* **2015**, *45*, 357–360. [CrossRef] [PubMed]
91. Dziedzic, M.; Marjańska, A.; Bąbol-Pokora, K.; Urbańczyk, A.; Grześk, E.; Młynarski, W.; Kołtan, S. Co-existence of Blau syndrome and NAID? Diagnostic challenges associated with presence of multiple pathogenic variants in NOD2 gene: A case report. *Pediatr. Rheumatol. Online J.* **2017**, *15*, 57. [CrossRef] [PubMed]
92. Morán-Villaseñor, E.; Saez-De-Ocariz, M.; Torrelo, A.; Arostegui, J.I.; Yamazaki-Nakashimada, M.A.; Alcántara-Ortigoza, M.A.; González-Del-Angel, A.; Velázquez-Aragón, J.A.; López-Herrera, G.; Berrón-Ruiz, L.; et al. Expanding the clinical features of autoinflammation and phospholipase Cγ2-associated antibody deficiency and immune dysregulation by description of a novel patient. *J. Eur. Acad. Dermatol. Venereol.* **2019**, *33*, 2334–2339. [CrossRef]
93. Aderibigbe, O.M.; Priel, D.L.; Lee, C.-C.R.; Ombrello, M.J.; Prajapati, V.H.; Liang, M.G.; Milner, J.D. Distinct Cutaneous Manifestations and Cold-Induced Leukocyte Activation Associated with PLCG2 Mutations. *JAMA Dermatol.* **2015**, *151*, 627–634. [CrossRef] [PubMed]
94. Milner, J.D. PLAID: A Syndrome of Complex Patterns of Disease and Unique Phenotypes. *J. Clin. Immunol.* **2015**, *35*, 527–530. [CrossRef] [PubMed]
95. Ombrello, M.; Remmers, E.F.; Sun, G.; Freeman, A.F.; Datta, S.; Torabi-Parizi, P.; Subramanian, N.; Bunney, T.D.; Baxendale, R.W.; Martins, M.; et al. Cold Urticaria, Immunodeficiency, and Autoimmunity Related to PLCG2 Deletions. *N. Engl. J. Med.* **2012**, *366*, 330–338. [CrossRef] [PubMed]

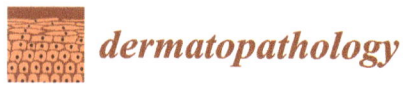 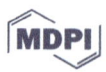

Review

Histological Patterns of Skin Lesions in Tuberous Sclerosis Complex: A Panorama

Marine Cascarino [1] and Stéphanie Leclerc-Mercier [2,*]

[1] Department of Pathology, Paris Saint-Joseph Hospital Group, 75014 Paris, France; marine.cascarino@gmail.com
[2] Reference Center for Genodermatoses (MAGEC Center), Department of Pathology, Necker-Enfants Malades Hospital, Paris Centre University, 75015 Paris, France
* Correspondence: stephanie.leclerc@aphp.fr

Abstract: Tuberous Sclerosis Complex (TSC) is a multisystem genetic disease characterized by cutaneous and extracutaneous hamartomas. The diagnosis is based on the association of major and minor criteria, defined by a consensus conference updated in 2012. The clinical examination of the skin is crucial because seven diagnostic criteria are dermatological: four major (hypomelanotic macules, angiofibroma or fibrous cephalic plaques, ungual fibromas, shagreen patches) and three minor criteria (confetti skin lesions, dental enamel pits, intraoral fibromas). Skin biopsy is commonly performed to assert the diagnosis of TSC when the clinical aspect is atypical. Histopathology of TSC cutaneous lesions have been poorly reported until now. In this article, we review the histologic features described in the literature and share our experience of TSC skin biopsies in our pediatric hospital specialized in genetic disorders. Both hypomelanotic lesions and cutaneous hamartomas (angiofibroma/fibrous cephalic plaques, ungual fibromas, shagreen patches) are discussed, including the recent entity called folliculocystic and collagen hamartoma, with a special emphasis on helpful clues for TSC in such lesions.

Keywords: tuberous sclerosis complex; hypomelanotic lesions; confetti skin lesions; shagreen patch; angiofibroma; cutaneous hamartoma; folliculocystic and collagen hamartoma; forehead fibrous plaque

Citation: Cascarino, M.; Leclerc-Mercier, S. Histological Patterns of Skin Lesions in Tuberous Sclerosis Complex: A Panorama. *Dermatopathology* **2021**, *8*, 236–252. https://doi.org/10.3390/dermatopathology8030029

Academic Editor: Gürkan Kaya

Received: 1 June 2021
Accepted: 1 July 2021
Published: 4 July 2021

Publisher's Note: MDPI stays neutral with regard to jurisdictional claims in published maps and institutional affiliations.

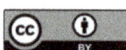

Copyright: © 2021 by the authors. Licensee MDPI, Basel, Switzerland. This article is an open access article distributed under the terms and conditions of the Creative Commons Attribution (CC BY) license (https://creativecommons.org/licenses/by/4.0/).

1. Introduction

Tuberous sclerosis complex (TSC) is a rare autosomal dominant disease characterized by cutaneous and extracutaneous hamartomas (kidney, eyes, heart, brain, lungs). The prevalence is around 1/20,000 in the general population and the incidence about 1/6000 to 1/10,000 live births [1]. Skin manifestations are present in almost 100% of the patients affected by TSC [2].

TSC results from an inactivating mutation in *TSC1* or *TSC2*, two genes encoding tumor suppressor proteins: hamartin and tuberin, respectively. These proteins belong to the m-TOR pathway. The *TSC1/TSC2* mutations lead to increased protein synthesis and cell growth [3]. Two third of the cases are sporadic forms. Mutations are not identified by conventional genetic testing in 10 to 25% of TSC patients, possibly be due to mosaicism: *TSC1/TSC2* mutation would be present in only some organs and only some cells within those organs, then a "second-hit" mutation inactivates the remaining wild-type copy of *TSC1/TSC2* [3].

The diagnosis is therefore based on the association of major and minor criteria, as defined by a consensus conference updated in 2012 [1] (Table 1).

The dermatologist has a central role in the diagnosis of TSC because cutaneous manifestations account for 4 (hypomelanotic macules, angiofibromas or fibrous cephalic plaques, ungual fibromas, shagreen patches) of 11 major and 3 (confetti skin lesions, dental enamel pits, intraoral fibromas) of 6 minor diagnostic criteria.

Table 1. Diagnostic criteria for tuberous sclerosis complex 2012. Reprinted from ref. [1].

A. Genetic diagnostic criteria
Identification of either *TSC1* or *TSC2* pathogenic mutation is sufficient to make a definitive diagnosis of TSC
B. Clinical diagnostic criteria **Major features:** 1. Hypomelanotic macules ($\geq$3, at least 5-mm diameter) 2. Angiofibromas ($\geq$3) or fibrous cephalic plaque 3. Ungueal fibromas ($\geq$2) 4. Shagreen patch 5. Multiple retinal hamartomas 6. Cortical dysplasia 7. Subependymal nodules 8. Subependymal giant cell astrocytoma 9. Cardiac rhabdomyoma 10. Lymphangioleiomyomatosis 11. Angiomyolipomas ($\geq$2) **Minor features:** 1. «Confetti» skin lesions 2. Dental enamel pits (>3) 3. Intraoral fibromas ($\geq$2) 4. Retinal achromic patch 5. Multiple renal cysts 6. Nonrenal hamartomas

Definite diagnosis: Two major features or one major feature with $\geq$2 minor features; Possible diagnosis: Either one major feature or $\geq$2 minor features.

An early diagnosis is crucial for a better management, and each lesion has a typical age of onset, but TSC diagnosis is sometimes challenging in pauci-symptomatic forms.

The cutaneous lesions of TSC can be classified into:

1. Hypomelanotic lesions:
    - hypomelanotic macules
    - confetti skin lesions
2. Connective tissue nevi (cutaneous hamartomas):
    - periungual fibromas (PF),
    - angiofibromas (AF),
    - shagreen patches (SP),
    - forehead fibrous plaques (FFP),
    - folliculocystic and collagen hamartomas (FCCH).

In this article, we will describe the histologic spectrum of TSC lesions reported in the literature, discuss the usefulness of skin biopsy in TSC and try to give clues for the diagnosis of TSC to avoid delayed diagnosis and allow an earlier management of the patient.

2. Hypomelanotic Lesions

Hypomelanotic lesions are the most frequent and earliest lesions (90% of the patients, often seen at birth). The three most common aspects are polygonal, lance-ovate (or ash leaf spot) and confetti (guttate) (Figure 1a,b). Woods lamp examination is helpful for detecting these macules in infants. Hypomelanotic macules are asymmetrically distributed over the entire skin surface, and most commonly on the trunk and buttock [4]. Confetti macules are usually numerous, well circumscribed, small (1 to 3 mm in diameter) and diffuse, particularly seen over the forearms and lower legs. The presence of confetti lesions must alert the physician about a possible diagnosis of TSC.

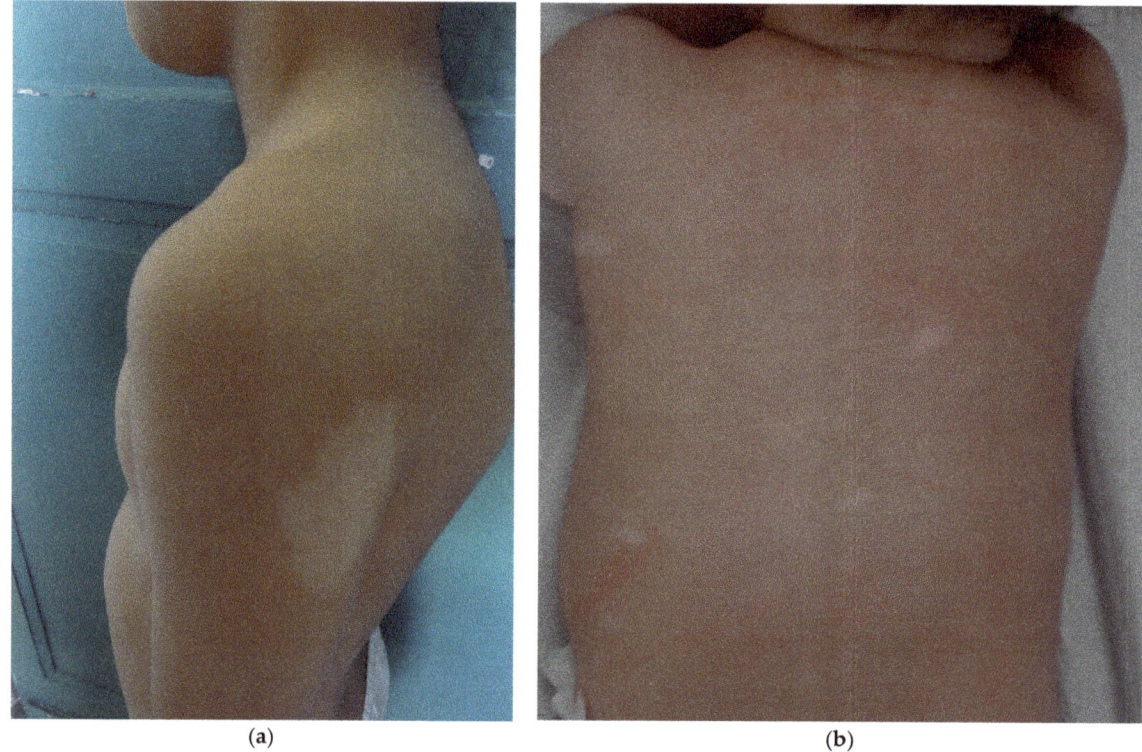

Figure 1. Hypomelanotic macules. (**a**): Ash leaf spot hypomelanotic lesion in a 7 year-old boy's arm; (**b**): lance-ovate hypomelanotic macules in a 4 months boy's back.

Histopathologic studies showed a normal density of active melanocytes contrasting with a significant decrease in the amount of melanin pigment in the epidermis [4,5].

Electron microscopy demonstrates a reduced number of smaller, immature, and less melanized melanosomes, both in melanocytes and keratinocytes, due to the target of rapamycin complex (mTOR) pathway alteration, which is normally implicated in melanogenesis.

Recently, hypopigmented macules have been evaluated after topical rapamycin application (an inhibitor of mTor). Topical rapamycin led to a substantial improvement of hypopigmented macules and normalization of melanosome abnormalities in the treated skin [6].

3. TSC-Associated Cutaneous Hamartomas (Connective Tissue Nevi)

This item encompasses periungueal fibromas (PF), angiofibromas (AF), shagreen patches (SP), forehead fibrous plaques (FFP) and folliculocystic and collagen hamartomas (FCCH).

3.1. Angiofibromas (AF)

Angiofibromas are skin-colored to red-brown papules, typically on the central face. They usually appear at 3-years-old and their prevalence increases with age (8% in children younger than 2-years-old, increasing to 75% in children of 9-years-old and older) [7,8] The lesions progress in number with age and multiple AF appearing in childhood are characteristic of TSC [1,8]. The lesions progress also in appearance with age: early lesions are vascular macules and with time the fibrous component becomes more prominent, with dome-shaped smooth papules.

At least three AF must be present to be considered to be a major criteria, because one or two isolated lesions can be a normal finding [1].

AF histopathology has been described in three main articles [9–11]. AF share histopathologic similarities with fibrous papules of the face [12]. It presents as a dome-shaped lesion with a normal or sometimes hyperplastic epidermis. In the dermis, there is an expanding hypertrophy of the collagen tissue and the vascular structures. In older lesions, the collagen becomes denser and more sclerotic.

There is a tendency for a perifollicular arrangement of collagen, compressing the adnexal structures sometimes replacing them with an aspect of concentric collagen bundles. The vascular component is represented by widely dilated venules throughout the lesion. Staining for elastic fibers reveals a lack or decrease of elastic tissue in the AF, as in Figure 2b,c.

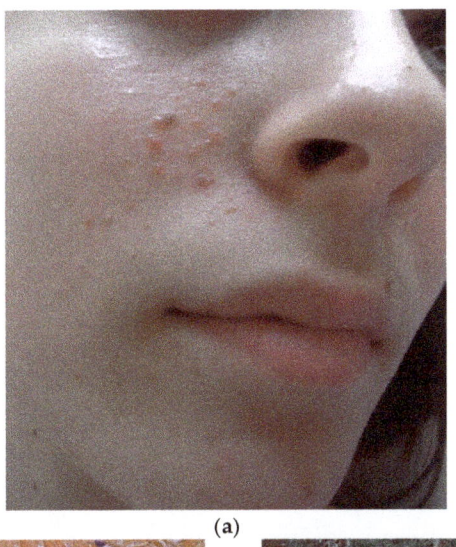

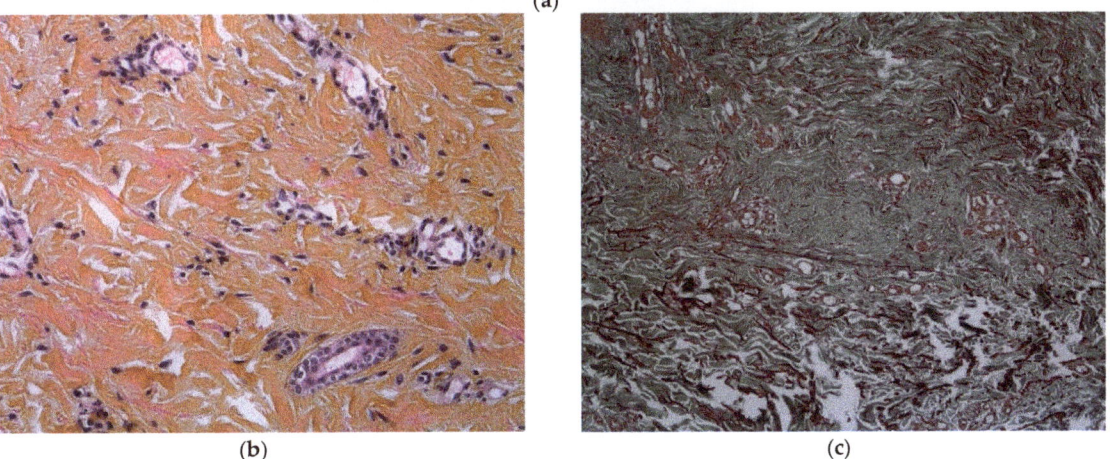

Figure 2. Angiofibroma. (**a**) Face's angiofibromas in a 14 year-old patient; (**b**) Hematein eosin ×40: hypertrophy of the collagen bundles and of the vascular elements represented by dilated venules; (**c**). Orcein staining ×40: decreased and fragmented elastic fibers.

The cellular component consists of increased oval or stellate cells, tending to make clusters around the dilated blood vessels. Sometimes, multinucleated giant cells can be seen. This stellate cells are probably descending from dendritic cells, with Factor XIIIa antibody positivity [11,12].

Recently, NGS was performed on AF sample of TSC patient and demonstrated that a somatic second-hit mutation of the form CC > TT occurs in TSC facial angiofibroma at a high frequency, indicative of sunlight-induced DNA damage. The authors suggest that sun exposure could be responsible for a second hit event in *TSC1/TSC2* and therefore be responsible for the development of facial AF [13]. Photoprotection should indeed be strongly advised to TSC patients.

3.2. Periungual Fibroma (PF)

PF should be multiple ($\geq$2) to be considered to be a TSC criteria, because post traumatic PF can also occur in the general population. They are located on the toes (90%) and/or fingers (56%) [14] (Figure 3a). Their frequency is 20 to 80% in older patients [1,7,8]. They are often painful and dysesthetic and then frequently removed.

In the literature, the histologic description is close to AF description and to idiopathic post traumatic PF [9,10]. The remarkable features distinguishing PF from AF are the vascular component and the arrangement of the collagen bundles. The vascular component is represented by an increased number of dilated venules lined by plumped endothelial cells. As in AF, the cellular component is made up of stellate cells with FXIIIa positivity (Figure 3e), usually not as numerous as in AF, and some multinucleate giant cells. Variable amounts of dense dermal collagen are present between the vascular spaces and collagen bundles, are vertically oriented and can even affect, in our experience, the hypodermis (Figure 3b,c). Elastic tissue is significantly decreased (Figure 3d).

3.3. Fibrous Cephalic Plaque (FCP)

Fibrous cephalic plaques are observed in about 25% of TSC patients [1]. Formerly called forehead plaque, although often located unilaterally, they may be present on other parts of the face or scalp (Figure 4a). They can occur at any age. FCP are not frequently biopsied.

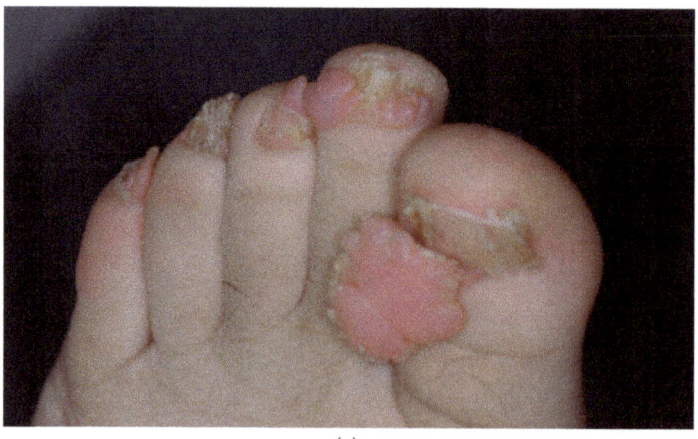

(a)

Figure 3. *Cont.*

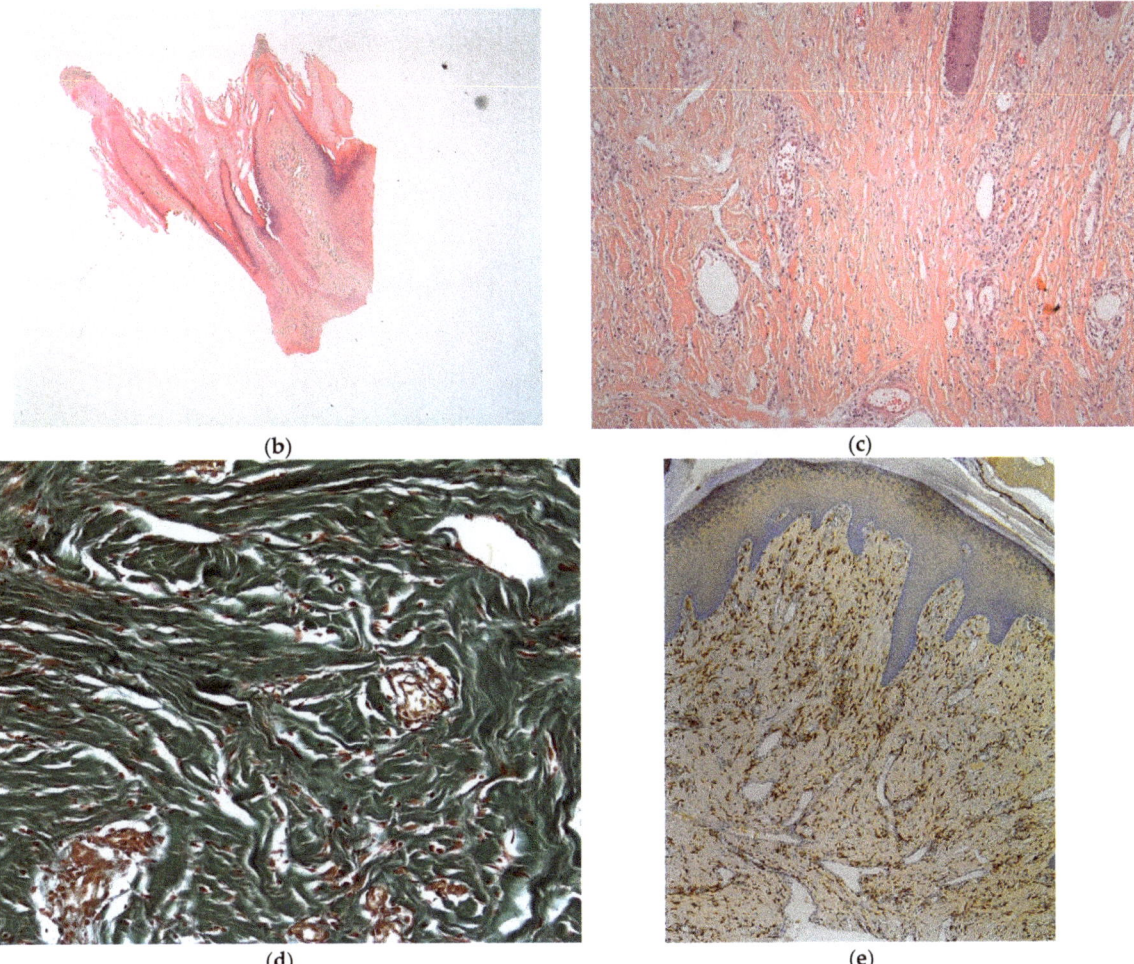

Figure 3. Periungual fibroma. (**a**). Clinical aspect of a toe periungual fibroma; (**b**). Hematein eosin ×5: exophytic dome-shaped lesion with hyperplastic epidermis; (**c**). Hematein eosin ×20: collagen bundles are vertically oriented; increased number of dilated venules; (**d**). Orcein staining × 40: decreased elastic fibers; (**e**). Immuno-histochemistry with anti-FXIIIa antibody showing positivity of stellate cells.

Pathological features of FCP described in the literature are similar to AF. The remarkable features distinguishing PF from AF are a more important prominent vascular dilatation and more sclerosis and hyalinization of the collagen with an aspect of concentric perifollicular fibrosis leading to atrophy and compression of the follicle [9] (Figure 4b,c). Recently, Traichel et al. described 13 FCP and noticed a FXIIIa positivity of the stromal cells and elastic fibers decreased [15].

3.4. Shagreen Patches (SP)

Shagreen patches commonly present as large plaques on the lower back, with a bumpy or orange-peel surface, and this clinical aspect is almost specific of TSC [1,14]. (Figure 5a). They appear commonly in children in the first decade of life [7].

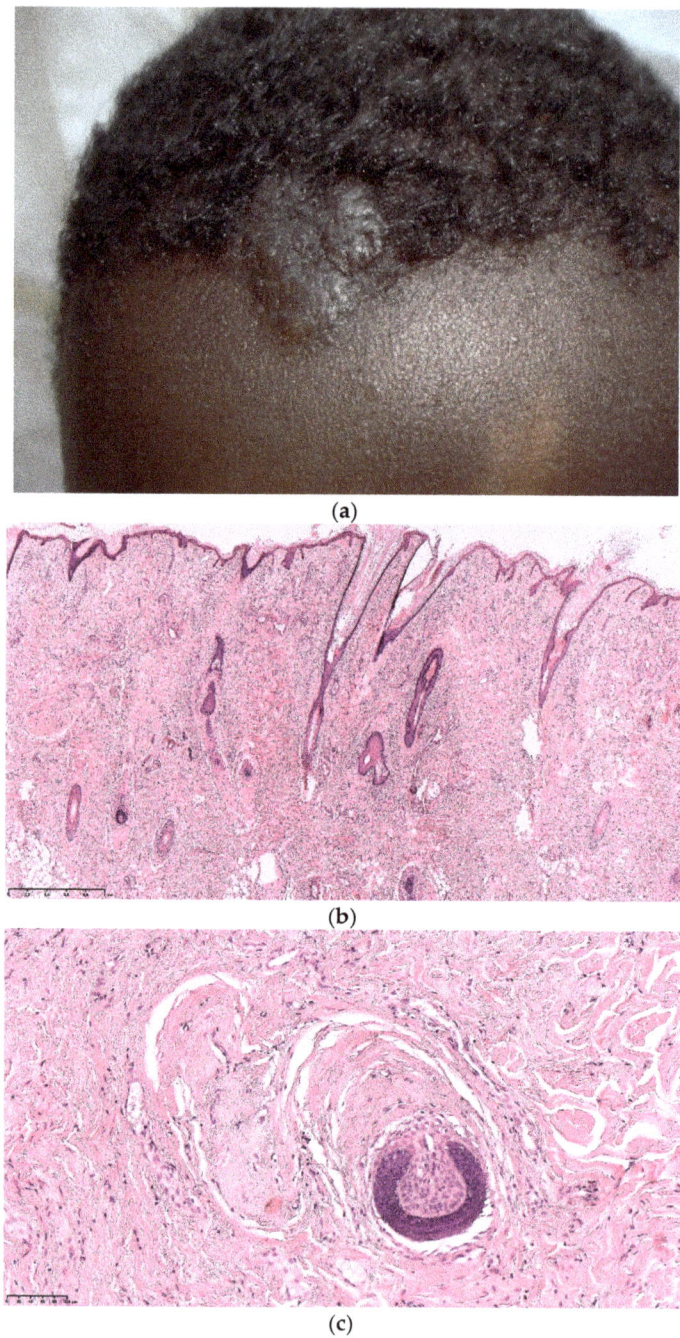

Figure 4. Fibrous cephalic plaque. (**a**): Clinical aspect of a fibrous cephalic plaque of the forehead; (**b**): Hematein eosin ×10: dense proliferation of collagen bundles in the dermis and the hypodermis; (**c**). Concentric perifollicular fibrosis leading to atrophy and compression of the follicle.

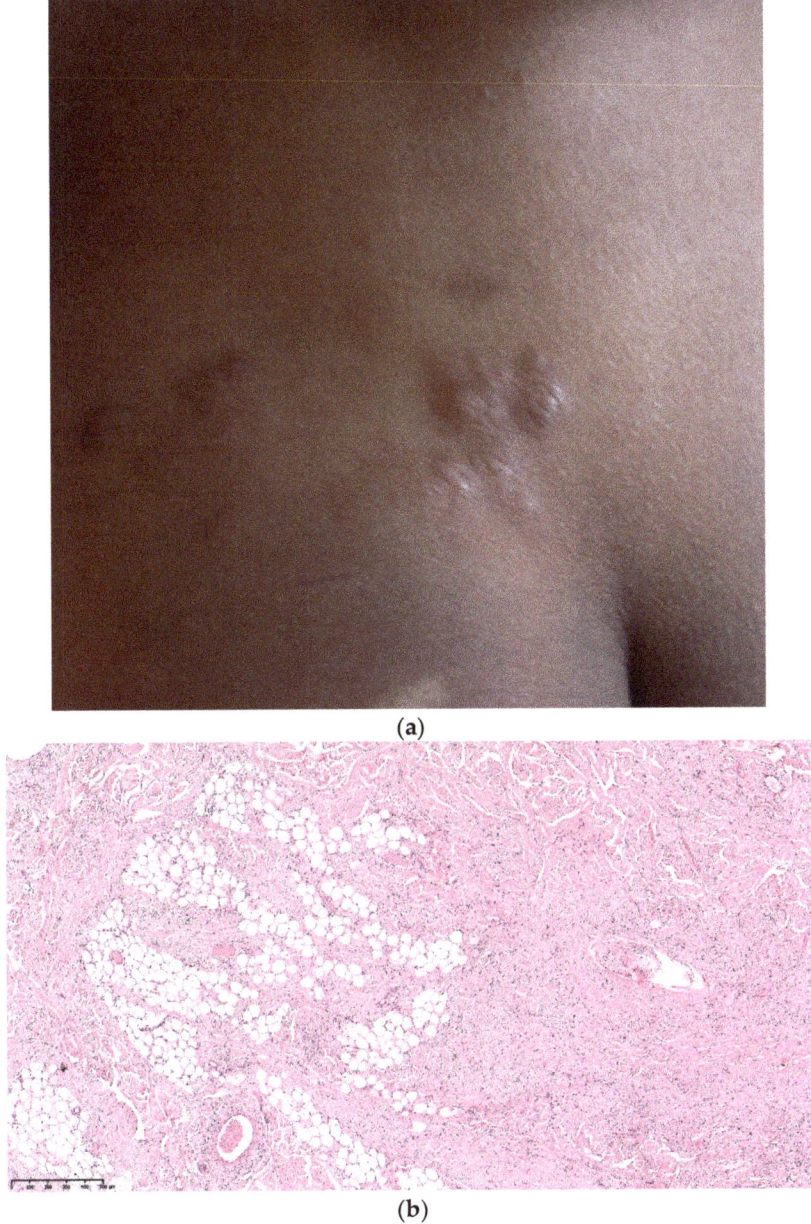

Figure 5. Cont.

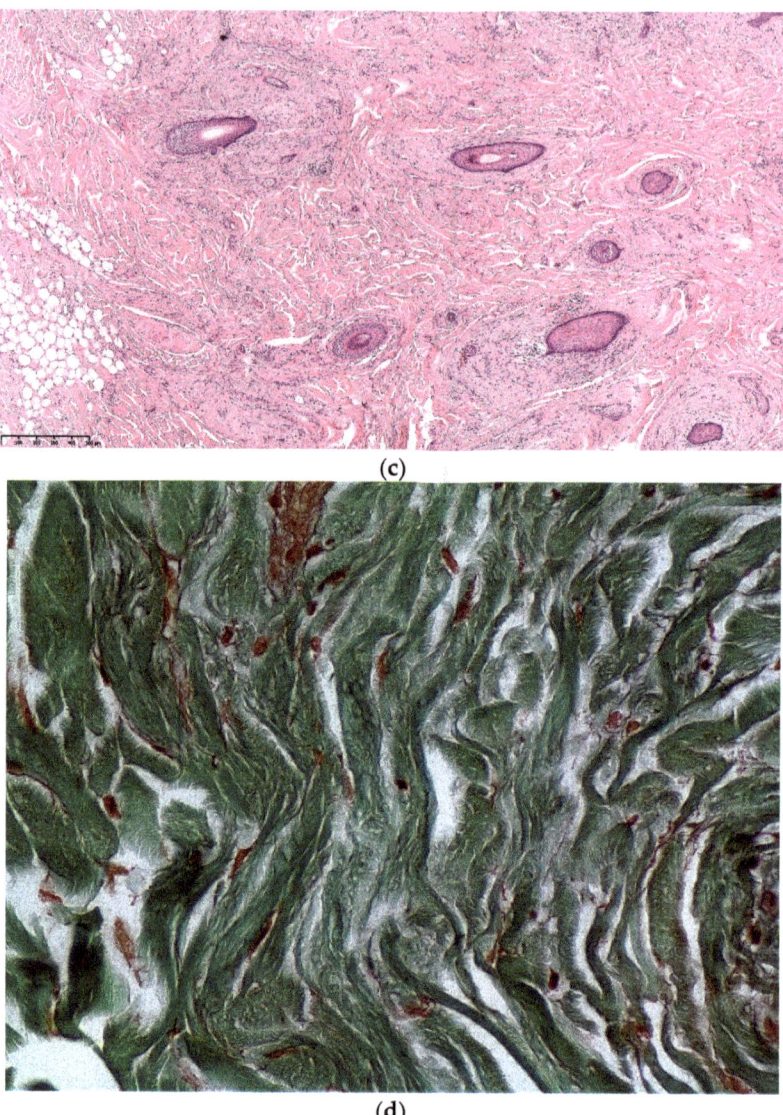

Figure 5. Shagreen patch. (**a**). Clinical aspect of a lumbar shagreen patch; (**b**). Hematein eosin ×20: extensive fibrosis with collagen bundles into the dermis and the hypodermis; (**c**). Hematein eosin ×20: concentric perifollicular fibrosis; (**d**). Orcein staining ×40: lack of elastic fibers.

SP correspond histologically to collagenomas (or collagenic hamartomas). The dermis is replaced by a dense, relatively acellular and hyaline collagen which extends down to the subcutaneous fat (Figure 5b). As in AF and FCP, follicles are also involved with a concentric perifollicular collagen, atrophy and compression (Figure 5c). Some follicles are abnormal in shape. Sometimes, they are entirely replaced by a fibrous collagenic column. Elastic fibers are thin, fragmented or absent (Figure 5d) [9,16].

3.5. Folliculocystic and Collagen Hamartoma (FCCH)

FCCH is a new entity described in 2012 by Torrelo et al. with six cases in male patients with TSC [17]. Six additional cases of FCCH were reported [18–23], all occurring in patients with TSC, suggesting a causal relationship.

The clinical examination shows a solitary, painless, and large (several centimeters) infiltrated exophytic tumor, with an elastic consistency and an irregular surface covered by comedo-like structures (Figure 6a). This hamartoma is noticed at birth or during early infancy, mainly in boys, tending to occur on the scalp and the trunk.

Histopathologic examination of FCCH shows abundant and thickened collagen bundles occupying the whole dermis and extending into the subcutaneous fat (Figure 6b). There is also a marked concentric perifollicular fibrosis, surrounding hair follicles. This concentric fibrosis also involves the eccrine glands and surrounds some small and medium vessels.

A distinctive feature of FCCH is the presence of comedo-like formation and cysts lined by an infundibular epithelium, containing intact keratin (Figure 6c,d). Occasionally a ruptured cyst with foreign body reaction has been seen [17,21]. A vascular component has also been noticed in two cases with increased and dilated blood vessels [19,23]. Elastic fibers were not studied in the reported cases but in our experience, they are decreased or absent.

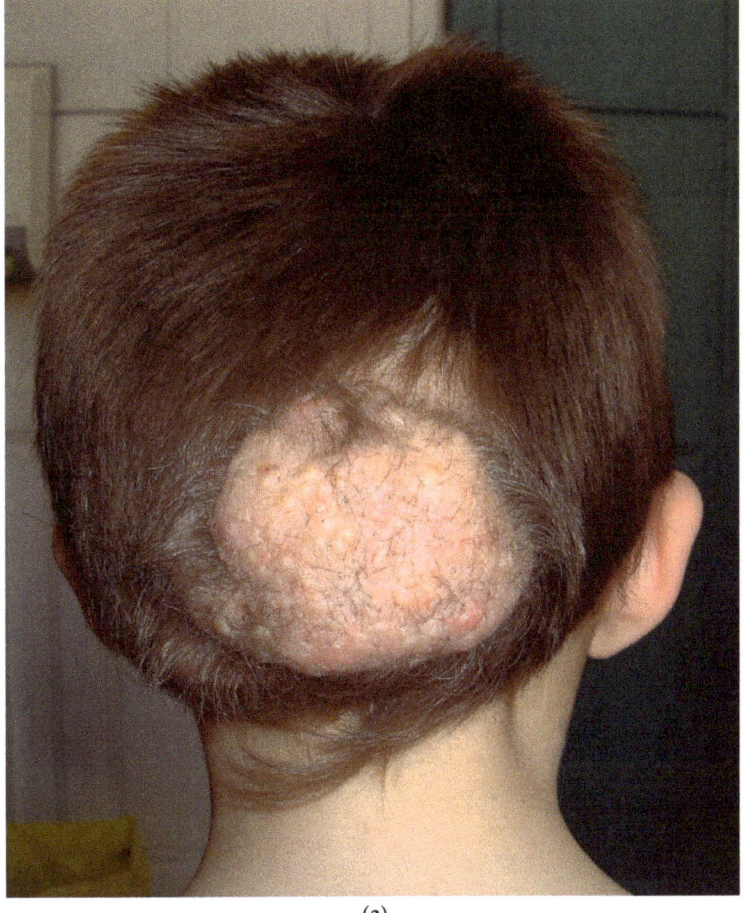

(a)

Figure 6. Cont.

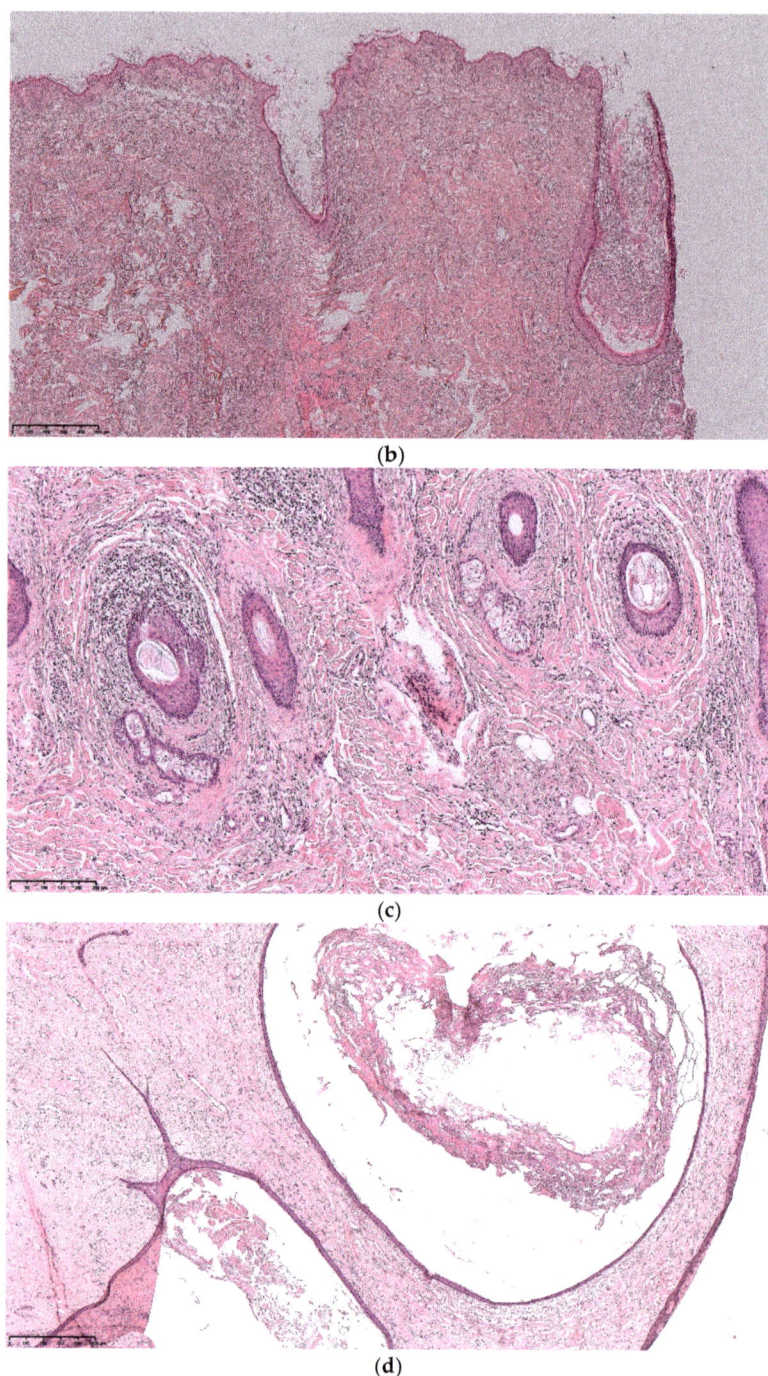

Figure 6. Folliculocystic Hamartoma. (**a**): clinical aspect of an occipital FCCH; (**b**): Hematein eosin ×10: extensive fibrosis and concentric perifollicular fibrosis; (**c**): Hematein eosin ×10: comedo openings; (**d**): Hematein eosin ×10: large infundibular cyst.

4. Other TSC-Associated Cutaneous Lesions

Café au lait spots are common, observed in 15 to 30% of CST patients, appearing in the first months of life. These lesions are not specific as they are seen in 16–19% of the general population [8,24,25].

Molluscum pendulum or acrochordons are found in 23% of patients with TSC [8]. However, these common lesions are also seen in the general population and have a non-specific histology (lesion with pedicle and fibrous axis without adnexa). Their necklace arrangement on the posterior neck could be a TSC sign [26].

Vascular cutaneous lesions, anemic nevus and Bier spots, are described in TSC patients in one study [27].

Recently, Lu et al. described the occurrence of juvenile xanthogranuloma in a 5 months old TSC patient [28]. Interestingly, Sirolimus (mTor inhibitor) had a significant effect on JXG and whole-exome sequencing in paraffin block tissue identified *TSC1* mutation.

5. Does TSC Cutaneous Hamartoma Belong to the Same Lesional Spectrum?

After the review of the literature and our retrospective examination of 20 lesions, we observed three common and constant components, more or less present in all varieties of TSC cutaneous hamartomas (AF, SP, FCP and FCCH):

- abundant thickened collagen, associated with adnexal involvement (concentric fibrosis)
- vascular hyperplasia,
- cellular proliferation of fibroblasts.

TSC1 or *TSC2* mutations cause a defect in mTOR inhibition and promote cell proliferation but also angiogenesis and vessel modification due to increased production of VEGF by fibroblastic cells carrying the mutation [3,29].

We also noticed the association of decreased elastic fibers.

Among those three components, the concentric peri-follicular fibrosis with concomitant atrophy and compression of the skin adnexa seems highly suggestive of TSC.

This finding is not present in other types of collagenomas (sporadic or hereditary) in the literature and in our personal experience [30–32] (i.e., familial cutaneous collagenomas [33,34], Cowden syndrome [35,36], Proteus syndrome, Bushkle-Ollendorff syndrome [37,38], multiple endocrine neoplasia type 1 (NEM1) [39]). However, interesting way, this pattern is present in sporadic angiofibromas of the face [12].

In Birt-Hogg-Dubbé syndrome, skin lesions close to TSC are seen: fibrofolliculomas, trichodiscosomas and acrochordons [40]. They are generally multiple small skin-colored to grayish papules on the face. Pathological examination shows important follicular changes more pronounced than those observed on TSC cutaneous hamartomas [41,42]. There is no vascular hyperplasia and abundant or thickened collagen bundles are seen only around the involved follicle. In addition, TSC cutaneous hamartoma are much larger.

The observation of epidermal inclusion/cysts is unusual and seems to be a distinctive feature of FCCH [9,17]. Some authors suggested that the cysts are a component of the hamartoma, but we believe that the cystic aspect could be a consequence of the marked perifollicular fibrosis with a progressive dilatation of the upper part of the hair follicle.

Therefore, we believe that (like Cardona et al. [21] and Treichel et al. [15]), TSC-hamartomas such as FCP, AF, SP, and FCCH belong to a same histopathologic spectrum with the predominance of one or another component (Table 2).

Table 2. Histopathological pattern of TSC cutaneous hamartoma.

	Fibrosis	Cellularity	Dilated Vessels	Perifollicular Fibrosis	Decreased or Fragmented Elastic Fibers
Angiofibroma	+ ++ in old AF	++	++	0 + in old AF	++
Periungueal fibroma	+ to ++	+++	+++	0	++
Fibrous cephalic plaque	+++	+ to ++	+	++	+++
Shagreen patches	+++	+ to ++	+	+	+++
Folliculocystic and collagen hamartoma	+++	+	+	+++	+++

Note. +: low; ++: moderate; +++: intense.

6. In Conclusion, Is Histopathological Examination Useful in TSC Diagnosis?

Histopathology of TSC cutaneous lesions have been poorly reported until now and histology did not appear to be helpful for routine diagnosis.

Interestingly, all TSC-associated hamartomas such as AF, FCP, SP and FCCH belong to a continuous spectrum with common and distinctive histologic findings: abundant thickened collagen, sometimes with follicular involvement (perifollicular concentric fibrosis, and infundibular cysts for FCCH), vascular hyperplasia, fibroblast hypercellularity, and decreased elastic fibers (Figure 7).

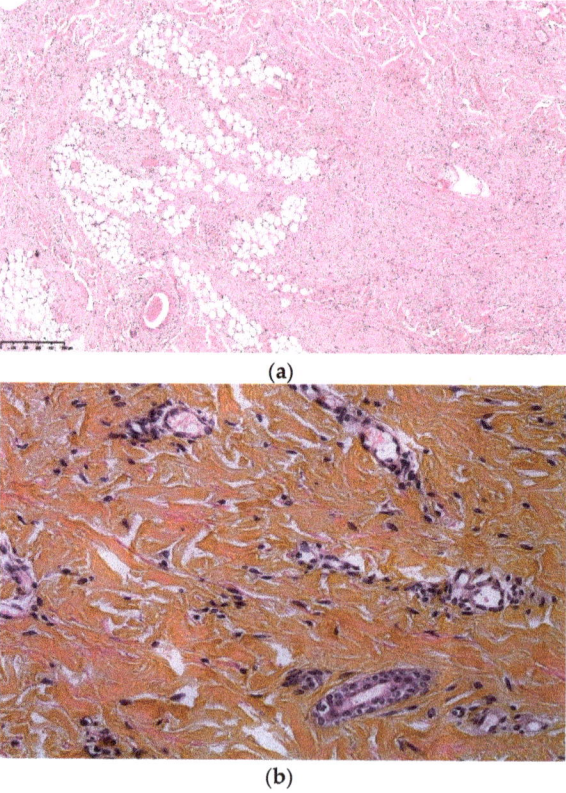

(a)

(b)

Figure 7. Cont.

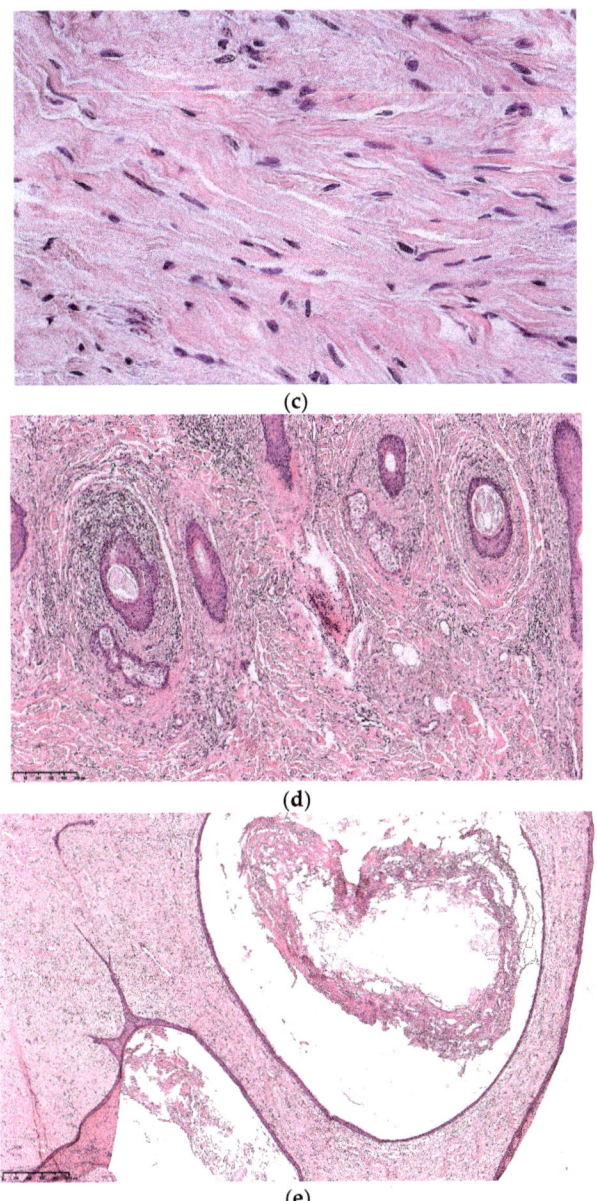

Figure 7. Cont.

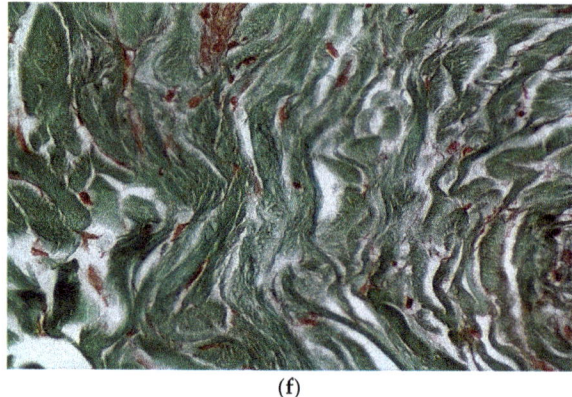

(f)

Figure 7. Common and distinctive histologic findings in TSC cutaneous hamartoma. (**a**): Hematein eosin ×10: fibrosis component: extensive fibrosis composed of thick collagen bundles; (**b**): Hematein eosin ×20: vascular component made of dilated vessels and thick collagen bundles; (**c**): Hematein eosin ×40: cellular component: stellate cells; (**d**): Hematein eosin ×10: Concentric perifollicular fibrosis; (**e**): Hematein eosin ×10: Dilated infundibular cyst; (**f**): Orcein staining: decreased or lack of elastic fibers.

FCCH seems to be specific entity of TSC, with a unique clinical aspect (irregular surface with comedo-like openings and cysts, a large size, occurring on the scalp or the trunk) and specific histologic findings (concentric fibrosis, infundibular cysts and comedo openings).

In pauci-symptomatic TSC, the histopathological features underlined above could be a strong argument for the diagnosis and allow the pathologist to suggest the diagnosis of TSC, conducting to an earlier diagnosis and a better management of the patient.

Author Contributions: Conceptualization, resources, writing—original draft preparation, writing—review and editing, visualization, supervision: M.C. and S.L.-M. All authors have read and agreed to the published version of the manuscript.

Funding: This research received no external funding.

Institutional Review Board Statement: Not applicable.

Informed Consent Statement: Not applicable.

Conflicts of Interest: The authors declare no conflict of interest.

References

1. Northrup, H.; Krueger, D.A. International Tuberous Sclerosis Complex Consensus Group. Tuberous sclerosis complex diagnostic criteria update: Recommendations of the 2012 Iinternational Tuberous Sclerosis Complex Consensus Conference. *Pediatr. Neurol.* **2013**, *49*, 243–254. [CrossRef] [PubMed]
2. Wataya-Kaneda, M.; Tanaka, M.; Hamasaki, T.; Katayama, I. Trends in the prevalence of tuberous sclerosis complex manifestations: An epidemiological study of 166 Japanese patients. *PLoS ONE* **2013**, *8*, e63910. [CrossRef]
3. Lam, H.C.; Nijmeh, J.; Henske, E.P. New developments in the genetics and pathogenesis of tumours in tuberous sclerosis complex. *J. Pathol.* **2017**, *241*, 219–225. [CrossRef] [PubMed]
4. Jimbow, K. Tuberous sclerosis and guttate leukodermas. *Semin. Cutan. Med. Surg.* **1997**, *16*, 30–35. [CrossRef]
5. Jimbow, K.; Fitzpatrick, T.B.; Szabo, G.; Hori, Y. Congenital circumscribed hypomelanosis: A characterization based on electron microscopic study of tuberous sclerosis, nevus depigmentosus, and piebaldism. *J. Investig. Dermatol.* **1975**, *64*, 50–62. [CrossRef]
6. Wataya-Kaneda, M.; Tanaka, M.; Yang, L.; Yang, F.; Tsuruta, D.; Nakamura, A.; Matsumoto, S.; Hamasaki, T.; Tanemura, A.; Katayama, I. Clinical and Histologic Analysis of the Efficacy of Topical Rapamycin Therapy Against Hypomelanotic Macules in Tuberous Sclerosis Complex. *JAMA Dermatol.* **2015**, *151*, 722–730. [CrossRef] [PubMed]
7. Jacks, S.K.; Witman, P.M. Tuberous Sclerosis Complex: An Update for Dermatologists. *Pediatr. Dermatol.* **2015**, *32*, 563–570. [CrossRef]

8. Jóźwiak, S.; Schwartz, R.A.; Janniger, C.K.; Michałowicz, R.; Chmielik, J. Skin lesions in children with tuberous sclerosis complex: Their prevalence, natural course, and diagnostic significance. *Int. J. Dermatol.* **1998**, *37*, 911–917. [CrossRef] [PubMed]
9. Nickel, W.R.; Reed, W.B. Tuberous Sclerosis: Special Reference to the Microscopic Alterations in the Cutaneous Hamartomas. *Arch. Dermatol.* **1962**, *85*, 209–226. [CrossRef]
10. Reed, R.J.; Ackerman, A.B. Pathology of the adventitial dermis. *Hum. Pathol.* **1973**, *4*, 207–217. [CrossRef]
11. Benjamin, D.R. Cellular composition of the angiofibromas in tuberous sclerosis. *Pediatr. Pathol. Lab. Med. J. Soc. Pediatr. Pathol. Affil. Int. Paediatr. Pathol. Assoc.* **1996**, *16*, 893–899.
12. de Cambourg, G.; Cribier, B. Fibrous papules of the face: A retrospective anatomoclinical study of 283 cases. *Ann. Dermatol. Venereol.* **2013**, *140*, 763–770. [CrossRef] [PubMed]
13. Tyburczy, M.E.; Wang, J.-A.; Li, S.; Thangapazham, R.; Chekaluk, Y.; Moss, J.; Kwiatkowski, D.J.; Darling, T.N. Sun exposure causes somatic second-hit mutations and angiofibroma development in tuberous sclerosis complex. *Hum. Mol. Genet.* **2014**, *23*, 2023–2029. [CrossRef] [PubMed]
14. Webb, D.W.; Clarke, A.; Fryer, A.; Osborne, J.P. The cutaneous features of tuberous sclerosis: A population study. *Br. J. Dermatol.* **1996**, *135*, 1–5. [CrossRef]
15. Treichel, A.M.; Pithadia, D.J.; Lee, C.-C.R.; Oyerinde, O.; Moss, J.; Darling, T.N. Histopathological Features of Fibrous Cephalic Plaques in Tuberous Sclerosis Complex. *Histopathology* **2021**. [CrossRef]
16. Bongiorno, M.A.; Nathan, N.; Oyerinde, O.; Wang, J.-A.; Lee, C.-C.R.; Brown, G.T.; Moss, J.; Darling, T.N. Clinical Characteristics of Connective Tissue Nevi in Tuberous Sclerosis Complex with Special Emphasis on Shagreen Patches. *JAMA Dermatol.* **2017**, *153*, 660–665. [CrossRef]
17. Torrelo, A.; Hadj-Rabia, S.; Colmenero, I.; Piston, R.; Sybert, V.P.; Hilari-Carbonell, H.; Hernández-Martín, A.; Ferreres, J.C.; Vañó-Galván, S.; Azorín, D.; et al. Folliculocystic and collagen hamartoma of tuberous sclerosis complex. *J. Am. Acad. Dermatol.* **2012**, *66*, 617–621. [CrossRef] [PubMed]
18. An, J.M.; Kim, Y.S.; Park, Y.L.; Lee, S. Folliculocystic and Collagen Hamartoma: A New Entity? *Ann. Dermatol.* **2015**, *27*, 593–596. [CrossRef] [PubMed]
19. Kaplan, L.; Kazlouskaya, V.; Ugorji, R.; Heilman, E.; Siegel, D.M.; Glick, S.A. Folliculocystic and collagen hamartoma of tuberous sclerosis: A new case in a female patient and review of literature. *J. Cutan. Pathol.* **2018**, *45*, 67–70. [CrossRef]
20. Brown, M.M.; Walsh, E.J.; Yu, L.; Smidt, A.C. Progressive Scalp Plaque in a Girl with Tuberous Sclerosis. *Pediatr. Dermatol.* **2014**, *31*, 249–250. [CrossRef]
21. Cardona, R.; Cancel-Artau, K.J.; Carrasquillo, O.Y.; Martin-Garcia, R.F. Folliculocystic and Collagen Hamartoma: A Distinct Hamartoma Associated with Tuberous Sclerosis Complex. *Am. J. Dermatopathol.* **2021**, *43*, 67–70. [CrossRef] [PubMed]
22. Bishnoi, A.; Tripathy, S.; Vinay, K.; De, D.; Parsad, D.; Chatterjee, D.; Saikia, U.N. Image Gallery: Folliculocystic and collagen hamartoma: A lesser-known presentation of tuberous sclerosis. *Br. J. Dermatol.* **2018**, *178*, e276. [CrossRef] [PubMed]
23. Reolid, A.; Navarro, R.; Daudén, E.; Alonso-Cerezo, M.C.; Fraga, J.; Llamas-Velasco, M. Facial folliculocystic and collagen hamartoma: A variant of fibrous cephalic plaque with prominent cyst formation? *J. Dtsch. Dermatol. Ges. J. Ger. Soc. Dermatol. JDDG* **2019**, *17*, 738–741. [CrossRef]
24. Santos, A.C.E.D.; Heck, B.; Camargo, B.D.; Vargas, F.R. Prevalence of Café-au-Lait Spots in children with solid tumors. *Genet. Mol. Biol.* **2016**, *39*, 232–238. [CrossRef]
25. Bell, S.D.; MacDonald, D.M. The prevalence of café-au-lait patches in tuberous sclerosis. *Clin. Exp. Dermatol.* **1985**, *10*, 562–565. [CrossRef]
26. Sachs, C.; Lipsker, D. The molluscum pendulum necklace sign in tuberous sclerosis complex: A case series A pathognomonic finding? *J. Eur. Acad. Dermatol. Venereol. JEADV* **2017**. [CrossRef] [PubMed]
27. Sachs, C.; Lipsker, D. Nevus Anemicus and Bier Spots in Tuberous Sclerosis Complex. *JAMA Dermatol.* **2016**, *152*, 217–218. [CrossRef]
28. Lu, Q.; Shi, X.-Y.; Wang, Y.-Y.; Zhang, M.-N.; Wang, W.-Z.; Wang, J.; Wang, Q.-H.; Chen, H.-M.; Chen, H.-M.; Zou, L.-P. Juvenile xanthogranuloma as a new type of skin lesions in tuberous sclerosis complex. *Orphanet J. Rare Dis.* **2020**, *15*, 147. [CrossRef] [PubMed]
29. Parker, W.E.; Orlova, K.A.; Heuer, G.G.; Baybis, M.; Aronica, E.; Frost, M.; Wong, M.; Crino, P.B. Enhanced epidermal growth factor, hepatocyte growth factor, and vascular endothelial growth factor expression in tuberous sclerosis complex. *Am. J. Pathol.* **2011**, *178*, 296–305. [CrossRef] [PubMed]
30. Uitto, J.; Santa Cruz, D.J.; Eisen, A.Z. Connective tissue nevi of the skin. Clinical, genetic, and histopathologic classification of hamartomas of the collagen, elastin, and proteoglycan type. *J. Am. Acad. Dermatol.* **1980**, *3*, 441–461. [CrossRef]
31. Arora, H.; Falto-Aizpurua, L.; Cortés-Fernandez, A.; Choudhary, S.; Romanelli, P. Connective Tissue Nevi: A Review of the Literature. *Am. J. Dermatopathol.* **2017**, *39*, 325–341. [CrossRef] [PubMed]
32. McCuaig, C.C.; Vera, C.; Kokta, V.; Marcoux, D.; Hatami, A.; Thuraisingam, T.; Marton, D.; Fortier-Riberdy, G.; Powell, J. Connective tissue nevi in children: Institutional experience and review. *J. Am. Acad. Dermatol.* **2012**, *67*, 890–897. [CrossRef]
33. Amato, L.; Mei, S.; Gallerani, I.; Moretti, S.; Cipollini, E.M.; Palleschi, G.M.; Fabbri, P. Familial cutaneous collagenoma: Report of an affected family. *Int. J. Dermatol.* **2005**, *44*, 315–317. [CrossRef] [PubMed]
34. Gurel, M.S.; Mulayim, M.K.; Ozardali, I.; Bitiren, M. Familial cutaneous collagenoma: New affected family with prepubertal onset. *J. Dermatol.* **2007**, *34*, 477–481. [CrossRef]

35. Stocchero, G.F. Storiform collagenoma: Case report. *Einstein Sao Paulo Braz.* **2015**, *13*, 103–105. [CrossRef] [PubMed]
36. Kieselova, K.; Santiago, F.; Henrique, M.; Cunha, M.F. Multiple sclerotic fibromas of the skin: An important clue for the diagnosis of Cowden syndrome. *BMJ Case Rep.* **2017**, *2017*. [CrossRef] [PubMed]
37. Tong, Y.; Schneider, J.A.; Coda, A.B.; Hata, T.R.; Cohen, P.R. Birt-Hogg-Dubé Syndrome: A Review of Dermatological Manifestations and Other Symptoms. *Am. J. Clin. Dermatol.* **2017**. [CrossRef] [PubMed]
38. Weintraub, R.; Pinkus, H. Multiple fibrofolliculomas (Birt-Hogg-Dubé) associated with a large connective tissue nevus. *J. Cutan. Pathol.* **1977**, *4*, 289–299. [CrossRef]
39. Pérez, A.D.A.; Yu, S.; North, J.P. Multiple cutaneous collagenomas in the setting of multiple endocrine neoplasia type 1. *J. Cutan. Pathol.* **2015**, *42*, 791–795. [CrossRef]
40. Birt, A.R.; Hogg, G.R.; Dubé, W.J. Hereditary multiple fibrofolliculomas with trichodiscomas and acrochordons. *Arch. Dermatol.* **1977**, *113*, 1674–1677. [CrossRef]
41. Spring, P.; Fellmann, F.; Giraud, S.; Clayton, H.; Hohl, D. Syndrome of Birt-Hogg-Dubé, a histopathological pitfall with similarities to tuberous sclerosis: A report of three cases. *Am. J. Dermatopathol.* **2013**, *35*, 241–245. [CrossRef] [PubMed]
42. Misago, N.; Narisawa, Y. Fibrofolliculoma in a patient with tuberous sclerosis complex. *Clin. Exp. Dermatol.* **2009**, *34*, 892–894. [CrossRef] [PubMed]

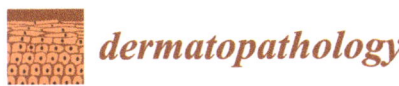

Review

Update on Superficial Spindle Cell Mesenchymal Tumors in Children

Philippe Drabent [1,2] and Sylvie Fraitag [1,3,*]

1. Department of Pathology, Necker-Enfants Malades Hospital, 75015 Paris, France; philippe.drabent@aphp.fr
2. Faculty of Medicine, Sorbonne University, 75006 Paris, France
3. Faculty of Medicine, University of Paris, 75006 Paris, France
* Correspondence: sylvie.fraitag@aphp.fr

Abstract: The diagnosis of cutaneous and subcutaneous spindle cell neoplasms in children is often challenging and has potential therapeutic and prognostic implications. Although correctly diagnosing dermatofibrosarcoma protuberans and infantile fibrosarcoma is paramount, pathologists should not ignore a number of diagnostic pitfalls linked to mostly rare tumors with completely different clinical outcomes. In the last decade, a spectrum of novel entities has been described; information from molecular biology has helped to shape this new landscape for spindle cell tumors. Here, we review the most noteworthy neoplasms in this spectrum, with a focus on their histological similarities: fibroblastic connective tissue nevus, medallion-like dermal dendrocyte hamartoma, or plaque-like CD34-positive dermal fibroma, which share features with fibrous hamartoma of infancy; lipofibromatosis and lipofibromatosis-like neural tumor; and plexiform myofibroblastoma, a recently described neoplasm that should be distinguished from plexiform fibrohistiocytic tumor. These tumors also have genetic similarities, particularly gene rearrangements involving *NTRK3* or *NTRK1*. These genetic features are not only essential for the differential diagnosis of infantile fibrosarcoma but are also of diagnostic value for lipofibromatosis-like neural tumors. The more recently described *RET*, *RAF*1, and *BRAF* gene fusions are also discussed.

Keywords: mesenchymal tumors; children; skin; subcutis; connective tissue nevus; plaque-like CD34-positive dermal fibroma; fibrous hamartoma of infancy; lipofibromatosis; lipofibromatosis-like neural tumor; plexiform myofibroblastoma; *NTRK*; *RET*; *RAF*1; *BRAF*

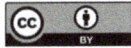

1. Introduction

Pediatric spindle cell mesenchymal neoplasms form a very diverse group of tumors with differing prognoses. Recently, a few entities in the skin and subcutis have been described in morphological and molecular terms. There has been particular interest in CD34-positive spindle cell neoplasms, in view of their importance as a differential diagnosis for dermatofibrosarcoma protuberans (DFSP). One of the first of these tumors to have been described was medallion-like dermal dendrocyte hamartoma (MLDDH) [1], a tumor with a peculiar clinical aspect characterized by a well-circumscribed erythematous atrophic plaque and (under the microscope) a dermal proliferation of CD34-positive, S100-negative spindle cells. This tumor was first considered to be a hamartoma but has since been classified as a neoplasm of fibroblastic lineage and not of dendrocytic lineage [2]. The term "plaque-like CD34-positive dermal fibroma" (PDF) has therefore been preferred in the more recent literature, and there is a tendency to consider MLDDH and PDF as one and the same entity. MLDDH/PDF shares clinical and pathological features with fibroblastic connective tissue nevus (FCTN), a variant of connective tissue nevus first characterized in 2012 by Fletcher and de Feraudy in a series of 25 cases [3]. Although lipofibromatosis (LPF) mainly involves the subcutis, it also contains a spindle cell component admixed with adipose tissue and can be a differential diagnosis for superficial spindle cell tumors in children. In 2016, a CD34-positive spindle cell neoplasm with an interesting, recurrent genetic anomaly was described: LPF-like neural tumor (LPF-NT), which was initially associated with *NTRK*1 gene fusions [4]. As indicated by its name, this tumor is very similar to LPF. It is usually located in the subcutis but infiltrates the surrounding adipose tissue, and it is composed of spindle cells arranged in fascicles. Immunohistochemically, LPF-NTs are positive for both CD34 and S100 protein. Importantly, LPF-NTs are characterized by gene fusions in the *NTRK* family of genes, or (less frequently) in the *RAF* family of genes [5] or *RET* [6]. The clinical course is benign in most but not all cases. The newest member of these pediatric spindle cell neoplasms is plexiform myofibroblastoma (PM), as described in 2020 by Papke and Fletcher [7]. This entity broadens the spectrum of superficial fibroblastic/myofibroblastic tumors and is particularly similar to plexiform fibrohistiocytic tumor (PFHT). However, the two must be distinguished because PFHT is a low-grade sarcoma and PM is benign.

Here, we review these interesting new entities and focus on their similarities and differences. We hope to demonstrate that most of these entities are part of clinical-pathological spectra. Despite valuable contributions from molecular pathology and genetics, a few gray zones nevertheless remain.

2. The "Connective Tissue Nevus/Medallion-Like Dermal Dendrocyte Hamartoma/Plaque-Like Cd34-Positive Dermal Fibroma/Superficial Fibrous Hamartoma of Infancy" Spectrum

Fibroblastic connective tissue nevus (FCTN) was described in 2012 in a series of 25 cases. This variant of connective tissue nevus has some clinical and histological particularities [3,8]. It typically appears during the first decade of life as a slowly growing, painless, plaque-like, or nodular skin lesion, and is mainly located on the trunk, head, and neck and less frequently on the limbs. Girls are more often affected than boys (sex ratio: 0.5–0.6). The lesions range from 0.18 to 2.0 cm in size, and FCTN is rarely diagnosed on the basis of clinical signs alone. Histologically, FCTN is a poorly circumscribed dermal lesion that arises in the reticular dermis and extends to the superficial subcutis. In 70% of cases, there is overlying papillomatosis of the epidermis. In about 60% of cases, abnormally superficial adipocytes are seen in the reticular dermis. The tumor is composed of short, intersecting fascicles of bland, spindle-shaped fibroblasts/myofibroblasts with weakly eosinophilic cytoplasm and elongated nuclei with no atypia and no mitoses. It extends between the collagen bundles, around the appendages and into the subcutaneous septa. The most useful immunostaining marker is CD34, which is positive in 87% of cases—albeit often weakly and in focal sites. Smooth muscle actin (SMA) is weakly and focally present in less than 50% of cases, and S100 is always absent (Figure 1).

The main differential diagnoses for FCTN are (i) plaque-stage DFSP and (ii) the fibroblast-predominant type of PFHT. DFSP differs from FCTN by its storiform architecture; the absence of epidermal papillomatous hyperplasia; the presence of a grenz-zone beneath the epidermis; the atypical nuclei; and the strong, widespread CD34 staining. If tested for, the presence of a *COL1A1–PDGFB* fusion transcript is pathognomic for DFSP. Furthermore, it should be borne in mind that other gene rearrangements have been found in the few cases of DFSP lacking the t(17; 22) translocation [9]. PFHT is discussed in more detail below, and its clinical features (an acral site) and morphological features (osteoclast-like giant cells or other histiocytoid component) will be of assistance in the differential diagnosis.

FCTN broadens the spectrum of connective tissue nevi (CTN), which are otherwise classified with regard to their most abundant component: collagen, elastin, or proteoglycans. In each of these categories, various entities have been described and differ in their clinical characteristics: inherited vs. acquired lesions, and an association with a genetic disorder (Buschke–Ollendorff syndrome, proteus syndrome, tuberous sclerosis complex, or multiple endocrine neoplasia type 1) [10]. A mixed pattern (in which both collagen and elastin are more abundant) appears to be more frequent than initially thought [8]. In line with this observation by Saussine et al., we suggest that the "connective tissue nevi spectrum" might be even broader and overlap with other entities.

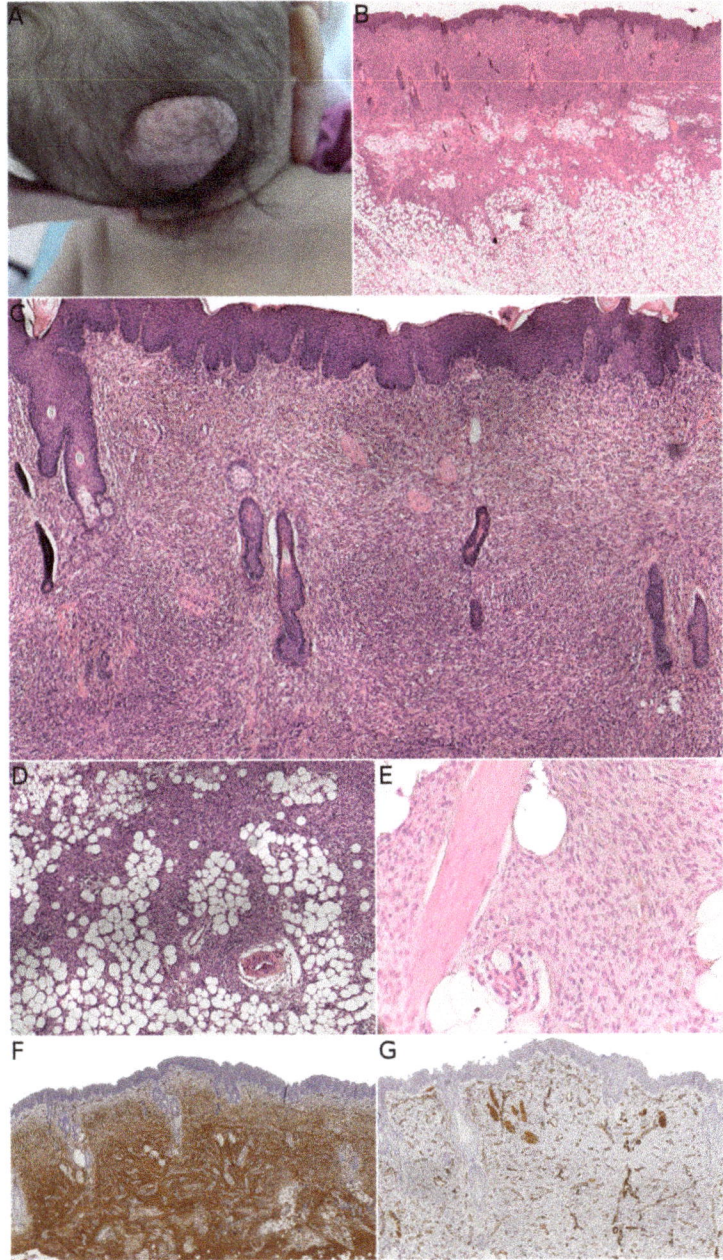

Figure 1. Fibroblastic connective tissue nevus. (**A**) Clinical presentation on the scalp of an infant (courtesy of the Department of Maxillofacial Surgery, Necker-Enfants Malades hospital, Paris, France). (**B**) Low-power view of the lesion showing infiltration of the dermis and subcutis (HE ×50). (**C**) Short intersecting fascicles surrounding the appendages and epidermal hyperplasia (HE ×100). (**D**) Extension into the subcutis (HE ×100). (**E**) High-power view showing the bland morphology of the spindle cells (HE ×200). (**F**) Diffuse positivity for CD34 (×50). (**G**) In this case, smooth muscle actin was negative, with internal controls on vessels and smooth muscles (×50).

MLDDH was the first of these entities to be described, in a series of three cases in 2004 [1]. The clinical presentation was characteristic: a medallion-like, well-circumscribed, brownish, erythematous lesion with a finely wrinkled, atrophodermic surface. The lesions were initially described as congenital, situated on the neck and the upper part of the trunk, and affecting girls. Some subsequently reported cases of MLDDH occurred in boys, appeared shortly after birth, or affected the limbs [11–14]. In 2010, Kutzner and colleagues described similar lesions on the limbs in four adults and a lesion of the neck in a 9-year-old boy [2]. The name "plaque-like CD34-positive dermal fibroma" (PDF) was suggested for these lesions because they appeared after birth and were more like tumors than hamartomas. The investigators also argued that dendrocytes are known to proliferate during wound healing and that PDF/MLDDH might be reactive lesions related to trauma. Histologically, MLDDH and PDF are indistinguishable [15]. The lesion consists of a superficial dermal spindle and sometimes ovoid cell proliferation, mainly occupying the reticular dermis but occasionally infiltrating the subcutis. The degree of epidermal atrophy is variable, and elastic fibers are often diminished or fragmented in the lesion. The stroma may contain mast cells and/or venules with a dilated lumen. The proliferating cells stain positive for CD34 (Figure 2). In their series of PDF cases, Kutzner et al. described a specific but inconstant pattern, with the fibroblasts in the upper part of the lesion oriented vertically to the epidermis and those in the lower part of the lesion oriented horizontally. The investigators also noted that PDF in adults never extended into the deep dermis and subcutaneous septa. Given this slight morphological distinction and the difference in clinical presentation between adults and children, it is still not clear whether PDF and MLDDH are one and the same lesion or if MLDDH is a congenital/infantile variant of PDF. It is noteworthy that MLDDH tends to extend into the subcutis, making it very challenging to differentiate between MLDDH and FCTN, as recently emphasized in a few case reports [15,16]. Both lesions may show slight infiltration clinically, although FCTN may be more irregular in shape [16]. Other differential diagnoses of MLDDH/PDF include dermatomyofibroma (which rather presents in young adults, shows fascicles preferentially oriented parallel to the epidermis, and is SMA-positive), non-pigmented cellular blue nevus (which is easily ruled out by immunophenotyping), plaque-like superficial neurofibroma (again, easily ruled out by immunophenotyping), and CD34-positive sclerotic fibroma of the skin (also known as "plywood fibroma", featuring a more nodular or stellate-like silhouette with characteristic clefts; it is extremely rare in children and is mainly associated with Cowden syndrome).

FCTN, MLDDH, and PDF can all contain cells that appear histologically similar to the fibroblastic component of fibrous hamartoma of infancy (FHI). Both the clinical and histological features must be examined when differentiating between FHI and the above-mentioned lesions. FHI arises in infants and young children—typically within the first two years of life—and is usually located in the axilla, upper limbs, and upper back [17,18]. It presents as a subcutaneous mass rather than a plaque, which is an important difference vs. MLDDH/PDF and some FCTNs. Histologically, it is essential to look for the three characteristic components of FHI: mature fibrous tissue, mature adipose tissue, and immature mesenchymal tissue (Figure 3). These three components are almost always present; if all components are seen, no other diagnosis should be sought. However, one or two of these components may be missing in biopsies or small samples. When the fibrous component alone is seen, misdiagnosis is possible. Furthermore, some FHI extend into the deep dermis and show a peri-eccrine and perivascular arrangement of bland spindle cells similar to those seen in MLDDH/PDF and FCTN [19]. An additional pseudoangiomatous pattern has been described in about half of cases and may be of diagnostic value [20]. Hyalinized zones with "cracking" artifacts mimicking giant cell fibroblastoma have also been observed, and the absence of a *PDGFB* gene rearrangement in these areas argues in favor of an FHI [18]. In the same report, the investigators discussed two interesting cases with sarcomatous-like foci, hyperdiploid or near tetraploid karyotypes, and segmental loss of heterozygosity (1p, 10p, 11p, chromosome 14, 22q). Amputation was decided in one of these cases, in view of extensive local disease and sarcomatous histological features. The investigators concluded that FHI is a complex neoplasm rather than a hamartoma. This is further supported by the results of Park et al. who found consistent *EGFR* exon 20 insertion/duplication mutations in FHI [21]. In difficult-to-diagnose cases, sequencing of *EGFR* exon 20 might be of value for diagnosing or ruling out FHI. Moreover, this raises the possibility of using tyrosine kinase inhibitors to treat large, non-resecable or relapsing FHI.

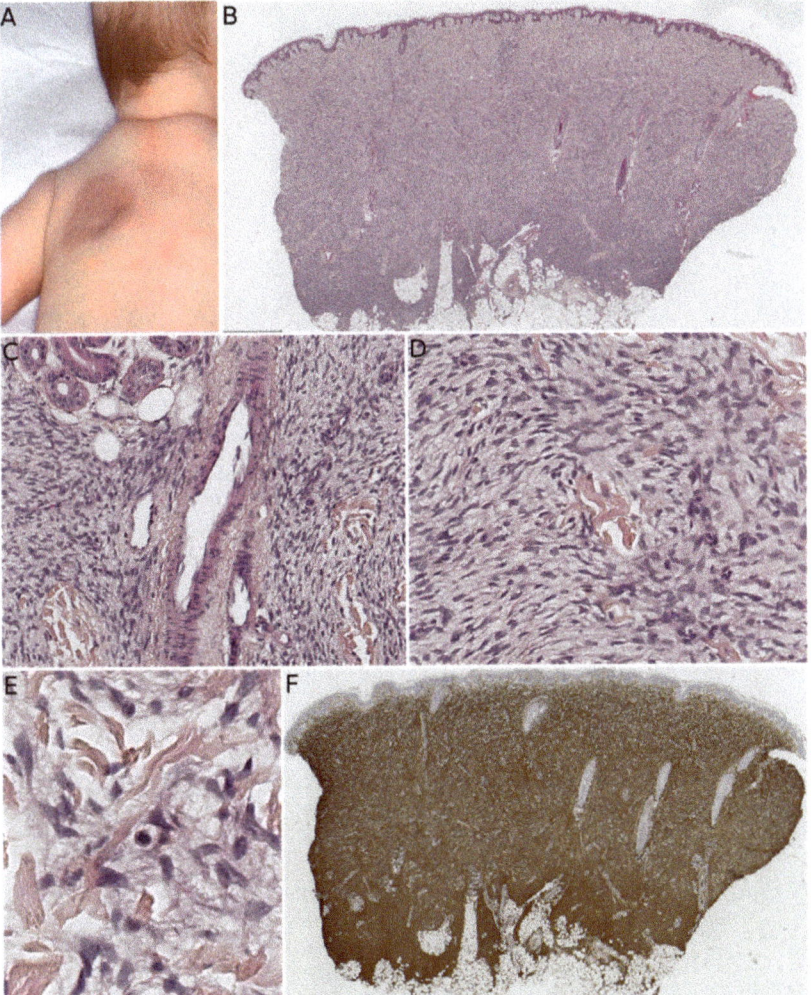

Figure 2. Medallion-like dermal dendrocyte hamartoma (MLDDH)/plaque-like CD34-positive dermal fibroma (PDF). (**A**) Clinical presentation as a medallion-like lesion on the upper back of an infant (courtesy of the Department of Maxillofacial Surgery, Necker-Enfants Malades hospital, Paris, France). (**B**) Low-power view of the lesion showing dermal location and slight extension into the subcutis (HES ×50). (**C**) Venules with dilated lumens (HES ×100). (**D**) Presence of both spindle cells and more ovoid cells (HES ×200). (**E**) High-power view showing the bland morphology of the spindle cells and a mast cell in the center of the picture (HES ×400). (**F**) Diffuse positivity for CD34 (×50).

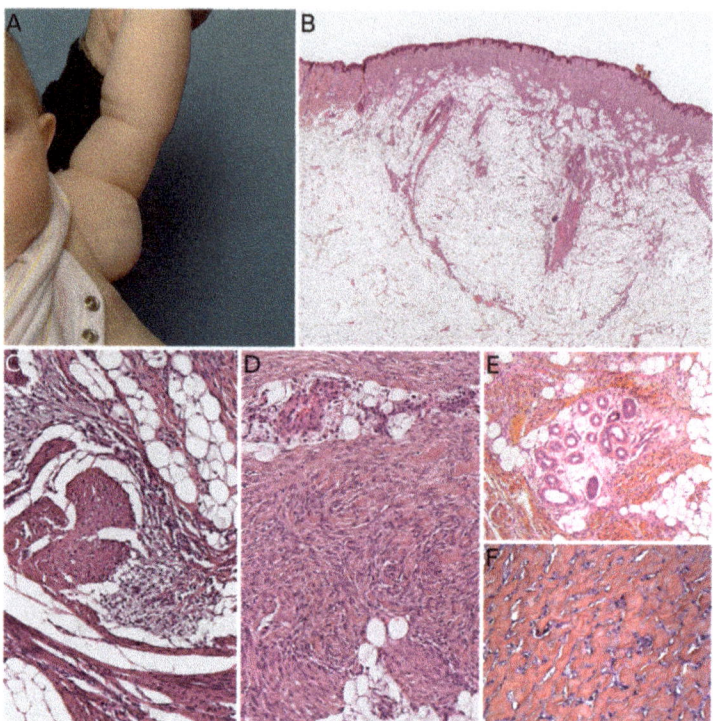

Figure 3. Fibrous hamartoma of infancy (FHI). (**A**) Typical clinical presentation as an axillary mass (courtesy of the Department of Maxillofacial Surgery, Necker-Enfants Malades hospital, Paris, France). (**B**) Low-power view of the lesion showing location in the subcutis and extension of the spindle-cell component into the dermis (HE ×50). (**C**) Presence of the three typical components (mature fibrous tissue, mature adipose tissue, immature mesenchymal tissue) (HE ×100). (**D**) In some cases, the immature mesenchymal tissue is not visible (HE ×100). (**E**) Peri-eccrine extension of the lesion (HES ×100). (**F**) Hyalinized zone reminiscent of giant cell fibroblastoma (HES ×100).

All the above-discussed lesions have similarities: they can be seen during infancy and can affect the upper back/trunk or upper limbs. Some present mostly as plaque-like lesions (MLDDH/PDF), some present as masses (FHI), and some present as both (FCTN). Under the microscope, all these lesions may show a proliferation of fibroblastic/myofibroblastic cells arranged in fascicles in the reticular dermis. For these reasons, it is important to consider all the available data (i.e., clinical; morphological; and, if necessary, molecular) when confronted with a lesion that belongs to this spectrum. In most cases, the presence of one or more of the characteristics described above will help the pathologist to make the right diagnosis (see Table 1). The most troublesome differential diagnosis is plaque-like DFSP, and therefore all equivocal cases should be screened for the *COL1A1-PDGFB* gene rearrangement. The literature data show that the combination of RT-PCR and FISH is the most sensitive diagnostic method [22]. For cases in which the *COL1A1-PDGFB* rearrangement is not found, our experience shows that it is best to take a closer look at the morphology: if there is any suspicion of DFSP, other gene rearrangements should be sought using RNA sequencing (RNA-seq) or next-generation sequencing techniques; if the morphology is not suggestive of DFSP, the most likely diagnosis will fall within the "FCTN-MLDDH/PDF" spectrum. Unfortunately, a characteristic, recurrent genetic abnormality has not yet been evidenced in cases of acquired CTN or MLDDH/PDF.

Table 1. The main clinical and pathological features of lesions from the "connective tissue nevus/medallion-like dermal dendrocyte hamartoma/plaque-like CD34-positive dermal fibroma/superficial fibrous hamartoma of infancy" spectrum and of dermatofibrosarcoma protuberans.

	Age	Sex	Site	Morphology	IHC	Genetic Abnormality
FCTN	<10 y	F > M	Trunk, head and neck, limbs	Poorly delimited, reticular dermis with extension into the subcutis; short bundles of (myo)fibroblasts	CD34+ weak, multifocal (87%) S100−	
MLDDH/ PDF	Infants and older children	F > M	Neck, upper trunk, limbs	Poorly delimited, reticular dermis with possible extension into the subcutis; spindle and/or ovoid cells; variable epidermal atrophy, elastic fibers diminished	CD34+ S100−	
Superficial FHI	<2 y	M > F	Axilla, upper limbs, upper back	Subcutis, three components: mature fibrous tissue, mature adipose tissue, and immature mesenchymal tissue; possible pseudoangiomatous or hyalinized areas	Not helpful	*EGFR* exon 20 ins/dup
DFSP	Older children	M > F	Trunk, proximal areas of the limbs, head and neck	Diffuse infiltration of the dermis and subcutis; high cellularity; spindle cells in a storiform pattern	CD34+ S100−	*COL1A1-PDGFB*, other rare fusions

FCTN: fibroblastic connective tissue nevus; MLDDH: medallion-like dermal dendrocyte hamartoma; PDF: plaque-like CD34-positive dermal fibroma; FHI: fibrous hamartoma of infancy; DFSP: dermatofibrosarcoma protuberans.

3. The "Lipofibromatosis/Lipofibromatosis-Like Neural Tumor" Spectrum—The "Lipofibromatosis-Like Pattern"

LPF was first described and named as such in 2000 [23], but this entity was already known and had been referred to by some as "infantile fibromatosis", which can cause confusion. LPF arises mainly in infants but can be present at birth. The initial series reported by Fetsch et al. showed male predominance (sex ratio: 2.7). The main sites involved are the distal parts of the upper limbs, followed by the lower limbs and (more rarely) the trunk or head. Microscopically, LPF is an infiltrative, poorly-circumscribed lesion, consisting of mature adipose tissue and spindled fibroblastic cells with focal, fascicular growth that extends mainly into the septa of fat and skeletal muscle. The fibroblastic cells show limited cytologic atypia and low mitotic activity. Cells with a single vacuole can sometimes be seen at the interface between the fibroblastic component and the mature adipocytes, which is suggestive of a transition between the two components (Figure 4). Immunohistochemistry is of limited value; it can show foci positive for CD34, SMA, and (more rarely) EMA. It is likely that the rare initial reports of a positivity for S100 protein correspond to another tumor (discussed below) that was unknown at that time. Recurrences are frequent.

LPF can be hard to differentiate histologically from FHI, especially in cases of FHI that lack a visible immature, mesenchymal component. Although immunohistochemistry is not helpful, LPF and FHI tend to occur in different sites.

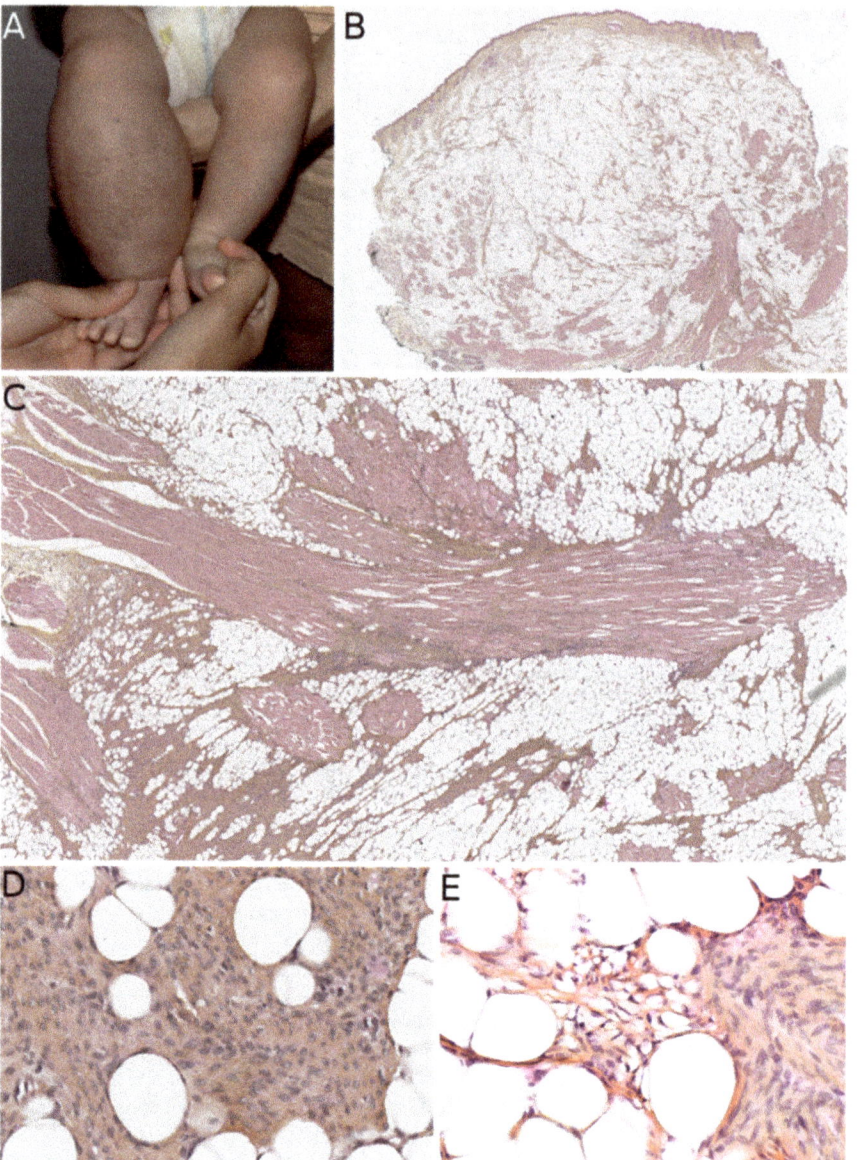

Figure 4. Lipofibromatosis (LPF). (**A**) Clinical presentation as a large mass of the right lower leg in an infant (courtesy of the Department of Maxillofacial Surgery, Necker-Enfants Malades hospital, Paris, France). (**B**) Low-power view of the lesion showing location in the subcutis (HES ×50). (**C**) Long fascicles of spindle cells admixed with adipose tissue (HES ×100). (**D**) High-power view showing the bland morphology of the cells (HES ×200). (**E**) Focus on cells with a single vacuole at the interface between the fibroblastic and the adipose components (HES ×200).

Recently, a spindle cell tumor with some similarities to LPF has been identified in adults and children and named "lipofibromatosis-like neural tumor" (LPF-NT) [4]. Interestingly, most of these tumors were first diagnosed as low-grade malignant peripheral nerve sheath tumors (LG-MPNSTs) in adults, which emphasizes the morphological similarity between these entities. However, LG-MPNSTs are almost always seen in adult or adolescent patients with neurofibromatosis type 1 (NF1), whereas this is never the case for LPF-NTs. In our experience, LPF-NTs in children were mostly misdiagnosed as LPF. LPF-NT can affect infants, older children, adolescents, and young adults, with a possible predominance in infants and adolescents. There is no obvious sex predominance. The presentation of LPF-NT appears to vary with age, due to differences in fat distribution. The limbs are affected more often than the trunk, and there appear to be more cases involving the trunk in infants and the chest in pubescent girls. LPF-NT presents as a subcutaneous tumor with a greatest dimension of 1 to 6 cm. Microscopically, the tumor has an infiltrative growth pattern within subcutaneous fat and can extend into skeletal muscle in some cases. It is composed of dense spindle cells arranged in streaming fascicles. The tumor cells have weakly eosinophilic cytoplasm with indistinct borders, elongated nuclei with mild atypia and hyperchromasia, and inconspicuous nucleoli. In rare cases, scattered pleomorphic cells may be present. The mitotic activity is low, with less than two mitoses per 10 high-power fields (HPFs) in most cases, and rarely more than 8 mitoses per 10 HPFs. One of the most striking characteristics of these tumors is the dual positivity for S100 protein and CD34 (sometimes focal) (Figure 5). A small proportion of cases can be positive for SMA. Melanocyte markers (SOX10, HMB45, melan A), desmin, STAT6, and GFAP are absent. H3K27me3 expression is retained, which can be useful in the differential diagnosis vs. MPNST. Local recurrences are possible, but metastases have not been reported. The key diagnostic element is the presence of recurrent gene fusions involving the *NTRK1* gene, which encodes the TRKA receptor tyrosine kinase (RTK), the high affinity receptor for the nerve growth factor. The various fusion partners include LMNA, TPM3, and TPR [4]. None of these gene rearrangements have been found in LPF [24]. However, no *NTRK1* gene partner can be identified in a subset of LPF-NTs [4,5]. Importantly, an anti-*NTRK1* antibody (or a panTRK antibody) can be used to immunohistochemically screen for NTRK1 expression. If this test is negative, molecular techniques must be used. Since the first description of LPF-NT, other gene rearrangements have been identified in children; they involve *NTRK3* (with *EML4* or *KHDRBS1* as partners) [5,25,26], *RAF1*, *BRAF* [5], or *RET* (with *CCDC6* or *NCOA4* as partners) [6]. These interesting molecular results require further explanation.

In a study reported in 2018, Suurmeijer et al. described a new group of spindle cell tumors with S100 and CD34 co-expression and recurrent gene fusions. In their series of 25 cases, 8 were located in subcutaneous tissue in children. Interestingly, there were four other pediatric cases involving visceral organs (the stomach and the rectum) or bones (the maxilla and the mandible). The remaining cases were in adults and featured a variety of superficial and deep sites. All the tumors had similar features: monomorphic cytology; stromal and perivascular hyalinization; immunopositivity for S100 and CD34; and *RAF1*, *BRAF*, or *NTRK1/2* fusions. Hence, it is likely that LPF-NT belongs to a wider group of spindle cell tumors sharing these characteristics. Moreover, some tumors showed possible signs of malignancy: scattered pleomorphic and/or multinucleate cells, highly cellular fascicular growth, or a primitive appearance. In fact, an 18-year-old patient in Suurmeijer et al.'s series died of metastatic disease, and other patients had metastases (in the lung and other sites) or disease recurrence. This aggressive clinical course was seen both for superficial and deep tumors, and in patients as young as 4 years old. It is most likely that tumors defined by *RAF1*, *BRAF*, or *NTRK1/2* fusions form a spectrum whose behavior can vary from benign to malignant.

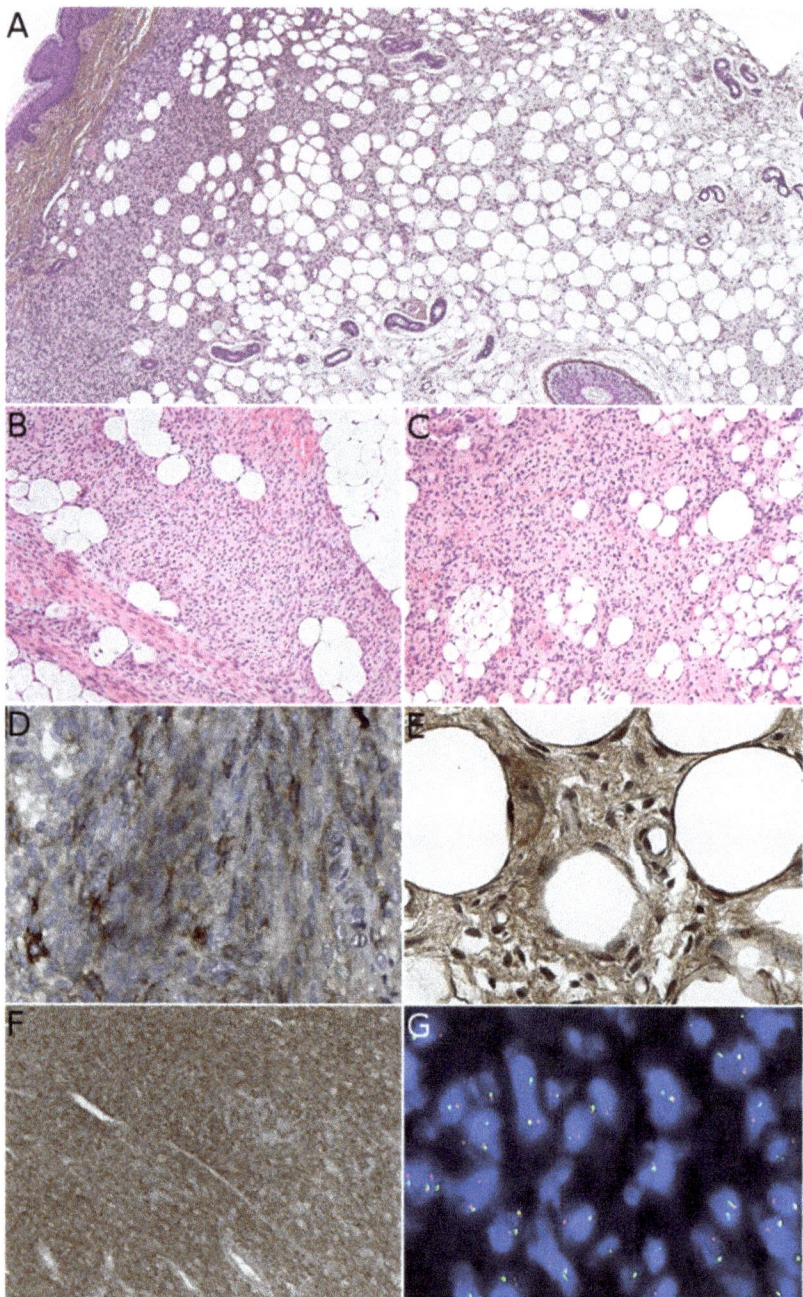

Figure 5. Lipofibromatosis-like neural tumor (LPF-NT). (**A**) Low-power view showing extension of the tumor in both the dermis and subcutis (HE ×50). (**B**) Spindle cells in fascicles admixed with adipose tissue (HE ×100). (**C**) Some areas can lack the typical fascicular growth (HE ×100). (**D**) Heterogeneous positivity for CD34 (×400). (**E**) Positivity for S100 (×400). (**F**) Diffuse positivity for NTRK1 (×200). (**G**) FISH showing fusion transcripts between *NTRK1* and *LMNA*. (Courtesy of Marie Karanian, Department of Pathology, Centre Léon Bérard, Lyon, France).

In 2019, Antonescu et al. reported on six cases with tumors that resembled LPF-NT but harbored *RET* gene rearrangements. Five of their cases occurred in children (including four infants): three of these were diagnosed as LPF-NT, one was diagnosed as an "infantile fibrosarcoma-like" tumor (involving the chest wall), and the last was diagnosed as infantile fibrosarcoma/cellular mesoblastic nephroma (involving the kidney with bilateral lung and brain metastases). Of the three cases of LPF-NT, one was a superficial tumor of the ankle, one was a deep tumor of the foot, and the last arose in the abdominal wall. None of the LPF-NTs recurred, although the tumor had an aggressive clinical course in the two cases with malignant histological features. These interesting results broadened the spectrum of spindle cell tumors with recurrent translocations and emphasized two important features of this group: (i) the predominant value of molecular characteristics (i.e., recurrent gene fusions) in the classification of these tumors with a wide range of morphologies (from LPF-NT to infantile fibrosarcoma to MPNST-like tumors), and (ii) the probable continuum in the degree of malignancy.

This second concept was already foreseen in the first description of LPF-NT by Agaram et al., who described a case of superficial LPF-NT of the leg in a young woman who developed lung metastases [4]. This tumor had the *LMNA–NTRK1* fusion, and its possible identity as a malignant counterpart of LPF-NT was mentioned by the researchers at the time.

The varying degrees of aggressiveness within this group of tumors warrant further investigation. To the best of our knowledge, no ancillary techniques (whether immunohistochemical or molecular) appear to be of value in this respect. At present, only the morphology seems to be related to the tumor's aggressiveness: elevated cellularity, presence of pleomorphic and/or multinucleate cells, and elevated mitotic activity are signs that should alert the pathologist and the clinician.

Besides the very similar FHI and LPF, the differential diagnoses of LPF-NT also include other entities, the most important of which is calcifying aponeurotic fibroma (CAF). This lesion is a superficial, slow-growing, ill-circumscribed tumor of the hands or feet that arises in children and adolescents. Histologically, CAF has a typically two-phase morphology that combines moderately cellular areas (with fibroblastic cells arranged in fascicles) and partly calcified nodules (with a fibrocartilage appearance, small epithelioid fibroblasts, and osteoclast-like giant cells). In 2016, a recurrent *FN1–EGF* fusion was found in eight out of nine cases, either by RNA-seq, RT-PCR, or FISH [27]. This fusion results in overexpression of epidermal growth factor (EGF), which is detected using immunohistochemistry in all cases, even when a gene fusion cannot be detected. Interestingly, in a report in 2019, the *FN1–EGF* fusion was found in four cases of apparently typical LPF that recurred as CAF [24]. In this study of 20 LPF cases, the other fusions involved genes that encode ligands for the EGF receptor (*EGF*, *TGFA*, *HBEGF*) or that encode RTKs as 3′-partners (*ROS1*, *PDGFRB*, *RET*). The researchers mentioned that these findings were strongly suggestive of a link between LPF and CAF; in some cases, LPF might correspond to "early" CAF characterized by a prominent adipocytic component and no calcification. It remains to be established whether the cases with a *FN1–EGF* fusion or another fusion constitute the same entity or whether the cases with *FN1–EGF* fusions are CAF and the cases with other fusions are LPF. However, this interesting study highlighted potential genetic variability in LPF, with a diverse range of gene fusions and proximity to CAF. Lastly, the differential diagnoses for LPF and LPF-NT in children include DFSP, which can be distinguished by its negativity for S100 protein and the presence of the characteristic gene fusions.

The most important features to look for when confronted with an "LPF-like lesion" are summarized in Table 2.

Table 2. The main clinical and pathological features of "LPF-like" lesions.

	Age	Sex	Site	Morphology	IHC	Genetic Abnormality
FHI	<2 y	M > F	Axilla, upper limbs, upper back	Subcutis, three components: mature fibrous tissue, mature adipose tissue, and immature mesenchymal tissue; pseudoangiomatous or hyalinized areas may be found	Not helpful	*EGFR* exon 20 ins/dup
LPF	Infants	M > F	Upper limbs (more than lower limbs), trunk, head	Subcutis, poorly delimited, mature fat and spindled fibroblasts, single-vacuole cells at the interface	Not helpful	Possible multiple gene fusions involving RTK or RTK ligands
LPF-NT	All ages	M = F	Limbs > trunk	Subcutis, infiltrative, "MPNST-like", possible scattered pleomorphic cells	CD34+ S100+ SOX10−	*NTRK1/3*, *RAF1*, *BRAF*, *RET* fusions
CAF	Children and adolescents	M > F (slight)	Hands, feet	Subcutis, aponeuroses, infiltrative growth, fibroblasts in fascicles, fibrocartilage-like nodules (sometimes absent), osteoclast-like giant cells (sometimes absent)	SMA+ (in most cases)	*FN1–EGF*

CAF: calcifying aponeurotic fibroma; FHI: fibrous hamartoma of infancy; LPF: lipofibromatosis; LPF-NT: lipofibromatosis-like neural tumor; RTK: receptor tyrosine kinase.

4. Plexiform Myofibroblastoma

Plexiform myofibroblastoma (PM) is a newly described entity. In a series of 36 cases, Papke et al. characterized this tumor; it had a broad age range and no male or female predominance (19 females and 17 males) [7]. PM can be congenital but may appear as late as the age of 50, although the median age at onset is 9.5 years. A total of 24 of Papke et al.'s 36 patients were children. In the pediatric population, the tumor was located (i) mostly in the neck and upper back; (ii) to a lesser extent in the lower back, axilla, chest wall and abdominal wall; and (iii) in one case in the left lower leg. The lesions were multifocal in three cases (all below the age of 2) and extended to the occiput in one case. Interestingly, two of the multifocal cases were brothers, raising the question of a genetically inherited anomaly (though not discussed by Papke et al.). None of the pediatric cases—even those with positive margins—showed any recurrence of the disease after surgical resection. Grossly, PM has a tan/white cut surface and ranges from 0.6 to 4 cm in size (in pediatric cases). Histologically, it is composed of fascicles in a plexiform pattern, which extend within the reticular dermis and subcutis. The tumor cells are fibroblastic/myofibroblastic, with a weakly eosinophilic, elongated cytoplasm and ovoid to tapered nuclei with no atypia. The characteristic collagenous stroma is reminiscent of mammary-like myofibroblastoma, with at least focal hyalinization in 35% of cases. Some cases show nodular fasciitis-like areas. The stroma may be focally myxoid. Mitoses are rare, with no more than 4 per 2 mm^2. There is no necrosis. The most frequently positive immunohistochemical markers are SMA (in 84% of cases), CD34 (in 54%), and desmin (in 43%) (Figure 6). The tumor is also negative for S100 protein, and there is no nuclear translocation of beta-catenin. To date, no recurrent genetic alterations have been identified. Only one case had a missense mutation in *FGFR2*, and another had a probable germline mutation in both *MUTYH* and *BRIP1*; the significance of these genetic abnormalities remains unclear.

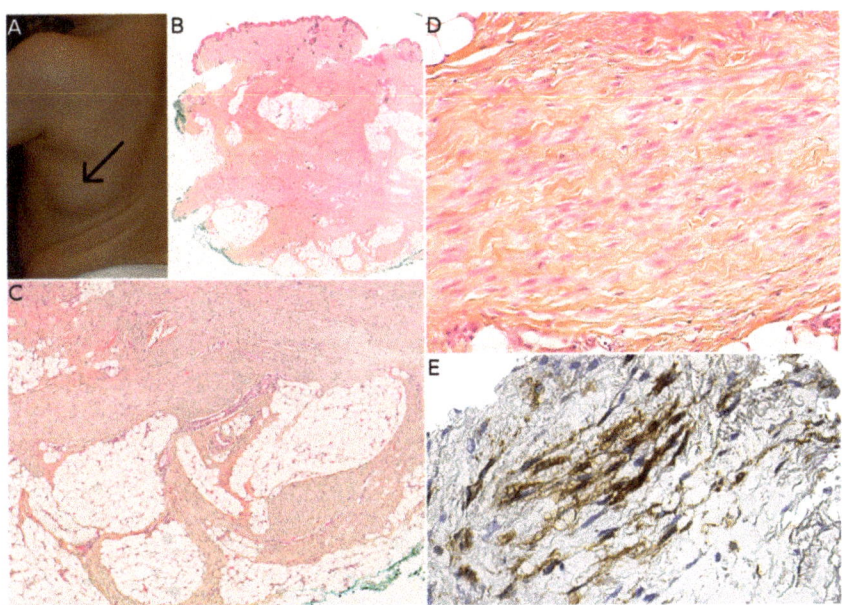

Figure 6. Plexiform myofibroblastoma (PM). (**A**) Clinical presentation as a sub-scapular subcutaneous mass in an infant (courtesy of the Department of Maxillofacial Surgery, Necker-Enfants Malades hospital, Paris, France). (**B**) Low-power view of the lesion showing location in the subcutis (HES ×50). (**C**) Typical plexiform architecture with extension into the subcutaneous septa (HES ×100). (**D**) High-power view showing the bland morphology of the cells and the characteristic collagenous stroma (HES ×200). (**E**) Positivity for smooth muscle actin in the spindle cells (SMA ×200).

There are many potential differential diagnoses for PM. The closest mimic is the fibroblastic variant of plexiform fibrohistiocytic tumor (PFHT), a superficial tumor of children and young adults (median age at onset: ≈15) that occurs mainly in the upper limbs but also in the axilla, back, neck, and chest wall [28]. Like PM, PFHT has a characteristic plexiform architecture. Most cases have a fibrohistiocytic or mixed fibroblastic–fibrohistiocytic morphology. Cases with a predominant fibroblastic component are the hardest to differentiate from PM, especially if no osteoclast-like giant cells or histiocytoid cells are present. CD68 immunostaining is useful for highlighting the histiocytoid component. PM is usually SMA-positive (which is not helpful for the differential diagnosis), and CD34 is usually negative. As discussed by Papke et al., it is possible that cases of purely fibroblastic PFHT are in fact PM. Interestingly, there are no reports of recurrence or metastasis in purely fibroblastic PFHT [7]. It is important to differentiate between PM and PFHT; the former is benign and does not seem to recur in children, whereas the latter is a low-grade sarcoma with metastatic potential.

Other differential diagnoses for PM lack the typical plexiform pattern and can thus be ruled out quite easily: desmoid fibromatosis, nodular fasciitis, dermatomyofibroma, plaque-like myofibroblastic tumor, FCTN, and FHI.

5. Conclusions

Superficial spindle cell mesenchymal tumors form a diverse group of lesions with benign and malignant entities that are often very similar clinically and/or histologically. In children, the patient's age; the lesion site; the presentation as a mass, nodule, or plaque; and the location in the dermis or subcutis are important features that will guide the dermatologist and the pathologist. The newest entities encompass two main histologic patterns.

The first pattern encompasses dermal, CD34-positive spindle cell lesions that can extend to the subcutis. The major differential diagnosis is DFSP. The distinction between FCTN, MLDDH/PDF, and the superficial variant of FHI can be challenging for the pathologist and the clinical utility of making this distinction is not obvious or well characterized. Indeed, all these entities probably fall within a common spectrum, which corresponds to a kind of fibroblastic-rich connective tissue nevus. Regardless of the type, all these lesions are benign and will be cured by excision with narrow margins. DFSP is the exception since it has an intermediate clinical behavior with frequent local recurrence. A wide excision is necessary, better achieved by either Mohs or slow-Mohs micrographic surgery [29]. A close follow-up is mandatory since rare cases of malignant transformation have been reported.

The second pattern encompasses subcutaneous lesions admixed with adipocytes and that are similar to LPF. It is important to consider other diagnoses when confronted with an LPF-like lesion: we have seen that CAF can mimic LPF and that this diagnosis can be confirmed by the presence of an *FN1–EGF* fusion. S100-protein-positive cases are likely to be LPF-NT and can be confirmed by the presence of gene fusions involving the *NTRK* family, the *RAF* family, or *RET*. In some relapsing cases or in overly superficial biopsies, a diagnosis of infantile fibrosarcoma could also be considered and then confirmed by the presence of the *ETV6–NTRK3* gene fusion [30]. MPNSTs are extremely rare in children and should be diagnosed with great caution.

The latest tumor to have been identified is PM, which is characterized by its plexiform architecture. Given the benign clinical course of PM, it is essential to distinguish this entity from PFHT.

The use of molecular techniques must be encouraged whenever the morphological and clinical data are insufficient, and especially when one of the differential diagnoses is a malignant condition. This is true for DFSP, some non-resectable or relapsing cases of FHI, LPF-NT, and other tumors with gene fusions in *NTRK*, *RAF*, or *RET*. Although the presence of a gene fusion is not essential for malignancy, it is an important element of diagnostic information and may provide a rationale for treatment with RTK inhibitors (e.g., larotrectinib for *NTRK*-rearranged tumors, and anti-EGFR agents for FHI) [31,32].

Author Contributions: Conceptualization, S.F.; investigation, P.D.; data curation, P.D.; writing—original draft preparation, P.D.; writing—review and editing, P.D. and S.F.; supervision, S.F.; funding acquisition, S.F. All authors have read and agreed to the published version of the manuscript.

Funding: The authors thank the Lions Club de Corrèze and Nicole Brousse for financial support.

Institutional Review Board Statement: Not applicable.

Informed Consent Statement: Not applicable.

Acknowledgments: The authors thank Marie Karanian (Centre Léon Bérard, Lyon, France) for providing pictures of one of the cases, and the Department of Maxillofacial Surgery at Necker-Enfants Malades hospital for providing clinical pictures.

Conflicts of Interest: The authors declare no conflict of interest.

References

1. Rodríguez-Jurado, R.; Palacios, C.; Durán-McKinster, C.; Mercadillo, P.; Orozco-Covarrubias, L.; Saez-De-Ocariz, M.D.M.; Ruiz-Maldonado, R. Medallion-like dermal dendrocyte hamartoma: A new clinically and histopathologically distinct lesion. *J. Am. Acad. Dermatol.* **2004**, *51*, 359–363. [CrossRef] [PubMed]
2. Kutzner, H.; Mentzel, T.; Palmedo, G.; Hantschke, M.; Rütten, A.; Paredes, B.E.; Schärer, L.; Guillen, C.S.; Requena, L. Plaque-like CD34-positive Dermal Fibroma ("Medallion-like Dermal Dendrocyte Hamartoma"). *Am. J. Surg. Pathol.* **2010**, *34*, 190–201. [CrossRef] [PubMed]
3. Wisell, J. Fibroblastic Connective Tissue Nevus: A Rare Cutaneous Lesion Analyzed in a Series of 25 Cases. *Yearb. Pathol. Lab. Med.* **2013**, *2013*, 97–98. [CrossRef]
4. Agaram, N.P.; Zhang, L.; Sung, Y.-S.; Chen, C.-L.; Chung, C.T.; Antonescu, C.R.; Fletcher, C.D. Recurrent NTRK1 Gene Fusions Define a Novel Subset of Locally Aggressive Lipofibromatosis-like Neural Tumors. *Am. J. Surg. Pathol.* **2016**, *40*, 1407–1416. [CrossRef]

5. Suurmeijer, A.; Dickson, B.C.; Swanson, D.; Zhang, L.; Sung, Y.-S.; Cotzia, P.; Fletcher, C.D.M.; Antonescu, C.R. A novel group of spindle cell tumors defined by S100 and CD34 co-expression shows recurrent fusions involving RAF1, BRAF, and NTRK1/2 genes. *Genes Chromosomes Cancer* **2018**, *57*, 611–621. [CrossRef]
6. Antonescu, C.R.; Dickson, B.C.; Swanson, D.; Zhang, L.; Sung, Y.-S.; Kao, Y.-C.; Chang, W.-C.; Ran, L.; Pappo, A.; Bahrami, A.; et al. Spindle Cell Tumors With RET Gene Fusions Exhibit a Morphologic Spectrum Akin to Tumors With NTRK Gene Fusions. *Am. J. Surg. Pathol.* **2019**, *43*, 1384–1391. [CrossRef]
7. Papke, D.J.; Al-Ibraheemi, A.; Fletcher, C.D. Plexiform Myofibroblastoma. *Am. J. Surg. Pathol.* **2020**, *44*, 1469–1478. [CrossRef]
8. Saussine, A.; Marrou, K.; Delanoé, P.; Bodak, N.; Hamel, D.; Picard, A.; Sassolas, B.; De Prost, Y.; LeMerrer, M.; Fraitag, S.; et al. Connective tissue nevi: An entity revisited. *J. Am. Acad. Dermatol.* **2012**, *67*, 233–239. [CrossRef]
9. Dadone-Montaudié, B.; Alberti, L.; Duc, A.; Delespaul, L.; Lesluyes, T.; Pérot, G.; Lançon, A.; Paindavoine, S.; Di Mauro, I.; Blay, J.-Y.; et al. Alternative PDGFD rearrangements in dermatofibrosarcomas protuberans without PDGFB fusions. *Mod. Pathol.* **2018**, *31*, 1683–1693. [CrossRef]
10. Arora, H.; Falto-Aizpurua, L.; Cortés-Fernandez, A.; Choudhary, S.; Romanelli, P. Connective Tissue Nevi: A Review of the Literature. *Am. J. Dermatopathol.* **2017**, *39*, 325–341. [CrossRef]
11. Marque, M.; Bessis, D.; Pedeutour, F.; Viseux, V.; Guillot, B.; Fraitag-Spinner, S. Medallion-like dermal dendrocyte hamartoma: The main diagnostic pitfall is congenital atrophic dermatofibrosarcoma. *Br. J. Dermatol.* **2008**, *160*, 190–193. [CrossRef]
12. Shah, K.N.; Anderson, E.; Junkins-Hopkins, J.; James, W.D. Medallion-Like Dermal Dendrocyte Hamartoma. *Pediatr. Dermatol.* **2007**, *24*, 632–636. [CrossRef]
13. Ducharme, E.E.; Baribault, K.E.; Husain, S.; Engler, D.E. Medallion-like dermal dendrocyte hamartoma in a 36-year-old male. *J. Am. Acad. Dermatol.* **2008**, *59*, 169–172. [CrossRef]
14. Restano, L.; Fanoni, D.; Colonna, C.; Gelmetti, C.; Berti, E. Medallion-Like Dermal Dendrocyte Hamartoma: A Case Misdiagnosed as Neurofibroma. *Pediatr. Dermatol.* **2010**, *27*, 638–642. [CrossRef]
15. Bouaoud, J.; Fraitag, S.; Soupre, V.; Mitrofanoff, M.; Boccara, O.; Galliot, C.; Bodemer, C.; Picard, A.; Khonsari, R.H. Congenital fibroblastic connective tissue nevi: Unusual and misleading presentations in three infantile cases. *Pediatr. Dermatol.* **2018**, *35*, 644–650. [CrossRef]
16. Horikawa, H.; Sato, T.; Gomi, H.; Yamazaki, K.; Ishida, Y.; Yuzaki, I.; Fukuzumi, S. Medallion-like dermal dendrocyte hamartoma: A rare congenital CD34-positive dermal lesion clinically and pathologically overlapping with fibroblastic connective tissue nevus. *Pediatr. Dermatol.* **2019**, *36*, 397–399. [CrossRef]
17. Dickey, G.E.; Sotelo-Avila, C. Fibrous Hamartoma of Infancy: Current Review. *Pediatr. Dev. Pathol.* **1999**, *2*, 236–243. [CrossRef]
18. Al-Ibraheemi, A.; Martinez, A.; Weiss, S.W.; Kozakewich, H.P.; Perez-Atayde, A.R.; Tran, H.; Parham, D.M.; Sukov, W.R.; Fritchie, K.J.; Folpe, A.L. Fibrous hamartoma of infancy: A clinicopathologic study of 145 cases, including 2 with sarcomatous features. *Mod. Pathol.* **2017**, *30*, 474–485. [CrossRef]
19. Grynspan, D.; Meir, K.; Senger, C.; Ball, N.J. Cutaneous changes in fibrous hamartoma of infancy. *J. Cutan. Pathol.* **2007**, *34*, 39–43. [CrossRef]
20. Saab, S.T.; McClain, C.M.; Coffin, C.M. Fibrous Hamartoma of Infancy. *Am. J. Surg. Pathol.* **2014**, *38*, 394–401. [CrossRef]
21. Park, J.Y.; Cohen, C.; Lopez, D.; Ramos, E.; Wagenfuehr, J.; Rakheja, D. EGFR Exon 20 Insertion/Duplication Mutations Characterize Fibrous Hamartoma of Infancy. *Am. J. Surg. Pathol.* **2016**, *40*, 1713–1718. [CrossRef]
22. Patel, K.U.; Szabo, S.S.; Hernandez, V.S.; Prieto, V.G.; Abruzzo, L.V.; Lazar, A.; López-Terrada, D. Dermatofibrosarcoma protuberans COL1A1-PDGFB fusion is identified in virtually all dermatofibrosarcoma protuberans cases when investigated by newly developed multiplex reverse transcription polymerase chain reaction and fluorescence in situ hybridization assays. *Hum. Pathol.* **2008**, *39*, 184–193. [CrossRef]
23. Fetsch, J.F.; Miettinen, M.; Laskin, W.B.; Michal, M.; Enzinger, F.M. A Clinicopathologic Study of 45 Pediatric Soft Tissue Tumors With an Admixture of Adipose Tissue and Fibroblastic Elements, and a Proposal for Classification as Lipofibromatosis. *Am. J. Surg. Pathol.* **2000**, *24*, 1491–1500. [CrossRef]
24. Al-Ibraheemi, A.; Folpe, A.L.; Perez-Atayde, A.R.; Perry, K.; Hofvander, J.; Arbajian, E.; Magnusson, L.; Nilsson, J.; Mertens, F. Aberrant receptor tyrosine kinase signaling in lipofibromatosis: A clinicopathological and molecular genetic study of 20 cases. *Mod. Pathol.* **2019**, *32*, 423–434. [CrossRef]
25. Davis, J.L.; Lockwood, C.; Albert, C.M.; Tsuchiya, K.; Hawkins, D.S.; Rudzinski, E.R. Infantile NTRK-associated Mesenchymal Tumors. *Pediatr. Dev. Pathol.* **2018**, *21*, 68–78. [CrossRef]
26. Tallegas, M.; Fraitag, S.; Binet, A.; Orbach, D.; Jourdain, A.; Reynaud, S.; Pierron, G.; Machet, M.-C.; Maruani, A. Novel KHDRBS1-NTRK3 rearrangement in a congenital pediatric CD34-positive skin tumor: A case report. *Virchows Arch.* **2018**, *474*, 111–115. [CrossRef]
27. Puls, F.; Hofvander, J.; Magnusson, L.; Nilsson, J.; Haywood, E.; Sumathi, V.P.; Mangham, D.C.; Kindblom, L.-G.; Mertens, F. FN1-EGFgene fusions are recurrent in calcifying aponeurotic fibroma. *J. Pathol.* **2016**, *238*, 502–507. [CrossRef]
28. Moosavi, C.; Jha, P.; Fanburg-Smith, J.C. An update on plexiform fibrohistiocytic tumor and addition of 66 new cases from the Armed Forces Institute of Pathology, in honor of Franz M. Enzinger, MD. *Ann. Diagn. Pathol.* **2007**, *11*, 313–319. [CrossRef]
29. Foroozan, M.; Sei, J.-F.; Amini, M.; Beauchet, A.; Saiag, P. Efficacy of Mohs Micrographic Surgery for the Treatment of Dermatofibrosarcoma Protuberans. *Arch. Dermatol.* **2012**, *148*, 1055–1063. [CrossRef]

30. Swiadkiewicz, R.; Galmiche, L.; Belhous, K.; Boccara, O.; Fraitag, S.; Pedeutour, F.; Dadone, B.; Buis, J.; Picard, A.; Orbach, D.; et al. Congenital Infantile Fibrosarcoma Associated With a Lipofibromatosis-Like Component: One Train May Be Hiding Another. *Am. J. Dermatopathol.* **2017**, *39*, 463–467. [CrossRef] [PubMed]
31. Dupuis, M.; Shen, Y.; Curcio, C.; Meis, J.M.; Wang, W.-L.; Amini, B.; Rhines, L.; Reuther, J.; Roy, A.; Fisher, K.E.; et al. Successful treatment of lipofibromatosis-like neural tumor of the lumbar spine with an NTRK-fusion inhibitor. *Clin. Sarcoma Res.* **2020**, *10*, 1–7. [CrossRef] [PubMed]
32. Hong, D.S.; DuBois, S.G.; Kummar, S.; Farago, A.F.; Albert, C.M.; Rohrberg, K.S.; van Tilburg, C.M.; Nagasubramanian, R.; Berlin, J.D.; Federman, N.; et al. Larotrectinib in patients with TRK fusion-positive solid tumours: A pooled analysis of three phase 1/2 clinical trials. *Lancet Oncol.* **2020**, *21*, 531–540. [CrossRef]

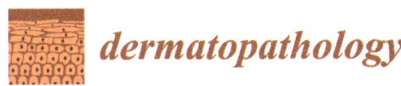

Review

Cutaneous Melanomas Arising during Childhood: An Overview of the Main Entities

Arnaud de la Fouchardière [1,2,*], Felix Boivin [1,2], Heather C. Etchevers [3] and Nicolas Macagno [1,3,4]

1 Department of Biopathology, Center Léon Bérard, 69008 Lyon, France; felix.boivin@etu.univ-lyon1.fr (F.B.); nicolas.macagno@lyon.unicancer.fr (N.M.)
2 Cancer Research Center of Lyon, Equipe Labellisée Ligue Contre le Cancer, Université de Lyon, Université Claude Bernard Lyon 1, INSERM 1052, CNRS 5286, 69008 Lyon, France
3 Marseille Medical Genetics, Institut MarMaRa, Aix-Marseille University, INSERM, U1251, 13005 Marseille, France; heather.etchevers@inserm.fr
4 Department of Pathology, APHM, Timone University Hospital, 13005 Marseille, France
* Correspondence: arnaud.delafouchardiere@lyon.unicancer.fr

Abstract: Cutaneous melanomas are exceptional in children and represent a variety of clinical situations, each with a different prognosis. In congenital nevi, the risk of transformation is correlated with the size of the nevus. The most frequent type is lateral transformation, extremely rare before puberty, reminiscent of a superficial spreading melanoma (SSM) ex-nevus. Deep nodular transformation is much rarer, can occur before puberty, and must be distinguished from benign proliferative nodules. Superficial spreading melanoma can also arise within small nevi, which were not visible at birth, usually after puberty, and can reveal a cancer predisposition syndrome (*CDKN2A* or *CDK4* germline mutations). Prognosis is correlated with classical histoprognostic features (mainly Breslow thickness). Spitz tumors are frequent in adolescents and encompass benign (Spitz nevus), intermediate (atypical Spitz tumor), and malignant forms (malignant Spitz tumor). The whole spectrum is characterized by specific morphology with spindled and epithelioid cells, genetic features, and an overall favorable outcome even if a regional lymph node is involved. Nevoid melanomas are rare and difficult to diagnose clinically and histologically. They can arise in late adolescence. Their prognosis is currently not very well ascertained. A small group of melanomas remains unclassified after histological and molecular assessment.

Keywords: congenital nevus; melanoma; childhood; skin; oncogenetics; SSM; malignant Spitz tumor

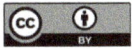

1. Introduction

Melanoma is a form of cancer arising from melanocytes that occurs mainly but not exclusively in the skin. Melanocytes are cells located in the basal layer of the epidermis that produce the melanin pigment responsible for skin color. They derive from neural crest progenitors (melanoblasts) that have migrated toward the skin during embryonic life. Melanocytes are nonadjacent and extend dendrites between the keratinocytes, through which a transcellular transfer of melanosomes encapsulating melanin occurs. This phenomenon *in fine* enables adjacent keratinocytes to protect their nuclei (i.e., DNA) from ultraviolet-induced mutations.

Nevi are benign melanocytic tumors of the skin defined by an abnormal number of melanocytes present in the epidermis and/or in the dermis, often arranged in "nests" where many melanocyte bodies are grouped in clusters and self-pigment. A small number of nevi can progressively undergo malignant transformation, usually through a multistep process that combines genetic (somatic and germline mutations), environmental (ultraviolet light exposure), and immunologic factors, to ultimately become malignant melanomas [1–4]. Children with a high count of nevi and a type I-II Fitzpatrick phototype or with a giant congenital melanocytic nevus (CMN) are the most at risk of developing melanoma. The

WHO classification of skin tumors (4th edition) separates melanocytic proliferations into nine separate classes according to clinical, morphological, and genetic criteria [5].

If nevi are quite common in children, melanomas remain exceptional. They cannot be grouped under a single entity as they represent a variety of clinical situations, each with different prognoses. We will present an illustrated review depicting the specificities of each of the various settings in which cutaneous melanoma can arise during childhood. Nailbed, uveal, and mucous melanomas, which can exceptionally occur in children, will not be discussed.

2. Superficial Spreading Melanoma (SSM)

The occurrence of superficial spreading melanoma (SSM) is exceptional during childhood. Most often, the clinical setting is an adolescent with a type I-II phototype who presents with a progressive modification of a small nevus located on a sun-exposed area. A history of sunburns is common, on par with the phototype. The classic ABCDE rule applies only to this type of melanoma in children. These lesions are very similar to most of the SSMs found in adults. Histologically, a portion of the preexisting nevus can be visible if it has not been replaced by the invasive phase. Distribution is usually asymmetrical and/or haphazard with intraepidermal nests and isolated large melanocytes with a wide foamy/hyperpigmented cytoplasm. Lateral pagetoid scatter of such melanocytes is the histological hallmark of these tumors (Figure 1). In advanced SSM, the dermis is invaded, often by nests of large melanocytes with similar morphology. A dense lymphocytic infiltrate is commonly present on the invasive front of the tumor. These tumor-infiltrating lymphocytes (TILs) are in close connection with melanocytes (with cell-to-cell protein interaction). Breslow thickness, dermal mitotic activity, and epidermal ulceration are to be assessed. A *BRAF*.pV600E mutation is frequently present (>80%) both in the melanoma and the nevus from which it arose [4,6–8]. The need for an oncogenetic consultation must be evaluated according to the clinical setting. This will be discussed in the paragraph related to melanomas arising in the setting of a germline predisposition syndrome. The main differential diagnosis when no nevus is present is a pagetoid Spitz nevus (Figure 1).

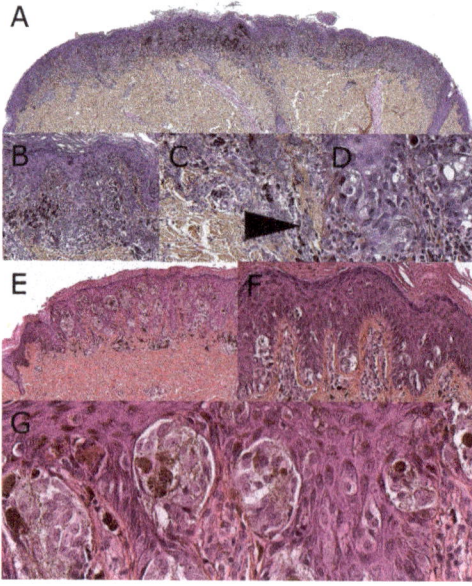

Figure 1. SSM melanoma and pagetoid Spitz nevus (hematoxylin, phloxin, safranin stain). (**A**): Low-magnification silhouette of SSM, 14-year-old: SSM melanoma and pagetoid Spitz nevus (hematoxylin,

phloxin, safranin stain). (**A**): Low-magnification silhouette of SSM, 14-year-old: mainly junctional disorganized melanocytic proliferation. (**B**): Close-up view showing dispersed junctional nests. Ascent of isolated cell. Numerous lymphocytes and melanophages clutter the upper dermis. (**C**): Invasive melanoma with "pseudo-maturation" and mitotic figure (arrow). (**D**): Large, junctional, foamy melanocytes. (**E**): Low-magnification silhouette of a pagetoid Spitz nevus, 6-year-old. Epidermal hyperplasia encasing numerous small nests with a regular distribution. (**F,G**): Close-up view with isolated cells and small nests. An important pericellular retraction is seen. Ascent of small, isolated cells. Arborescent vascular structure in the upper dermis surrounded by small lymphocytes.

3. Malignant Spitz Tumor (Melanoma with a Spitzoid Morphology and Specific Genetic Features)

Melanocytic neoplasms of the Spitz group show distinctive features and encompass benign, intermediate, and malignant tumors, all of which are characterized by prototypic enlarged spindle or epithelioid cells. Benign Spitz nevi are frequent during childhood, especially after puberty, and constitute a diagnostic pitfall of melanoma, mostly of the SSM-type. They often appear located on the lower limbs, especially the knee area, or on the face. Most are unique lesions, although rare cases of eruptive nevi have been described, notably in the clinical setting of a nevus spilus [9]. These lesions grow rapidly, and their important vascularization and lack of pigmentation clinically suggest a benign vascular tumor, such as a botryomycoma or an angioma. Spitz tumors encompass many morphological subtypes (pigmented, hyperpigmented spindle (Reed), plexiform, pagetoid, desmoplastic, angiomatoid...) and have specific, mutually exclusive genetic anomalies. These include *HRAS* mutations, receptor tyrosine kinase fusions, and serine-threonine kinase mutations and fusions, described in Table 1. For benign cases, the most common fusions involve *NTRK1/3*, *ALK1*, and *ROS1*, whereas MAP3K8 and ALK1 predominate in atypical and malignant Spitz tumors [6].

Table 1. Summary of the main genes involved in Spitz tumors, molecular alteration, and their function.

Gene	Molecular Alteration	Function	Frequence	References
NTRK1	Gene fusion	Receptor tyrosine kinase	Common	[10–12]
HRAS	Mutation amplification	Serine/Threonine kinase	Common	[13]
ROS1	Gene fusion	Receptor tyrosine kinase	Common	[14–17]
ALK	Gene fusion	Receptor tyrosine kinase	Common	[10,12,18,19]
RET	Gene fusion	Receptor tyrosine kinase	Rare	[10]
NTRK3	Gene fusion	Receptor tyrosine kinase	Common	[20,21]
NTRK2	Gene fusion	Receptor tyrosine kinase	Rare	[22]
MAP3K8	Gene fusion	Serine/Threonine kinase	Common	[23–26]
BRAF	Gene fusion	Serine/Threonine kinase	Uncommon	[12,25,27–29]
MET	Gene fusion	Receptor tyrosine kinase	Rare	[30,31]
ERBB4	Gene fusion	Receptor tyrosine kinase	Rare	[24]
FGFR1	Gene fusion	Receptor tyrosine kinase	Rare	[24]
LCK	Gene fusion	Tyrosine kinase	Rare	[9]
MAP2K1	Missense mutation	Serine/Threonine kinase	Rare	[32]
MAP3K3	Gene fusion	Serine/Threonine kinase	Rare	[24]
MERTK	Gene fusion	Receptor tyrosine kinase	Rare	[16]
PRKDC	Gene fusion	Serine/Threonine kinase	Rare	[24]

Histologically, Spitz nevi are symmetrical compound lesions with either a pediculated or elevated silhouette. The junctional component is arranged in nests that are often large, coalescent, and vertically oriented, intermingled with a hyperplastic epidermis, bearing pseudo-epitheliomatous changes. Depending on the histological subtype, cytology can range from small hyperpigmented spindled cells (Reed nevus prototypic morphology) to large epithelioid melanocytes with a glassy eosinophilic cytoplasm (Spitz nevus prototypic morphology), with every intermediate possibility. The dermal component is often of similar cytology with variable deep maturation according to the subtype. A fibrotic background with multiple dilated blood vessel lumens is commonly present in the upper dermis. Dermal mitotic activity is frequent (including atypical mitotic figures) on par with the rapid clinical growth.

In a small subset of cases and at all ages, a progression toward malignant melanoma can occur. Clinically, such lesions become rapidly bulky with heterochromatic melanocytic pigmentation. Histologically, a dermal clone appears, showing severe cytological atypia, increased mitotic activity, higher dermal density, a sheet-like pattern, and destructive extension to the subcutis (Figure 2). Importantly, Breslow thickness and nodal metastases do not carry the same weight in predicting outcome in pediatric Spitzoid neoplasms as in adult conventional melanoma. Indeed, regional nodal extension of a Spitz group neoplasm can commonly be observed without a dismal prognosis [33–35]. The diffuse widespread disease remains exceptional in cases with canonical genetic mutations. Homozygous deletions of *CDKN2A* and *TERT* promoter mutations are the most frequent secondary events observed during this progression [36].

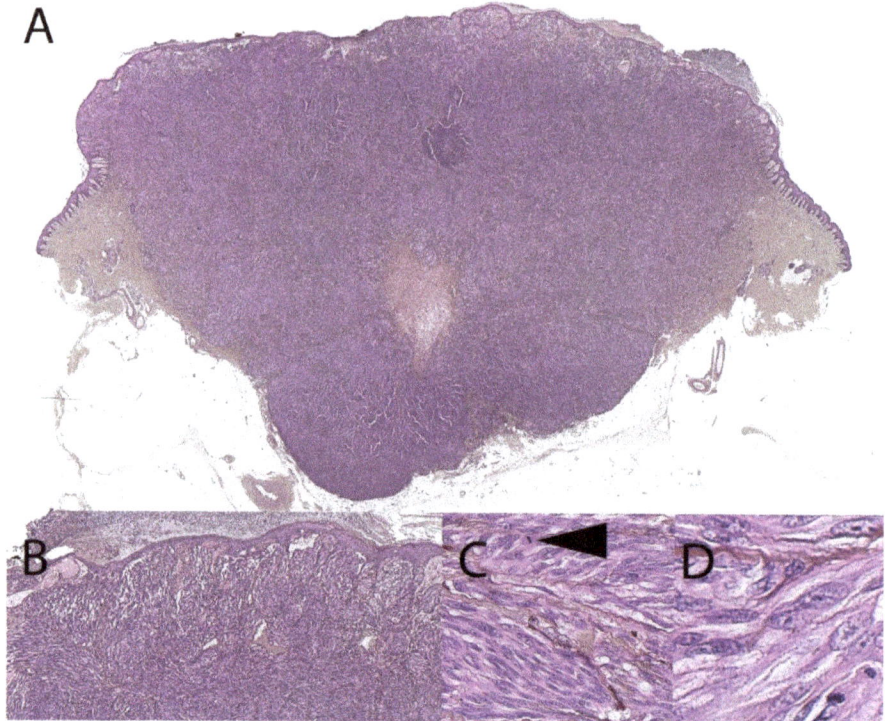

Figure 2. Malignant Spitz tumor, with *MYO5A-RET* fusion, 4-year-old (hematoxylin, phloxin, safranin stain). (**A**): Low-magnification silhouette: massive, sheet-like, destructive dermal expansion elevating the epidermis and invading the subcutis. Central dermal tumoral necrosis patch. (**B**): Close-up view of junction with a thinned epidermis covered by a crust. Obscuration of the grenz zone by dense fascicules. (**C,D**): High-power view of the dermal fascicules made of large spindled atypical melanocytes with mitotic activity (arrow).

The majority of pediatric melanomas arising from such lesions are associated with a good prognosis, even in cases with nodal extension [23]. Recent investigations recommend conservative management for pediatric Spitzoid tumors due to the extremely low associated death rate [33,37]. However, these studies were not always associated with a genetic analysis of the tumors. In the future, the identification of genetic Spitz-driving anomalies for each lesion could reveal itself useful to avoid overdiagnosis in pediatric populations while identifying the tumors the most at risk of a negative outcome. The recent advances in the knowledge of genetic alterations present in this group need to be explored in larger series. Indeed, there appears to be significant morphological overlap in lesions with similar genetic anomalies, including specificities related to the 5′ fusion partners, enhancing the complexity of this group. In our current vision, there could be significantly different outcomes in malignant Spitz tumors with tyrosine kinase fusion (*ALK, ROS1, NTRK1/3*) and serine-threonine fusion (*BRAF, MAP3K8*) with fatal cases published in the latter group only [23,36].

As a side note, the "Spitzoid" terminology is used inconsistently and currently refers to cases with a Spitz-like cytomorphology, i.e., composed of large spindled or epithelioid melanocytes, but for which the specific genetic background linking it to the Spitz group has not been confirmed yet. Previous data have indicated that the Spitzoid histomorphology *per se* is an unreliable predictor of Spitz lineage, also encompassing *BRAF* or *NRAS*-mutated melanoma [38]. In other words, it means uncertainty about whether the prognosis will be good (*bona fide* Spitz, with tyrosine kinase fusion), or conversely, the evolution could be more aggressive and eventually lethal (*BRAF* or *NRAS* melanoma) (Figure 3). However, this morphological uncertainty has been dramatically reduced by various ancillary techniques aiming to reveal their genetic backgrounds, such as immunohistochemistry, FISH, and sequencing techniques (Table 1).

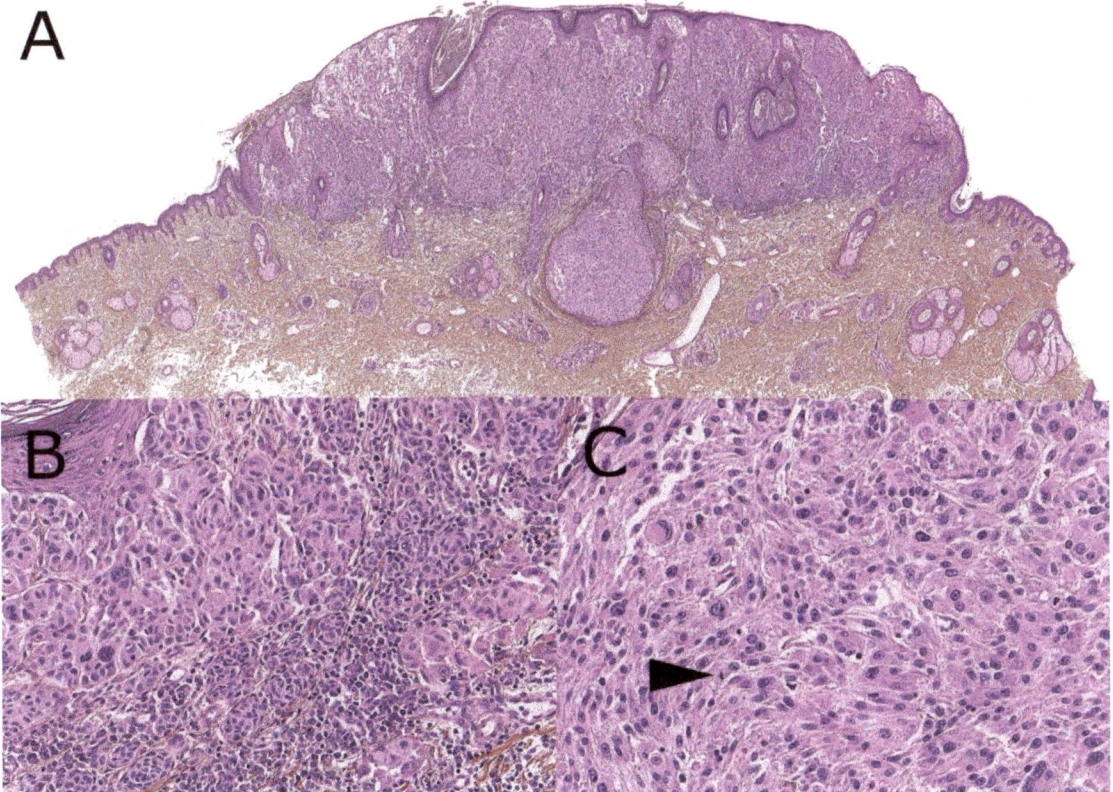

Figure 3. Spitzoid melanoma, 9-year-old (hematoxylin, phloxin, safranin stain). (**A**): Low-magnification silhouette: mainly dermal clonal proliferation, without pigmentation, elevating a slightly verrucous epidermis. Central vertical periadnexial expansion. (**B**): Confluent nests are present in the junction. Abrupt cytological hiatus and lymphocytes are seen in the dermis below. (**C**): Close-up view of the dermal component with spindled and epithelioid large melanocytes with mitotic figure (arrow).

4. Melanoma Arising from a Congenital Nevus

Congenital melanocytic nevi (CMNi) are benign melanocytic tumors that can be present at birth or become apparent in early childhood. The size of these nevi ranges from a few millimeters to whole body segments. Genetic events occurring in melanoblasts or their immediate progenitors can explain the development of such lesions.

During embryogenesis, highly multipotent cells undergo a complex selective triage leading to the formation of a variety of cell lineages in the transient neural crest. Among these, melanoblasts later colonize the epidermis in which they become melanocytes, following earlier dorsal and later ventral migration schemes. Therefore, a single, multipotent neural crest stem cell bearing a somatic mutation can differentiate into a melanoblast-competent progenitor that, after population expansion and dissemination along peripheral nerves, will cause the formation of CMNi at the periphery. Due to the potentially early nature of this developmental anomaly, the resulting nevus may involve up to the whole thickness of the skin, but also the central nervous system (CNS). The risk of nevus deposits in leptomeninges increases when multiple lesions are observed in a newborn, a phenomenon sometimes called nevus satellitosis or neurocutaneous melanocytosis (NCM), but these are, in fact, simply disseminated nevi of identical genetic makeup to the largest CMN [39].

Activating missense mutations of *NRAS* (predominantly *NRAS* Q61K/L/R) are the most frequent genetic alterations associated with CMNi, found in 60% to 80% of the largest lesions [40,41]. Other anomalies such as the V600E mutation of *BRAF* and rarer gene rearrangements (*ZEB2-ALK, SOX5-RAF1, SAA6-RAF1,* and *BRAF*) have also been described [41–43].

Nonetheless, despite affecting the phenotype of the lesion, these alterations are not predictive of patient outcome [41]. Rather than genotype, the number of satellites (disseminated lesions) and the projected adult size (PAS) of the largest tumor are both linked to the risk of developing melanoma [44]. Therefore, small, solitary congenital nevi carry a lower risk of transformation than larger and multiple lesions. It is estimated that 1% of children worldwide are born with a visible nevus, but only 1/20,000 births will have a nevus over 10 cm, and as few as 1/500,000 births will have a nevus over 40 cm in PAS [45].

Both cutaneous and CNS sites can potentially give rise to melanomas in early childhood. The risk of transformation is most important in the first few years [46–48], but remains present throughout the whole patient's life, with a lifetime risk of transformation estimated at up to 5% [49], thus requiring patient education about clinical and auto-evaluation methods on a regular basis.

Melanoma can develop from epidermal or dermal melanocytes of CMNi through lateral or deep nodular transformation, respectively.

The most frequent is lateral transformation, which is fully reminiscent of a superficial spreading melanoma (SSM) *ex*-nevus (as described above). Such melanoma is virtually absent before puberty, except in patients with *xeroderma pigmentosum* (see below). Its low-magnification silhouette is typically asymmetrical: on one side of the nevus, an intraepidermal melanoma arises, first extending superficially, increasing the surface of the lesion in an asymmetrical and variably pigmented clinical pattern. Secondly, the proliferation will invade the dermis during the vertical phase. The prognosis of such melanoma parallels the prognosis of adult-type SSMs of identical Breslow thickness. Early recognition by regular skin screening is the most preventive method (Figure 4).

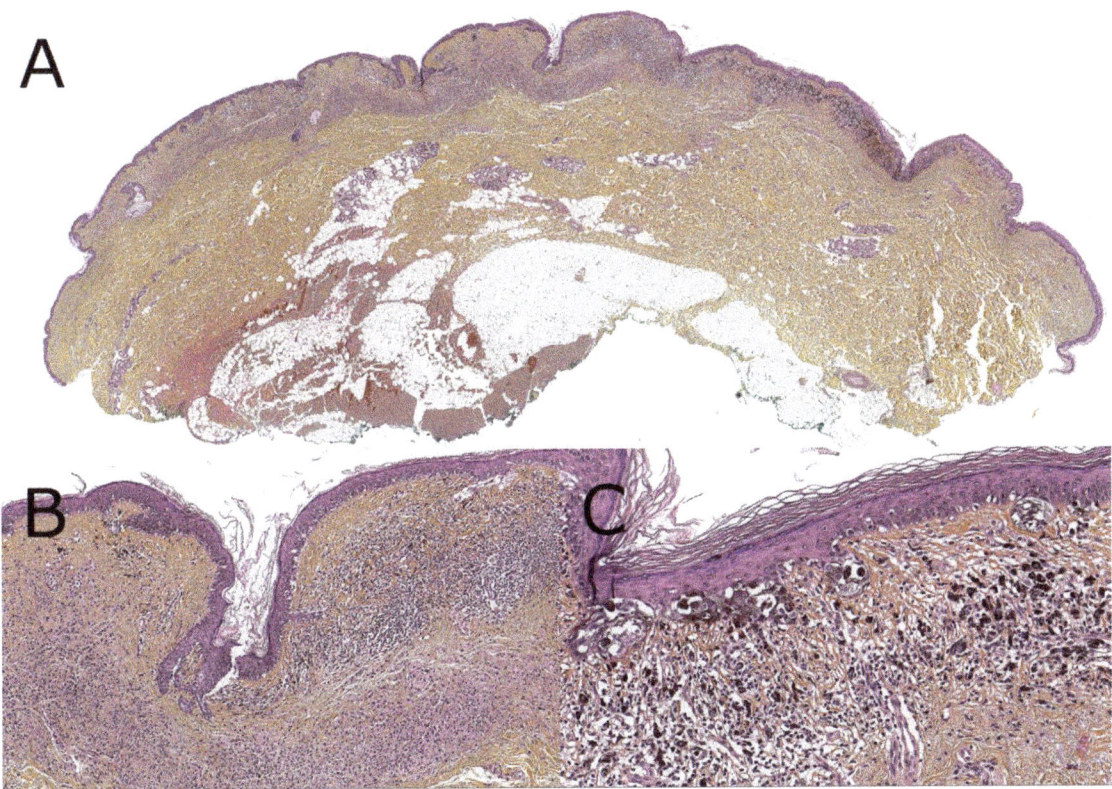

Figure 4. Superficial spreading melanoma ex-congenital nevus, 13-year-old (hematoxylin, phloxin, safranin stain). (**A**): Low-magnification silhouette: asymmetrical lesion with on the left side a compound, mainly dermal, congenital nevus with a loose horizontal band of melanocytes under a slightly verrucous epidermis, and on the right side a mainly junctional melanocytic proliferation underlined by a pigmented inflammatory reaction. (**B**): Close-up view on the transition between the nevus and melanoma. (**C**): Close-up view disorganized confluent junctional nests of large spindled hyperpigmented melanocytes in a slightly atrophic epidermis with numerous.

Deep nodular transformation can occur before puberty and is much rarer. Nodular transformation must be distinguished from benign proliferative nodules, which are more frequent. Indeed, rapidly growing, variably pigmented, and often multiple nodules can arise from giant CMNi during childhood before either stabilizing or becoming malignant. Nodular transformation usually shows higher mitotic activity and ulceration [48]. Moreover, melanoma and proliferative nodules seem to harbor different DNA-methylation patterns, suggesting a role for these studies in the differential diagnosis of such tumors [44]. In this context, epigenetic loss of H3K27me3 or 5-hmC expression, detected by immunohistochemistry, suggests a melanoma rather than a benign proliferative nodule [50–52]. Array-CGH can also be used to discriminate melanoma and proliferative nodules [53,54]. On prognostic grounds, the metastatic potential is greater in these melanomas, with a dismal prognosis and high mortality [50,55] (Figure 5).

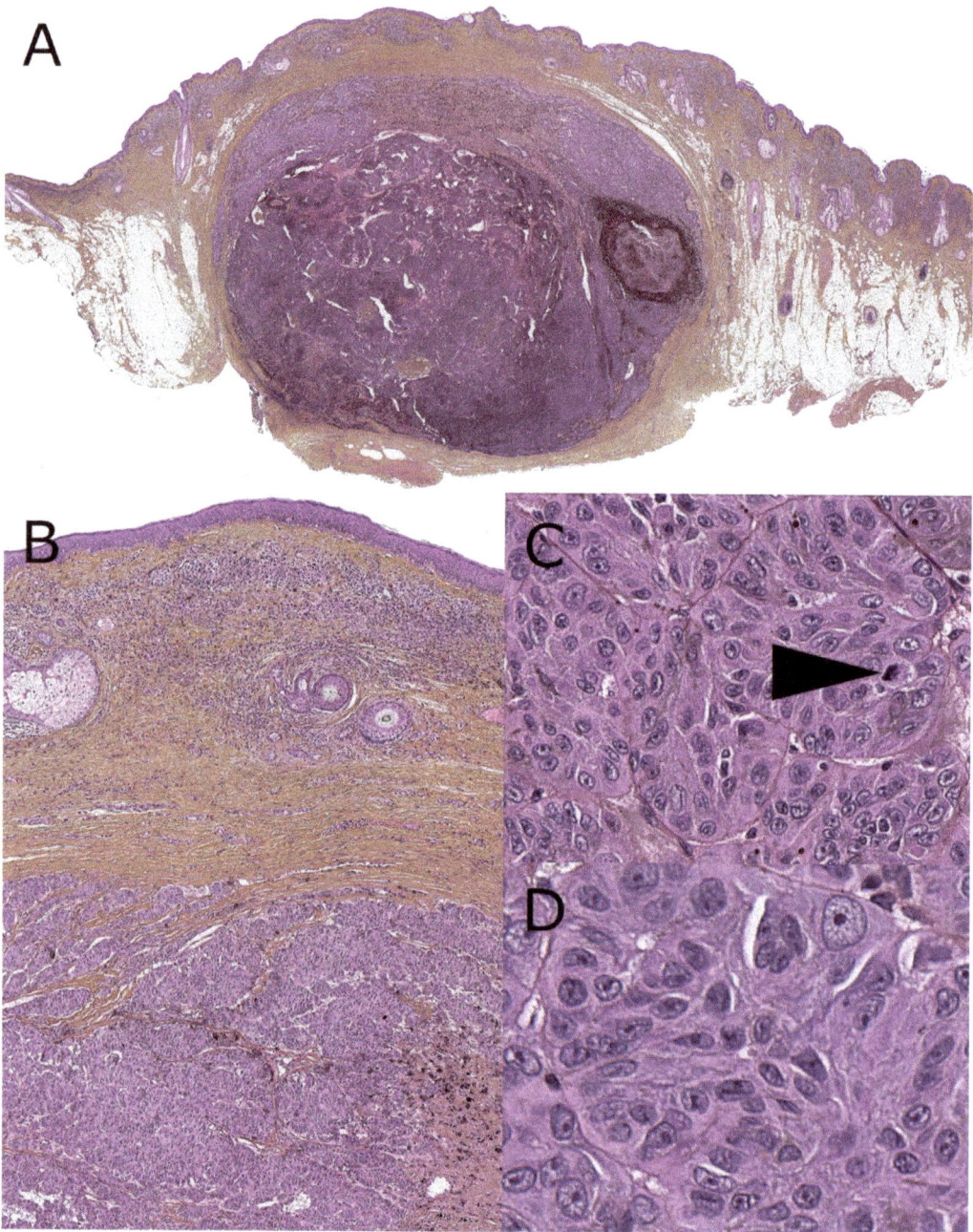

Figure 5. Melanoma ex-giant congenital nevus, 8-year-old (hematoxylin, phloxin, safranin stain). (**A**): Low-magnification silhouette: loose horizontal band of melanocytes under a verrucous epidermis elevated by a large cellular dermal nodule with hyperpigmented areas and patch of tumoral necrosis. (**B**): Close-up view on transition area with the congenital nevus made of loose bland melanocytes in the upper dermis separated by fibrous collagen from the dense nests of the melanoma underneath. (**C**,**D**): High-power view of the melanoma with confluent nests of large epithelioid and nevoid melanocytes; mitotic figure (arrow).

Malignant transformation can also occur in the leptomeningeal CNS nevus deposits of NCM. They are usually detected at an advanced stage when neurological symptoms are triggered by tumor compression of adjacent structures and can be associated with hydrocephalus. At such stages of development, these melanomas are most often unresectable with a rapidly fatal outcome, and can disseminate through ventriculo-peritoneal shunts placed to treat the intracranial pressure [56–58]. However, CNS melanoma in a child with a large or giant CMN is not always fatal, and can develop in the presence of other brain malformations [59]. In evolved lesions, the presence of pigmented spindled and/or epithelioid cells in the cytology of cerebrospinal fluid is diagnostic [60].

5. Nevoid Melanomas

Nevoid melanoma is rare and difficult to diagnose clinically as it usually grows slowly, simulating an exophytic, verrucous, warty nevus. Nevoid melanoma can, however, reach large clinical sizes. Histologically, nevoid melanoma constitutes an important diagnostic pitfall as it mimics a benign compound nevus, especially at low power. Indeed, nevoid melanoma provides the most important share of false-negative diagnoses of malignancy. A high density of melanocytes, an asymmetrical distribution of melanocytes, a perivascular and horizontal dermal extension that extends beyond the limit of the epidermal component are all suggestive of nevoid melanoma. Mitotic activity and Ki67 staining are frequently limited to the upper dermis. The immunophenotype is usually aberrant regarding the expression of Melan-A, HMB45, and p16. Nevoid melanoma mostly arises in adults, but it can also be observed in late adolescence (Figure 6). Their prognosis is currently not very well ascertained [61–64].

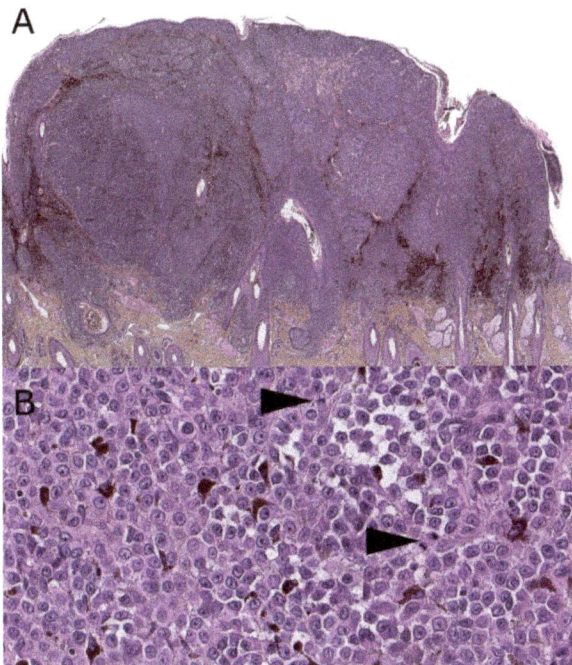

Figure 6. Nevoid melanoma, 17-year-old (hematoxylin, phloxin, safranin stain). (**A**): Low-magnification silhouette: massive dermal invasion by a pigmented clonal proliferation with the destruction of hair follicles. The grenz zone is obscured, and the epidermis is elevated. (**B**): Close-up view displaying sheets of large epithelioid melanocytes with mitotic figures (arrows) and dispersed melanophages.

6. Melanomas Arising in the Setting of a Germline Predisposition Syndrome

A personal or familial history of previous melanoma is present in less than 10% of melanoma cases. Oncogenetic studies have identified several germline mutations that predispose to melanoma, even during childhood. Anomalies that only predispose adults to melanoma will, however, not be discussed.

Germline mutations in *CDKN2A* (encoding for the p16ink and p14arf proteins) are the most frequently (38%) found anomalies [65,66]. *CDKN2A* mutations are responsible for dysplastic nevus syndrome (OMIM #155601) in patients presenting a clinically large number of atypical nevi. In this setting, the risk of developing melanoma nears 100% during the person's lifetime. This justifies recommending solar exposition avoidance as much as possible and skin surveillance starting at age 10. These melanomas occur mainly after puberty, as superficial spreading melanomas (SSM) arising from a preexisting compound nevus. This anomaly also predisposes to pancreatic adenocarcinoma, glioblastomas, sarcomas, and head and neck squamous cell carcinomas, but these arise in adults [67]. *CDK4* germline mutations are much less frequent and give rise to a similar clinical phenotype (multiple nevi with melanoma risk).

The terminology *xeroderma pigmentosum* encompasses a significant number of germline mutations impairing cellular DNA-repair functions to various degrees. In the most severe forms, children, who are exposed to sunlight, develop predominantly multiple basal cell and spindle cell skin carcinomas but also melanomas related both to chronic (*lentigo maligna* melanoma) and non-chronic sun exposure (SSM-type melanoma).

The germline mutations of *BAP1* predispose to multiple cancers, including cutaneous and uveal melanomas. Most of these occur in adults. Carriers frequently develop benign BAP1-inactivated melanocytic nevi during childhood, which often helps identify the disease. Immunohistochemical studies can easily assess a loss of nuclear BAP1 expression. Exceptional transformations of such lesions can occur, including during childhood. The presence of a dense, possibly pigmented, clonal sheet-like area within a BAP1-inactivated nevus is evocative of this diagnosis (Figure 7).

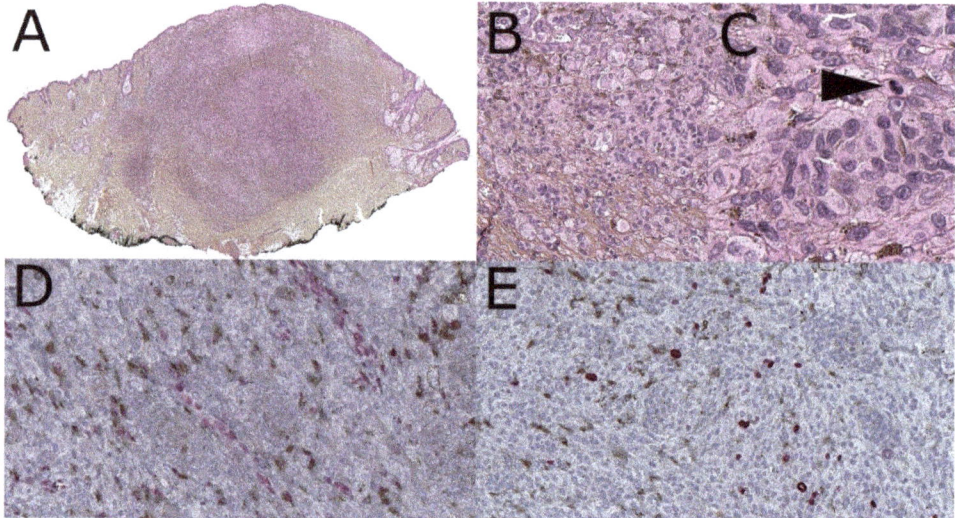

Figure 7. Melanoma *ex* BAP1 inactivated nevus; relapse, initial lesion at age 11(hematoxylin, phloxin, safranin stain). (**A**): Low-magnification silhouette: compound melanocytic proliferation with dense dermal nodular areas including pigmented clones. (**B**): Intermediate view of a cellular area with admixed small and large cells. (**C**): Close-up view of a deep dermal nodule with mixed small nevocytoid and large epithelioid melanocytes. A few of them show a pigmented cytoplasm; mitotic figure (arrow). (**D**): BAP1 immunohistochemistry (clone C4; 1/50): loss of nuclear staining with positive controls of endothelial cells. (**E**): Ki67 immunohistochemistry: variable dermal staining with clonal areas showing a 10% positivity.

Exceptional cases of melanomas and atypical melanocytic tumors have been described in children in the setting of a Li-Fraumeni syndrome (*TP53* mutation) [68,69].

7. Unclassified Melanomas

Despite the expansion of the histological and molecular classification of melanocytic tumors, some pediatric lesions do not fit in any of the categories due to their intradermal origin or as the consequence of undescribed clinical or genetic features. Such cases must be thoroughly explored on molecular grounds and clinically monitored. Research data are currently lacking in this field.

8. Melanoma Risk in Children with Impaired Immunity

It is now well known that immunosuppression, whatever the cause, is a risk factor for melanoma. Several studies have assessed the risk of developing melanoma in patients receiving immunomodulating drugs following organ or bone marrow transplantation. A case was recently reported where malignant leptomeningeal melanoma developed in an adolescent with CMNi, asymptomatic NCM and inflammatory bowel disease, following treatment with TNFα inhibitors [70]. Most such melanomas arise in adults, but skin and neurological surveillance is advised early on in this setting [71,72].

9. Conclusions

Numerous recent genetic discoveries and the WHO classification of skin tumors have restructured our vision of melanocytic tumors. Given the low frequency of pediatric melanoma, it may take some time for genetically well-characterized cohorts to be followed up and published. Nonetheless, this should encourage all teams involved in such rare cases to collaborate and work further to assess the presence of specific genetic markers that will ensure later more precise diagnosis, treatment, and follow-up.

Author Contributions: Writing—original draft preparation, A.d.l.F., F.B., N.M.; writing—review and editing, A.d.l.F., F.B., H.C.E., N.M. All authors have read and agreed to the published version of the manuscript.

Funding: This research received no external funding.

Institutional Review Board Statement: Not applicable.

Informed Consent Statement: Not applicable.

Conflicts of Interest: All authors declare no conflict of interest to disclose.

References

1. Gamble, R.G.; Asdigian, N.L.; Aalborg, J.; Gonzalez, V.; Box, N.F.; Huff, L.S.; Barón, A.E.; Morelli, J.G.; Mokrohisky, S.T.; Crane, L.A.; et al. Sun damage in ultraviolet photographs correlates with phenotypic melanoma risk factors in 12-year-old children. *J. Am. Acad. Dermatol.* **2012**, *67*, 587–597. [CrossRef]
2. Duffy, D.L.; Lee, K.J.; Jagirdar, K.; Pflugfelder, A.; Stark, M.S.; McMeniman, E.K.; Soyer, H.P.; Sturm, R.A. High naevus count and MC1R red hair alleles contribute synergistically to increased melanoma risk. *Br. J. Dermatol.* **2019**, *181*, 1009–1116. [CrossRef] [PubMed]
3. Tannous, Z.S.; Mihm, M.C.; Sober, A.J.; Duncan, L.M. Congenital melanocytic nevi: Clinical and histopathologic features, risk of melanoma, and clinical management. *J. Am. Acad. Dermatol.* **2005**, *52*, 197–203. [CrossRef]
4. Shain, A.H.; Yeh, I.; Kovalyshyn, I.; Sriharan, A.; Talevich, E.; Gagnon, A.; Dummer, R.; North, J.; Pincus, L.; Ruben, B.; et al. The Genetic Evolution of Melanoma from Precursor Lesions. *N. Engl. J. Med.* **2015**, *373*, 1926–1936. [CrossRef]
5. Elder, D.E.; Massi, D.; Scolyer, R.A.; Willemze, R. *WHO Classification of Skin Tumours*; International Agency for Research on Cancer: Lyon, France, 2018.
6. Pappo, A.S.; McPherson, V.; Pan, H.; Wang, F.; Wang, L.; Wright, T.; Hussong, M.; Hawkins, D.; Kaste, S.C.; Davidoff, A.M.; et al. A prospective, comprehensive registry that integrates the molecular analysis of pediatric and adolescent melanocytic lesions. *Cancer* **2021**. [CrossRef]
7. Seynnaeve, B.; Lee, S.; Borah, S.; Park, Y.; Pappo, A.; Kirkwood, J.M.; Bahrami, A. Genetic and Epigenetic Alterations of TERT Are Associated with Inferior Outcome in Adolescent and Young Adult Patients with Melanoma. *Sci. Rep.* **2017**, *7*, 45704. [CrossRef] [PubMed]

8. Bahrami, A.; Barnhill, R.L. Pathology and genomics of pediatric melanoma: A critical reexamination and new insights. *Pediatr. Blood Cancer* **2018**, *65*, e26792. [CrossRef]
9. Goto, K.; Pissaloux, D.; Durand, L.; Tirode, F.; Guillot, B.; de la Fouchardière, A. Novel three-way complex rearrangement of TRPM1-PUM1-LCK in a case of agminated Spitz nevi arising in a giant congenital hyperpigmented macule. *Pigment. Cell Melanoma Res.* **2020**, *33*, 767–772. [CrossRef] [PubMed]
10. Wiesner, T.; He, J.; Yelensky, R.; Esteve-Puig, R.; Botton, T.; Yeh, I.; Lipson, D.; Otto, G.; Brennan, K.; Murali, R.; et al. Kinase fusions are frequent in Spitz tumours and spitzoid melanomas. *Nat. Commun.* **2014**, *5*, 3116. [CrossRef] [PubMed]
11. Yeh, I.; Busam, K.J.; McCalmont, T.H.; LeBoit, P.E.; Pissaloux, D.; Alberti, L.; de la Fouchardière, A.; Bastian, B.C. Filigree-like Rete Ridges, Lobulated Nests, Rosette-like Structures, and Exaggerated Maturation Characterize Spitz Tumors With NTRK1 Fusion. *Am. J. Surg. Pathol.* **2019**, *43*, 737–746. [CrossRef]
12. Amin, S.M.; Haugh, A.M.; Lee, C.Y.; Zhang, B.; Bubley, J.A.; Merkel, E.A.; Verzì, A.E.; Gerami, P. A Comparison of Morphologic and Molecular Features of BRAF, ALK, and NTRK1 Fusion Spitzoid Neoplasms. *Am. J. Surg. Pathol.* **2017**, *41*, 491–498. [CrossRef]
13. Bastian, B.C.; LeBoit, P.E.; Pinkel, D. Mutations and copy number increase of HRAS in Spitz nevi with distinctive histopathological features. *Am. J. Pathol.* **2000**, *157*, 967–972. [CrossRef]
14. Donati, M.; Kastnerova, L.; Martinek, P.; Grossmann, P.; Sticová, E.; Hadravský, L.; Torday, T.; Kyclova, J.; Michal, M.; Kazakov, D.V. Spitz Tumors With ROS1 Fusions: A Clinicopathological Study of 6 Cases, Including FISH for Chromosomal Copy Number Alterations and Mutation Analysis Using Next-Generation Sequencing. *Am. J. Dermatopathol.* **2020**, *42*, 92–102. [CrossRef]
15. Gerami, P.; Kim, D.; Compres, E.V.; Zhang, B.; Khan, A.U.; Sunshine, J.C.; Quan, V.L.; Busam, K. Clinical, morphologic, and genomic findings in ROS1 fusion Spitz neoplasms. *Mod. Pathol.* **2021**, *34*, 348–357. [CrossRef] [PubMed]
16. Goto, K.; Pissaloux, D.; Kauer, F.; Huriet, V.; Tirode, F.; de la Fouchardière, A. GOPC-ROS1 mosaicism in agminated Spitz naevi: Report of two cases. *Virchows Arch.* **2021**. [CrossRef]
17. Wiesner, T.; Murali, R.; Fried, I.; Cerroni, L.; Busam, K.; Kutzner, H.; Bastian, B.C. A distinct subset of atypical Spitz tumors is characterized by BRAF mutation and loss of BAP1 expression. *Am. J. Surg. Pathol.* **2012**, *36*, 818–830. [CrossRef]
18. Yeh, I.; de la Fouchardiere, A.; Pissaloux, D.; Mully, T.W.; Garrido, M.C.; Vemula, S.S.; Busam, K.J.; LeBoit, P.E.; McCalmont, T.H.; Bastian, B.C. Clinical, histopathologic, and genomic features of Spitz tumors with ALK fusions. *Am. J. Surg. Pathol.* **2015**, *39*, 581–591. [CrossRef] [PubMed]
19. Kastnerova, L.; Martinek, P.; Grossmann, P.; Steiner, P.; Vanecek, T.; Kyclova, J.; Ferak, I.; Zalud, R.; Slehobr, O.; Svajdler, P.; et al. A Clinicopathological Study of 29 Spitzoid Melanocytic Lesions With ALK Fusions, Including Novel Fusion Variants, Accompanied by Fluorescence In Situ Hybridization Analysis for Chromosomal Copy Number Changes, and Both TERT Promoter and Next-Generation Sequencing Mutation Analysis. *Am. J. Dermatopathol.* **2020**, *42*, 578–592.
20. De la Fouchardière, A.; Tee, M.K.; Peternel, S.; Valdebran, M.; Pissaloux, D.; Tirode, F.; Busam, K.J.; LeBoit, P.E.; McCalmont, T.H.; Bastian, B.C.; et al. Fusion partners of NTRK3 affect subcellular localization of the fusion kinase and cytomorphology of melanocytes. *Mod. Pathol.* **2021**, *34*, 735–747. [CrossRef]
21. Yeh, I.; Tee, M.K.; Botton, T.; Shain, A.H.; Sparatta, A.J.; Gagnon, A.; Vemula, S.S.; Garrido, M.C.; Nakamaru, K.; Isoyama, T.; et al. NTRK3 kinase fusions in Spitz tumours. *J. Pathol.* **2016**, *240*, 282–290. [CrossRef] [PubMed]
22. Goto, K.; Pissaloux, D.; Tirode, F.; de la Fouchardière, A. Spitz nevus with a novel TFG-NTRK2 fusion: The first case report of NTRK2-rearranged Spitz/Reed nevus. *J. Cutan. Pathol.* **2021**. [CrossRef] [PubMed]
23. Newman, S.; Pappo, A.; Raimondi, S.; Zhang, J.; Barnhill, R.; Bahrami, A. Pathologic Characteristics of Spitz Melanoma With MAP3K8 Fusion or Truncation in a Pediatric Cohort. *Am. J. Surg. Pathol.* **2019**, *43*, 1631–1637. [CrossRef] [PubMed]
24. Quan, V.L.; Zhang, B.; Zhang, Y.; Mohan, L.S.; Shi, K.; Wagner, A.; Kruse, L.; Taxter, T.; Beaubier, N.; White, K.; et al. Integrating Next Generation Sequencing with Morphology Improves Prognostic and Biologic Classification of Spitz Neoplasms. *J. Investig. Dermatol.* **2020**, *140*, 1599–1608. [CrossRef]
25. Quan, V.L.; Zhang, B.; Mohan, L.S.; Shi, K.; Isales, M.C.; Panah, E.; Taxter, T.J.; Bealubier, N.; White, K.; Gerami, P. Activating Structural Alterations in MAPK Genes Are Distinct Genetic Drivers in a Unique Subgroup of Spitzoid Neoplasms. *Am. J. Surg. Pathol.* **2019**, *43*, 538–548. [CrossRef]
26. Houlier, A.; Pissaloux, D.; Masse, I.; Tirode, F.; Karanian, M.; Pincus, L.B.; McCalmont, T.H.; LeBoit, P.E.; Bastian, B.C.; Yeh, I.; et al. Melanocytic tumors with MAP3K8 fusions: Report of 33 cases with morphological-genetic correlations. *Mod. Pathol.* **2020**, *33*, 846–857. [CrossRef]
27. Donati, M.; Kastnerova, L.; Ptakova, N.; Michal, M.; Kazakov, D.V. Polypoid Atypical Spitz Tumor With a Fibrosclerotic Stroma, CLIP2-BRAF Fusion, and Homozygous Loss of 9p21. *Am. J. Dermatopathol.* **2020**, *42*, 204–207. [CrossRef] [PubMed]
28. Perron, E.; Pissaloux, D.; Neub, A.; Hohl, D.; Tartar, M.D.; Mortier, L.; Alberti, L.; de la Fouchardière, A. Unclassified sclerosing malignant melanomas with AKAP9-BRAF gene fusion: A report of two cases and review of BRAF fusions in melanocytic tumors. *Virchows Arch.* **2018**, *472*, 469–476. [CrossRef]
29. Wu, G.; Barnhill, R.L.; Lee, S.; Li, Y.; Shao, Y.; Easton, J.; Dalton, J.; Zhang, J.; Pappo, A.; Bahrami, A. The landscape of fusion transcripts in spitzoid melanoma and biologically indeterminate spitzoid tumors by RNA sequencing. *Mod. Pathol.* **2016**, *29*, 359–369. [CrossRef]
30. VandenBoom, T.; Quan, V.L.; Zhang, B.; Garfield, E.M.; Kong, B.Y.; Isales, M.C.; Panah, E.; Igartua, C.; Taxter, T.; Beaubier, N.; et al. Genomic Fusions in Pigmented Spindle Cell Nevus of Reed. *Am. J. Surg. Pathol.* **2018**, *42*, 1042–1051. [CrossRef]

31. Yeh, I.; Botton, T.; Talevich, E.; Shain, A.H.; Sparatta, A.J.; de la Fouchardiere, A.; Mully, T.W.; North, J.P.; Garrido, M.C.; Gagnon, A.; et al. Activating MET kinase rearrangements in melanoma and Spitz tumours. *Nat. Commun.* **2015**, *6*, 7174. [CrossRef] [PubMed]
32. Donati, M.; Nosek, D.; Waldenbäck, P.; Martinek, P.; Jonsson, B.A.; Galgonkova, P.; Hawawrehova, M.; Berouskova, P.; Kastnerova, L.; Persichetti, P.; et al. MAP2K1-Mutated Melanocytic Neoplasms With a SPARK-Like Morphology. *Am. J. Dermatopathol.* **2021**, *43*, 412–417. [CrossRef] [PubMed]
33. Bartenstein, D.W.; Fisher, J.M.; Stamoulis, C.; Weldon, C.; Huang, J.T.; Gellis, S.E.; Liang, M.G.; Schmidt, B.; Hawryluk, E.B.; Bartenstein, D.W.; et al. Clinical features and outcomes of spitzoid proliferations in children and adolescents. *Br. J. Dermatol.* **2019**, *181*, 366–372. [CrossRef] [PubMed]
34. Lallas, A.; Kyrgidis, A.; Ferrara, G.; Kittler, H.; Apalla, Z.; Castagnetti, F.; Longo, C.; Moscarella, E.; Piana, S.; Zalaudek, I.; et al. Atypical Spitz tumours and sentinel lymph node biopsy: A systematic review. *Lancet Oncol.* **2014**, *15*, e178–e183. [CrossRef]
35. Pol-Rodriquez, M.; Lee, S.; Silvers, D.N.; Celebi, J.T. Influence of age on survival in childhood spitzoid melanomas. *Cancer* **2007**, *109*, 1579–1583. [CrossRef]
36. Lee, S.; Barnhill, R.L.; Dummer, R.; Dalton, J.; Wu, J.; Pappo, A.; Bahrami, A. TERT Promoter Mutations Are Predictive of Aggressive Clinical Behavior in Patients with Spitzoid Melanocytic Neoplasms. *Sci. Rep.* **2015**, *5*, 11200. [CrossRef]
37. Davies, O.M.T.; Majerowski, J.; Segura, A.; Kelley, S.W.; Sokumbi, O.; Humphrey, S.R. A sixteen-year single-center retrospective chart review of Spitz nevi and spitzoid neoplasms in pediatric patients. *Pediatr. Dermatol.* **2020**, *37*, 1073–1082. [CrossRef]
38. Raghavan, S.S.; Peternel, S.; Mully, T.W.; North, J.P.; Pincus, L.B.; LeBoit, P.E.; McCalmont, T.H.; Bastian, B.C.; Yeh, I. Spitz melanoma is a distinct subset of spitzoid melanoma. *Mod. Pathol.* **2020**, *33*, 1122–1134. [CrossRef] [PubMed]
39. Kinsler, V. Satellite lesions in congenital melanocytic nevi—Time for a change of name. *Pediatr. Dermatol.* **2011**, *28*, 212–213. [CrossRef]
40. Kinsler, V.A.; Thomas, A.C.; Ishida, M.; Bulstrode, N.W.; Loughlin, S.; Hing, S.; Chalker, J.; McKenzie, K.; Abu-Amero, S.; Slater, O.; et al. Multiple congenital melanocytic nevi and neurocutaneous melanosis are caused by postzygotic mutations in codon 61 of NRAS. *J. Investig. Dermatol.* **2013**, *133*, 2229–2236. [CrossRef] [PubMed]
41. Polubothu, S.; McGuire, N.; Al-Olabi, L.; Baird, W.; Bulstrode, N.; Chalker, J.; Josifova, D.; Lomas, D.; O'Hara, J.; Ong, J.; et al. Does the gene matter? Genotype-phenotype and genotype-outcome associations in congenital melanocytic naevi. *Br. J. Dermatol.* **2020**, *182*, 434–443. [CrossRef] [PubMed]
42. Martins da Silva, V.; Martinez-Barrios, E.; Tell-Martí, G.; Dabad, M.; Carrera, C.; Aguilera, P.; Brualla, D.; Esteve-Codina, A.; Vicente, A.; Puig, S.; et al. Genetic Abnormalities in Large to Giant Congenital Nevi: Beyond NRAS Mutations. *J. Investig. Dermatol.* **2019**, *139*, 900–908. [CrossRef] [PubMed]
43. Baltres, A.; Salhi, A.; Houlier, A.; Pissaloux, D.; Tirode, F.; Haddad, V.; Karanian, M.; Dahlouk, S.Y.; Boukendakdji, F.; Dahlouk, D.; et al. Malignant melanoma with areas of rhabdomyosarcomatous differentiation arising in a giant congenital nevus with RAF1 gene fusion. *Pigment. Cell Melanoma Res.* **2019**, *32*, 708–713. [CrossRef]
44. Kinsler, V.A.; O'Hare, P.; Bulstrode, N.; Calonje, J.E.; Chong, W.K.; Hargrave, D.; Jacques, T.; Lomas, D.; Sebire, N.; Slater, O. Melanoma in congenital melanocytic naevi. *Br. J. Dermatol.* **2017**, *176*, 1131–1143. [CrossRef]
45. Castilla, E.E.; da Graça Dutra, M.; Orioli-Parreiras, I.M. Epidemiology of congenital pigmented naevi: I. Incidence rates and relative frequencies. *Br. J. Dermatol.* **1981**, *104*, 307–315. [CrossRef] [PubMed]
46. Paradela, S.; Fonseca, E.; Prieto, V.G. Melanoma in children. *Arch. Pathol. Lab. Med.* **2011**, *135*, 307–316. [CrossRef] [PubMed]
47. Vourc'h-Jourdain, M.; Martin, L.; Barbarot, S. Large congenital melanocytic nevi: Therapeutic management and melanoma risk: A systematic review. *J. Am. Acad. Dermatol.* **2013**, *68*, 493–498. [CrossRef]
48. Yélamos, O.; Arva, N.C.; Obregon, R.; Yazdan, P.; Wagner, A.; Guitart, J.; Gerami, P. A comparative study of proliferative nodules and lethal melanomas in congenital nevi from children. *Am. J. Surg. Pathol.* **2015**, *39*, 405–415. [CrossRef]
49. Price, H.N.; Schaffer, J.V. Congenital melanocytic nevi—When to worry and how to treat: Facts and controversies. *Clin. Dermatol.* **2010**, *28*, 293–302. [CrossRef]
50. Busam, K.J.; Shah, K.N.; Gerami, P.; Sitzman, T.; Jungbluth, A.A.; Kinsler, V. Reduced H3K27me3 Expression Is Common in Nodular Melanomas of Childhood Associated With Congenital Melanocytic Nevi But Not in Proliferative Nodules. *Am. J. Surg. Pathol.* **2017**, *41*, 396–404. [CrossRef]
51. Lian, C.G.; Xu, Y.; Ceol, C.; Wu, F.; Larson, A.; Dresser, K.; Xu, W.; Tan, L.; Hu, Y.; Zhan, Q.; et al. Loss of 5-hydroxymethylcytosine is an epigenetic hallmark of melanoma. *Cell* **2012**, *150*, 1135–1146. [CrossRef]
52. Pavlova, O.; Fraitag, S.; Hohl, D. 5-Hydroxymethylcytosine Expression in Proliferative Nodules Arising within Congenital Nevi Allows Differentiation from Malignant Melanoma. *J. Investig. Dermatol.* **2016**, *136*, 2453–2461. [CrossRef]
53. Lacoste, C.; Avril, M.-F.; Frassati-Biaggi, A.; Dupin, N.; Chrétien-Marquet, B.; Mahé, E.; Bodemer, C.; Vergier, B.; Fouchardière, A.; Fraitag, S. Malignant Melanoma Arising in Patients with a Large Congenital Melanocytic Naevus: Retrospective Study of 10 Cases with Cytogenetic Analysis. *Acta Derm. Venereol.* **2015**, *95*, 686–690. [CrossRef]
54. Feito-Rodríguez, M.; de Lucas-Laguna, R.; Bastian, B.C.; Leboit, P.; González-Beato, M.J.; López-Gutiérrez, J.C.; Requena, L.; Pizarro, A. Nodular lesions arising in a large congenital melanocytic naevus in a newborn with eruptive disseminated Spitz naevi. *Br. J. Dermatol.* **2011**, *165*, 1138–1142. [CrossRef]

55. Macagno, N.; Etchevers, H.C.; Malissen, N.; Rome, A.; Hesse, S.; Mallet, S.; Degardin, N.; Gaudy, C. Reduced H3K27me3 Expression is Common in Nodular Melanomas of Childhood Associated With Congenital Melanocytic Nevi But Not in Proliferative Nodules. *Am. J. Surg. Pathol.* **2018**, *42*, 701–704. [CrossRef] [PubMed]
56. Hayes-Jordan, A.; Green, H.; Prieto, V.; Wolff, J.E. Unusual cases: Melanomatosis and nephroblastomatosis treated with hyperthermic intraperitoneal chemotherapy. *J. Pediatr. Surg.* **2012**, *47*, 782–787. [CrossRef]
57. Cajaiba, M.M.; Benjamin, D.; Halaban, R.; Reyes-Múgica, M. Metastatic peritoneal neurocutaneous melanocytosis. *Am. J. Surg. Pathol.* **2008**, *32*, 156–161. [CrossRef]
58. Faillace, W.J.; Okawara, S.H.; McDonald, J.V. Neurocutaneous melanosis with extensive intracerebral and spinal cord involvement. Report of two cases. *J. Neurosurg.* **1984**, *61*, 782–785. [CrossRef] [PubMed]
59. Ramaswamy, V.; Delaney, H.; Haque, S.; Marghoob, A.; Khakoo, Y. Spectrum of central nervous system abnormalities in neurocutaneous melanocytosis. *Dev. Med. Child Neurol.* **2012**, *54*, 563–568. [CrossRef] [PubMed]
60. Reyes-Mugica, M.; Chou, P.; Byrd, S.; Ray, V.; Castelli, M.; Gattuso, P.; Gonzalez-Crussi, F. Nevomelanocytic proliferations in the central nervous system of children. *Cancer* **1993**, *72*, 2277–2285. [CrossRef]
61. Cassarino, D.S.; Fullen, D.R.; Sondak, V.K.; Duray, P.H. Metastatic nevoid melanoma in a 4 1/2-year-old child. *J. Cutan. Pathol.* **2003**, *30*, 647–651. [CrossRef]
62. Knöpfel, N.; Martín-Santiago, A.; Del Pozo, L.J.; Saus, C.; Pascual, M.; Requena, L. Amelanotic naevoid melanoma in a 16-month-old albino infant. *Clin. Exp. Dermatol.* **2017**, *42*, 84–88. [CrossRef]
63. Moyer, A.B.; Diwan, A.H. "Puffy shirt appearance": Cell crowding at low magnification may represent nevoid melanoma. *J. Cutan. Pathol.* **2019**, *46*, 805–809. [CrossRef]
64. Idriss, M.H.; Rizwan, L.; Sferuzza, A.; Wasserman, E.; Kazlouskaya, V.; Elston, D.M. Nevoid melanoma: A study of 43 cases with emphasis on growth pattern. *J. Am. Acad. Dermatol.* **2015**, *73*, 836–842. [CrossRef]
65. Goldstein, A.M.; Chan, M.; Harland, M.; Hayward, N.K.; Demenais, F.; Bishop, D.T.; Azizi, E.; Bergman, W.; Scarrà, G.B.; Bruno, W.; et al. Features associated with germline CDKN2A mutations: A GenoMEL study of melanoma-prone families from three continents. *J. Med. Genet.* **2007**, *44*, 99–106. [CrossRef]
66. Casula, M.; Paliogiannis, P.; Ayala, F.; De Giorgi, V.; Stanganelli, I.; Mandalà, M.; Colombino, M.; Manca, A.; Sini, M.C.; Caracò, C.; et al. Germline and somatic mutations in patients with multiple primary melanomas: A next generation sequencing study. *BMC Cancer* **2019**, *19*, 772. [CrossRef] [PubMed]
67. Jouenne, F.; de Beauchene, I.C.; Bollaert, E.; Avril, M.-F.; Caron, O.; Ingster, O.; Lecesne, A.; Benuisiglio, P.; Terrier, P.; Caumette, V.; et al. Germline CDKN2A/P16INK4A mutations contribute to genetic determinism of sarcoma. *J. Med. Genet.* **2017**, *54*, 607–612. [CrossRef] [PubMed]
68. Kollipara, R.; Cooley, L.D.; Horii, K.A.; Hetherington, M.L.; Leboit, P.E.; Singh, V.; Zwick, D.L. Spitzoid melanoma in a child with Li-Fraumeni syndrome. *Pediatr. Dev. Pathol.* **2014**, *17*, 64–69. [CrossRef]
69. Jacquemus, J.; Perron, E.; Pissaloux, D.; Alberti, L.; de la Fouchardière, A. Atypical cutaneous melanocytic tumours arising in two patients with Li-Fraumeni syndrome. *Pathology* **2017**, *49*, 801–805. [CrossRef]
70. Schaff, L.R.; Marghoob, A.; Rosenblum, M.K.; Meyer, R.; Khakoo, Y. Malignant transformation of neurocutaneous melanosis (NCM) following immunosuppression. *Pediatr. Dermatol.* **2019**, *36*, 497–500. [CrossRef] [PubMed]
71. Berge, L.A.M.; Andreassen, B.K.; Stenehjem, J.S.; Heir, T.; Karlstad, Ø.; Juzeniene, A.; Ghiasvand, R.; Larsen, I.K.; Green, A.C.; Veierød, M.B.; et al. Use of Immunomodulating Drugs and Risk of Cutaneous Melanoma: A Nationwide Nested Case-Control Study. *Clin. Epidemiol.* **2020**, *12*, 1389–1401. [CrossRef] [PubMed]
72. Fattouh, K.; Ducroux, E.; Decullier, E.; Kanitakis, J.; Morelon, E.; Boissonnat, P.; Sebbag, L.; Jullien, D.; Euvrard, S. Increasing incidence of melanoma after solid organ transplantation: A retrospective epidemiological study. *Transpl. Int.* **2017**, *30*, 1172–1180. [CrossRef] [PubMed]

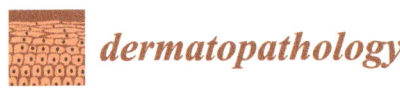

Review

Panniculitis in Children

Isabelle Moulonguet [1,2,*] and Sylvie Fraitag [3]

1. Cabinet de Dermatopathologie Mathurin Moreau, 75019 Paris, France
2. Dermatology Department, Hôpital Saint Louis, 75010 Paris, France
3. Dermatopathology Department, Hospital Necker Enfants-Malades, 75006 Paris, France; sylvie.fraitag@aphp.fr
* Correspondence: imoulonguetmichau@gmail.com

Abstract: Panniculitides form a heterogenous group of inflammatory diseases that involve the subcutaneous adipose tissue. These disorders are rare in children and have many aetiologies. As in adults, the panniculitis can be the primary process in a systemic disorder or a secondary process that results from infection, trauma or exposure to medication. Some types of panniculitis are seen more commonly or exclusively in children, and several new entities have been described in recent years. Most types of panniculitis have the same clinical presentation (regardless of the aetiology), with tender, erythematous subcutaneous nodules. Although the patient's age and the lesion site provide information, a histopathological assessment is sometimes required for a definitive diagnosis and classification of the disorder. In children, most panniculitides are lobular. At present, autoimmune inflammatory diseases and primary immunodeficiencies have been better characterised; panniculitis can be the presenting symptom in some of these settings. Unexplained panniculitis in a young child should prompt a detailed screen for monogenic immune disorders because the latter usually manifest themselves early in life. Here, we review forms of panniculitis that occur primarily in children, with a focus on newly described entities.

Keywords: panniculitis; histopathology; autoinflammatory diseases

1. Introduction

Panniculitides comprise a heterogenous group of inflammatory diseases that involve the subcutaneous adipose tissue. In children, these disorders are rare but can be difficult to diagnose. In the present review, "adult" types of panniculitis that occasionally occur in children will only be cited or just briefly described. Certain subtypes of panniculitis (such as Rothmann-Makai syndrome, Weber-Christian disease, and cytophagic histiocytic panniculitis) are no longer considered to be specific entities. Furthermore, genetic lipodystrophies characterised by the loss of adipose tissue at some body sites will not be described here.

Most types of panniculitis have the same clinical appearance (regardless of the aetiology), with tender, erythematous subcutaneous nodules that occur mostly where fatty tissue is prominent (i.e., on the legs, thighs, buttocks, and cheeks) [1,2]. The histopathologic assessment of panniculitis is often difficult and requires adequate tissue samples—including subcutaneous fat. As non-specific histopathologic findings are common for late panniculitis lesions, it is necessary to sample early lesions [3]. With an appropriate biopsy specimen and an adequate clinical-pathological correlation, a specific diagnosis can be made in most cases of panniculitis [4].

Panniculitis are classified as lobular or septal, depending on where the inflammatory infiltrate is mainly located. However, the lobular or septal pattern is not related to the clinical findings; here, we will use the aetiological classification [4,5]. Most paediatric panniculitides have a lobular pattern (Table 1).

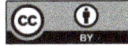

Table 1. The histopathologic classification of lobular panniculitis in children.

No Vasculitis	
When lymphocytes are predominant:	
With superficial and deep perivascular dermal infiltrate	Cold panniculitis
With lymphoid follicles, plasma cells, and lymphocyte nuclear dust	Lupus panniculitis
With lymphocytes and plasma cells	Dermatomyositis
	TRAPS
With small to medium-sized pleomorphic lymphocytes	Cytotoxic T-cell panniculitis
With histiocytes, eosinophils, plasma cells, and neutrophils	Recurrent lipoatrophic panniculitis of children along with variable degrees of lipoatrophy
When neutrophils are predominant:	
With extensive fat necrosis and saponification of adipocytes	Pancreatic panniculitis
With neutrophils between collagen bundles in the deep reticular dermis	Alpha1-antitrypsin deficiency
With bacteria, fungi, or protozoa identified by specific stains	Infective panniculitis
With foreign bodies	Factitial panniculitis
	Panniculitis during vemurafenib treatment
	Familial Mediterranean fever
When mononuclear atypical cells are predominant	
With neutrophils	CANDLE syndrome
When histiocytes are predominant	
Histiocytes with enlarged, amphophilic cytoplasm	Post-vaccination subcutaneous aluminium granuloma
No crystals in adipocytes	Blau syndrome
With crystals in histiocytes or adipocytes	SFN, post-steroid panniculitis
With interstitial monocyte-derived cells and fibrosis in the dermis and hypodermis	H syndrome.
With Vasculitis	
	Deficiency in ADA2
	Otulopenia

2. Specific Paediatric Panniculitides

2.1. Subcutaneous Fat Necrosis of the Newborn (SFN)

SFN is a rare variant of lobular panniculitis that appears in term or post-term newborns during the first days of life. The lesions are characterised clinically by indurated plaques and subcutaneous nodules that are primarily located on the buttocks, shoulders, cheeks, and thighs (Figure 1A). In some cases, the nodules and plaques can ulcerate and exude purulent material [6–8] (Figure 1B). The cause of SFN is unknown, although many cases are associated with perinatal asphyxia and meconium aspiration. The pathogenesis of SFN might be related to a greater saturated/unsaturated fatty acid ratio in the newborn, since saturated fatty acids have a greater tendency to crystallise in adipose tissue. SFN has an excellent prognosis, and spontaneous resolution within several weeks is common. However, delayed-onset hypercalcemia may occur, and so prolonged calcium monitoring is advisable. A biopsy is not always necessary because the clinical diagnosis is often straightforward. However, a biopsy can be useful in clinically misleading cases (such as multinodular cases, in particular) because the histological findings are specific.

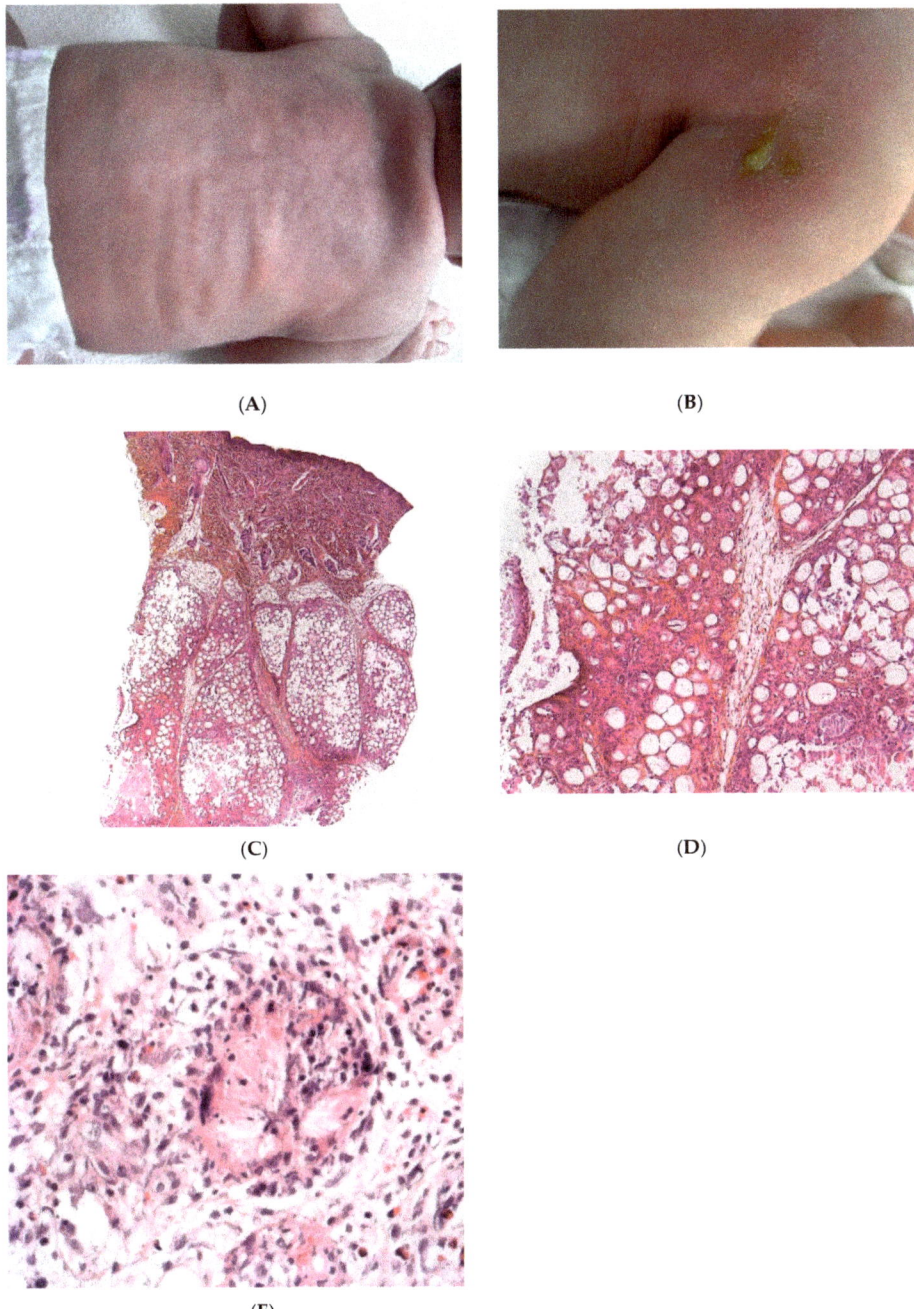

Figure 1. Subcutaneous fat necrosis of the newborn. (**A**) Indurated plaques on the neck and on the back of a newborn. (**B**) Significant purulent material of the shoulder *Photo Dermatology Department Hopital Necker Enfants Malades. Paris France.* (**C**) Lobular panniculitis without involvement of the dermis (original magnification ×20) (**D**) Many adipocytes are replaced by cells with finely eosinophilic granular cytoplasm that contain narrow needle-shaped clefts (original magnification ×100). (**E**) Needle-shaped crystals in radial fashion surrounded by histiocytes (original magnification ×400).

2.1.1. Histopathology

Most cases of SFN show characteristic features and are immediately recognisable as lobular panniculitis with necrosis of the fat lobule. It is a purely panniculitis, and the dermis is never affected. A high proportion of the adipocytes are replaced by cells with a finely eosinophilic, granular cytoplasm that contains radially arranged, narrow, needle-shaped clefts (Figure 1C–E). These clefts are characteristic of SFN and correspond to fatty acid crystals that have dissolved during sample processing. The adiponecrosis is associated with infiltration by inflammatory cells (lymphocytes, lipophages, and multinucleated giant cells), which can also contain these. Eosinophils and neutrophils can also be present. The neutrophil-rich variant of SFN can be difficult to distinguish from an infection [9]. Late-stage lesions can show septal fibrosis and areas of calcification within the fat lobule.

2.1.2. Differential Diagnoses

Intracytoplasmic, needle-shaped fatty acid crystals are quite characteristic of SFN but can be also observed in post-steroid panniculitis and in "sclerema neonatorum" (SN). This very rare disorder manifests itself within a few days of birth in premature newborns, with comorbidities such as congenital heart disease and other major developmental defects [10]. From a histopathologic point of view, it is notorious that, despite striking clinical features, histopathology usually minimal changes. In the subcutaneous fat, the inflammatory infiltrate is sparse or even absent [2]. Given that (i) no new cases of SN have been reported in the last few years and (ii) SFN and SN have clinical and pathological similarities, they are now considered to be variants of the same disease. Hence, SN may be a severe form of SFN that primarily manifests itself in premature newborns [2].

2.2. Post-Steroid Panniculitis

Post-steroid panniculitis is a very rare form of lobular panniculitis that has only been observed in children in whom systemic treatment with high-dose corticosteroids has been suddenly withdrawn. One to ten days after this withdrawal, erythematous subcutaneous nodules measuring 0.5 to 4 cm appear on the cheeks, the arms, or trunk (Figure 2A). The nodules may ulcerate, with scarring. The sudden withdrawal of corticosteroids might cause an increase in the saturated:unsaturated fatty acid ratio, and thus, crystal formation.

Histopathology

The findings are similar to SFN: a mostly lobular panniculitis features an inflammatory infiltrate of foamy histiocytes, with lymphocytes in the fat lobules. Some of the histiocytes show needle-shaped clefts in the cytoplasm (Figure 2B,C). In most cases, the inflammation is less intense and the crystals are less numerous than in SFN [11].

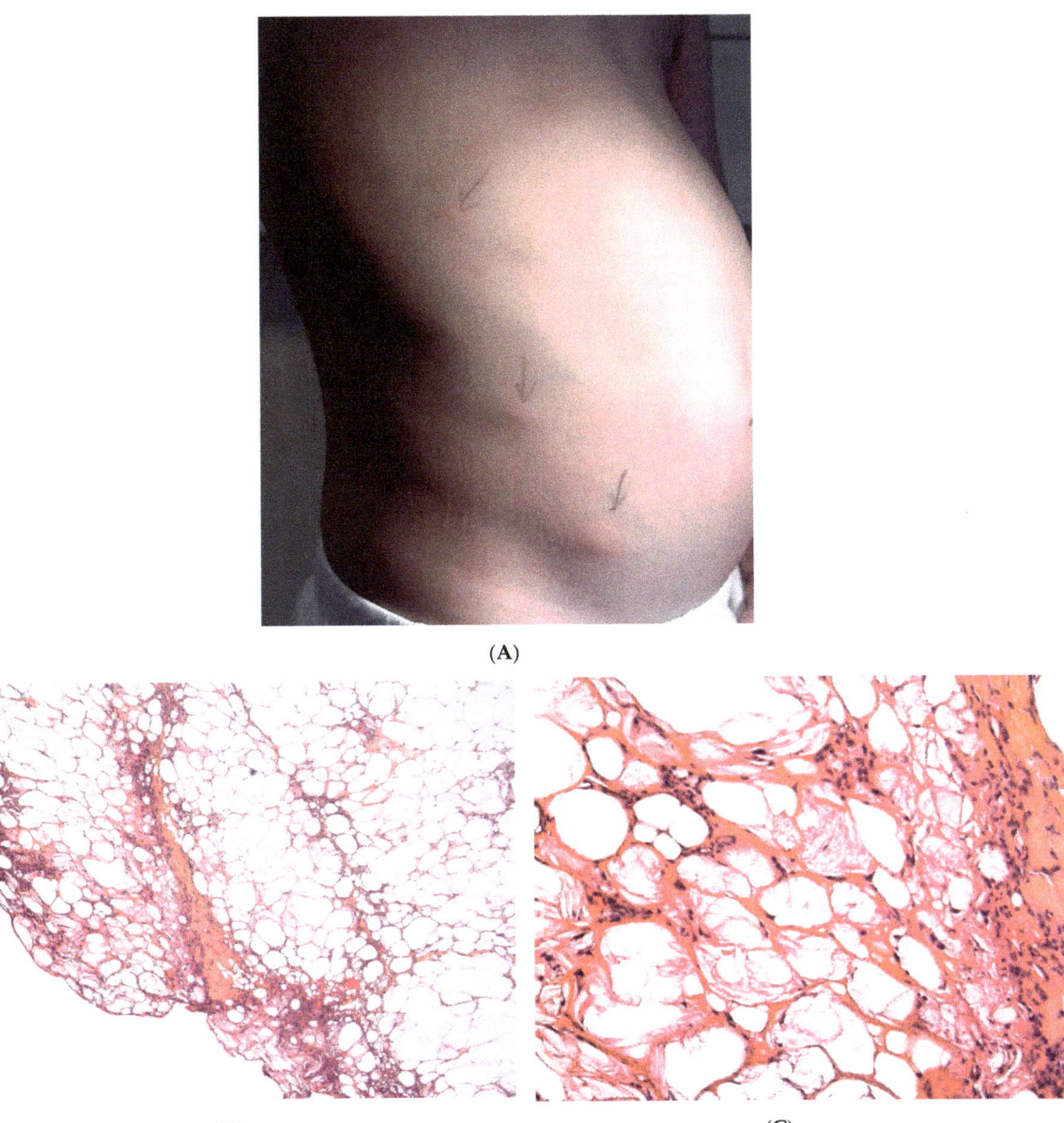

Figure 2. Post-steroid panniculitis. (**A**) Clinical presentation: subcutaneous nodules with overlying erythema. (**B**) Histopathologic features of post-steroid panniculitis: mostly lobular panniculitis with an inflammatory infiltrate of foamy histiocytes involving the fat lobules (original magnification ×40). (**C**) Needle-shaped clefts (original magnification ×400).

2.3. Cold Panniculitis

Cold panniculitis is related to cold exposure. It is more frequent in infants and children than in adults—probably because of age-related differences in fat composition. Cold panniculitis usually affects the cheeks and chin and appear 48 to 72 h after cold exposure. In particular, cold panniculitis is reported in infants after the application of ice bags for the treatment of supraventricular tachycardia [12] and as "popsicle panniculitis" in children sucking ice cubes or popsicles.

The clinic features include firm, indurated erythematous nodules or plaques with ill-defined margins on the cheeks and the submental region. The prognosis is excellent, and the disorder resolves spontaneously over a period of weeks to months. A biopsy is not usually required if the history of a cold exposure is reported. However, distinguishing clearly between SFN and cold panniculitis is difficult in some cases [2]. Given that SFN requires prolonged calcium monitoring, a biopsy may be needed if direct exposure to cold has not been reported.

Histopathology

Cold panniculitis is a mostly lobular form of panniculitis. The infiltrate mostly comprises lymphocytes and histiocytes in the fat lobules. The inflammation can affect both the interlobular septa and lobules, and is most intense at the dermal-subcutaneous junction. The dermis usually shows both superficial and deep perivascular infiltrates composed mostly of lymphocytes, in the absence of vasculitis.

2.4. Autoinflammatory Diseases

Early-onset panniculitis with systemic inflammation had been reported in cases of autoinflammatory diseases with or without an associated immunodeficiency [13,14]. Most cases have variable, non-specific histopathologic features: lobular or septal panniculitis with a mixture of cells or with a predominance of neutrophils or lymphocytes (Figures 3 and 4). However, the histopathologic features can sometimes have diagnostic value, such as the granulomatous infiltrate characteristic of Blau syndrome (BS) or the polyarteritis-nodosa-like vasculitis in deficiency of adenosine deaminase 2 (DADA2). The presence of early-onset panniculitis with systemic inflammation should prompt the physician to screen for autoinflammatory disorders.

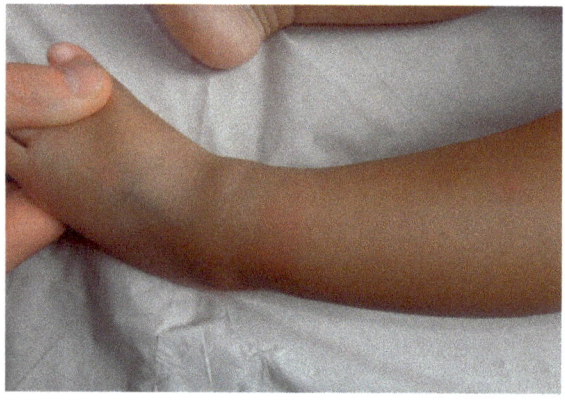
(A)

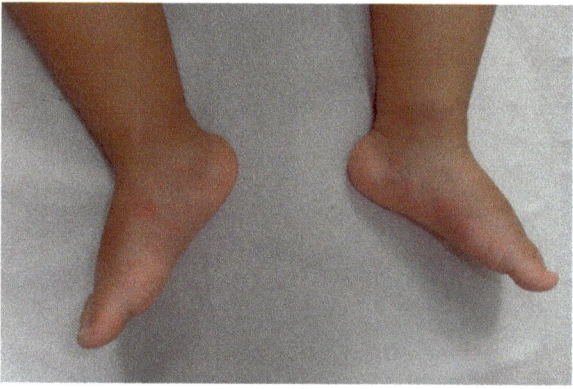
(B)

Figure 3. Cont.

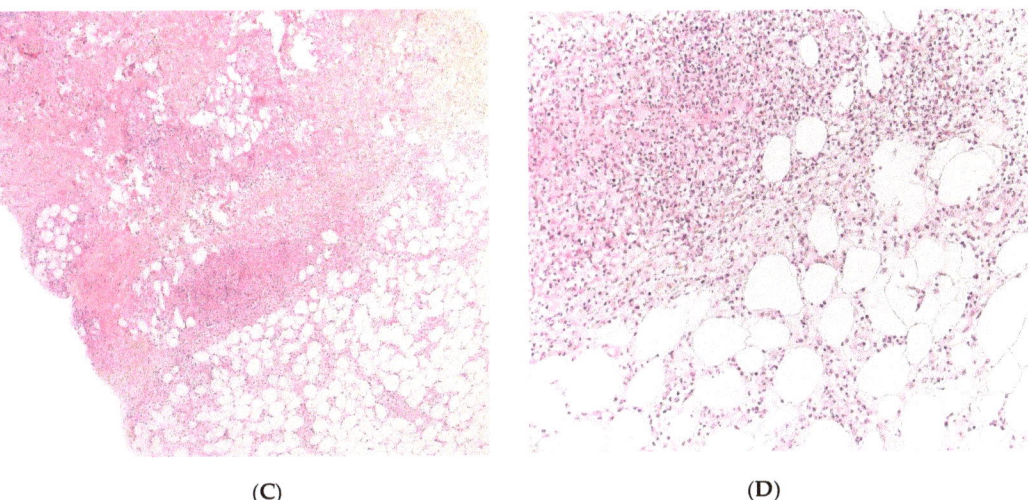

Figure 3. Panniculitis associated with inherited immunodeficiency. (**A,B**) Clinical presentation: Erythematous nodules of the leg of a 20 month-old boy *Photo Dermatology Department Hopital Necker Enfants Malades. Paris France* (**C,D**) Histopathology: inflammation of the deep dermis and the subcutis localised in the septa and the lobules composed of mixed infiltrate. (**C**) Original magnification ×80, (**D**) original magnification ×200.

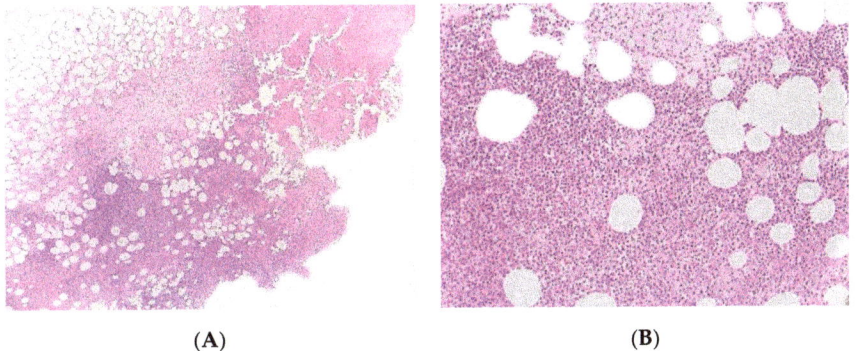

Figure 4. Panniculitis associated with inherited immunodeficiency. (**A**) Lobular panniculitis with dense neutrophilic infiltrate replacing part of the subcutis (original magnification ×80). (**B**) Closer view of showing entrapped adipocytes within the neutrophilic infiltrate (original magnification ×200).

2.4.1. Autoinflammatory Diseases in the Absence of Immunodeficiency
Proteasome-Associated Autoinflammatory Syndromes (PRAAS)

PRAAS (OMIM 256040) are a group of distinct clinical entities that have recently been recognised to share a common molecular cause. They include joint contractures, muscle atrophy, microcytic anemia and panniculitis-induced lipodystrophy syndrome (JMP), Nakajo-Nishimura syndrome (NNS, also referred to as Japanese autoinflammatory syndrome with lipodystrophy, JASL), and chronic atypical neutrophilic dermatosis with lipodystrophy and elevated temperature syndrome (CANDLE). All these syndromes are characterised by the early onset of nodular, pernio-like, violaceous skin lesions with atypical neutrophil infiltrates, muscle atrophy, lipodystrophy, failure to thrive, and deformities of the hands and feet due to joint contractures. Recurrent periodic fever episodes and elevated acute phase reactant levels are usually present [15–17].

Histopathology

CANDLE is not a true panniculitis, since the reticular dermis and the hypodermis are affected and contain a perivascular and interstitial mononuclear inflammatory infiltrate. Many of the mononuclear cells exhibit large, vesicular, irregularly shaped nuclei, and thus, resemble atypical myeloid cells. Scattered mature neutrophils, some mature lymphocytes, and (in some cases) eosinophils are also present. Although leukocytoclasis is often present, there is no vasculitis [18]. Immunohistological studies have indicated that the cutaneous inflammatory infiltrate in CANDLE syndrome is polymorphous; it includes a mixture of immature myeloid cells that are strongly positive for myeloperoxidase, macrophages that are strongly positive for CD68 and CD163, and a moderate number of CD123-positive plasmacytoid dendritic cells.

Familial Mediterranean Fever

Familial Mediterranean fever classically consists of short, recurrent episodes of fever, serositis, arthritis, and erysipelas-like-erythema. The disorder results from mutations in the gene coding for pyrin (also known as marenostrin). Lobular panniculitis has been reported in adults but also in children, where tender, erythematous, bruise-like, warm, irregularly shaped nodules on the limbs and face coincide with the episodes of fever. The skin lesions heal as greyish macules without lipoatrophy. Panniculitis may be the main clinical manifestation, along with periods of fever [19].

Histopathology

Familial Mediterranean fever is a predominantly lobular neutrophilic panniculitis. Neither necrosis nor vasculitis is present [20].

Otulipenia

Otulipenia (also known as OTULIN-related autoinflammatory syndrome) is an autosomal recessive autoinflammatory disease caused by mutations in the *FAM105B* gene coding for OTU deubiquitinase with linear linkage specificity (OTULIN, a Met-1-specific deubiquitinase that downregulates the NF-kB signalling pathway). In clinical terms, patients present with early-onset, prolonged, recurrent episodes of fever, joint pain, abdominal pain, diarrhoea, and lymphadenopathy. A painful erythematous rash with nodules first noted in the neonatal period is the most frequent cutaneous manifestation.

Histopathology

Otulipenia is predominantly a septal form panniculitis with occasional vasculitis of small and medium-sized blood vessels [21].

BS

BS (also known as paediatric granulomatous arthritis) is usually caused by inherited dominant mutations in the *NOD2/CARD15* gene. The disorder can also present sporadically as "early-onset sarcoidosis" after an acquired gene mutation. The skin, eyes, and joints are commonly involved, although some BS patients do not exhibit the full clinical triad. Skin involvement is most prominent and typically appears before joint symptoms and then eye involvement. Together with a histological analysis, a detailed clinical exploration of skin lesions by an expert dermatologist may enable the diagnosis of this orphan disease in early childhood. Early-onset skin lesions have a homogeneous, stereotypical clinical presentation as non-confluent erythematous or pigmented millimetre-size papules. In contrast, late-stage skin lesions have a more heterogeneous clinical presentation and may be wrongly diagnosed as erythema nodosum (EN), ichthyosiform dermatosis, livedoid lesions, or vasculitis [22]. Vouters et al. reported four children with infantile onset lobular panniculitis, high fever, uveitis, arthritis, and systemic granulomatous inflammation without CARD15 mutation [23].

Histopathology

BS is a granulomatous panniculitis, with an inflammatory infiltrate of typical, non-necrotising, non-caseating "sarcoid type" epithelioid and multinucleated giant cell granulomas.

Tumour Necrosis Factor Receptor-Associated Periodic Syndrome (TRAPS)

TRAPS is the most frequent autosomal dominant autoinflammatory disease. Mutations in the *TNFRSF1A* gene (coding for the tumour necrosis factor receptor 1) induce the overproduction of interleukin-1b. In children, variants of TRAPS usually occur as recurrent, irregular febrile episodes with generalised myalgia, joint pain, abdominal pain, ocular lesions, and (in about 80% of cases) skin involvement. The most frequent skin lesions are painful, migratory, centrifugal, tender, non-purpuric, well-demarcated erythematous plaques. Other manifestations include urticaria-like plaques, generalised serpiginous plaques, and small-vessel vasculitis [24,25].

Histopathology

TRAPS is mostly a lymphocytic, lobular form of panniculitis.

2.4.2. Autoinflammatory Syndromes with Inherited Immunodeficiency

Early-onset childhood panniculitis may reveal inherited immunodeficiency, and patients who present with unexplained panniculitis must undergo a detailed immunological screen because the clinical manifestations of immunodeficiency may not yet have emerged. An association with aseptic panniculitis was initially reported in infants with inherited immunodeficiency caused by mutations in the *GATA2* gene (coding for a zinc finger transcription factor) or *ADA2*. Other mutations (in *TRNT1*, *NFKB2*, and *LCK*) have since been reported [13] (Figures 4–6).

Panniculitis in *GATA2* Deficiency

The transcription factor *GATA2* regulates haematopoietic differentiation, lymphatic development, and vascular development. Nearly 100 different *GATA2* mutations have been described. Germline mutations arise spontaneously but are then transmitted via autosomal dominant inheritance. Patients with *GATA2* mutations have very heterogeneous clinical presentations. The level of severity ranges from asymptomatic disease to life-threatening infections with respiratory failure and leukaemia. Up to 70% of patients with *GATA2* mutations have dermatological features (mainly genital or extragenital warts) and up to a third have EN or panniculitis (usually on the lower limbs). These conditions can have several causes (nontuberculous mycobacterial infections, bacterial infections, or autoimmune phenomena) and may constitute the first manifestation of disease [26,27].

Histopathology

Panniculitis in *GATA2* deficiency may be lobular or septal. Scleroderma-like changes deep in the subcutis (resembling deep morphoea) have been described [27].

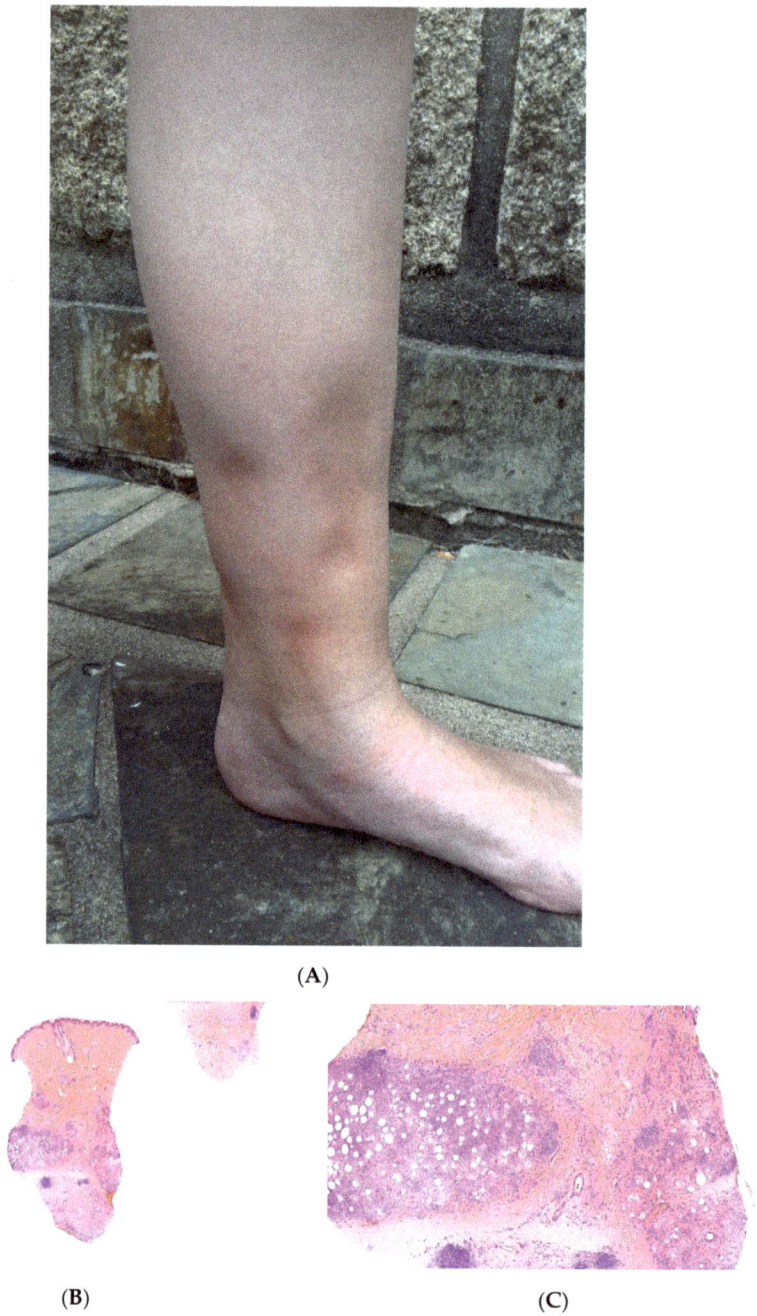

Figure 5. A Recurrent lipoatrophic panniculitis of children. (**A**) Areas of lipoatrophy in the leg *Photo Dermatology Department Hopital Necker Enfants Malades. Paris France*. (**B**,**C**) Lobular panniculitis with a mixed infiltrate, including neutrophils, as well as lymphocytes and macrophages. (**B**) Original magnification ×10, (**C**) original magnification ×40. *Photo Courtesy of Christina Mittledorf Dermatologie, Venerologie und Allergologie Göttingen Germany.*

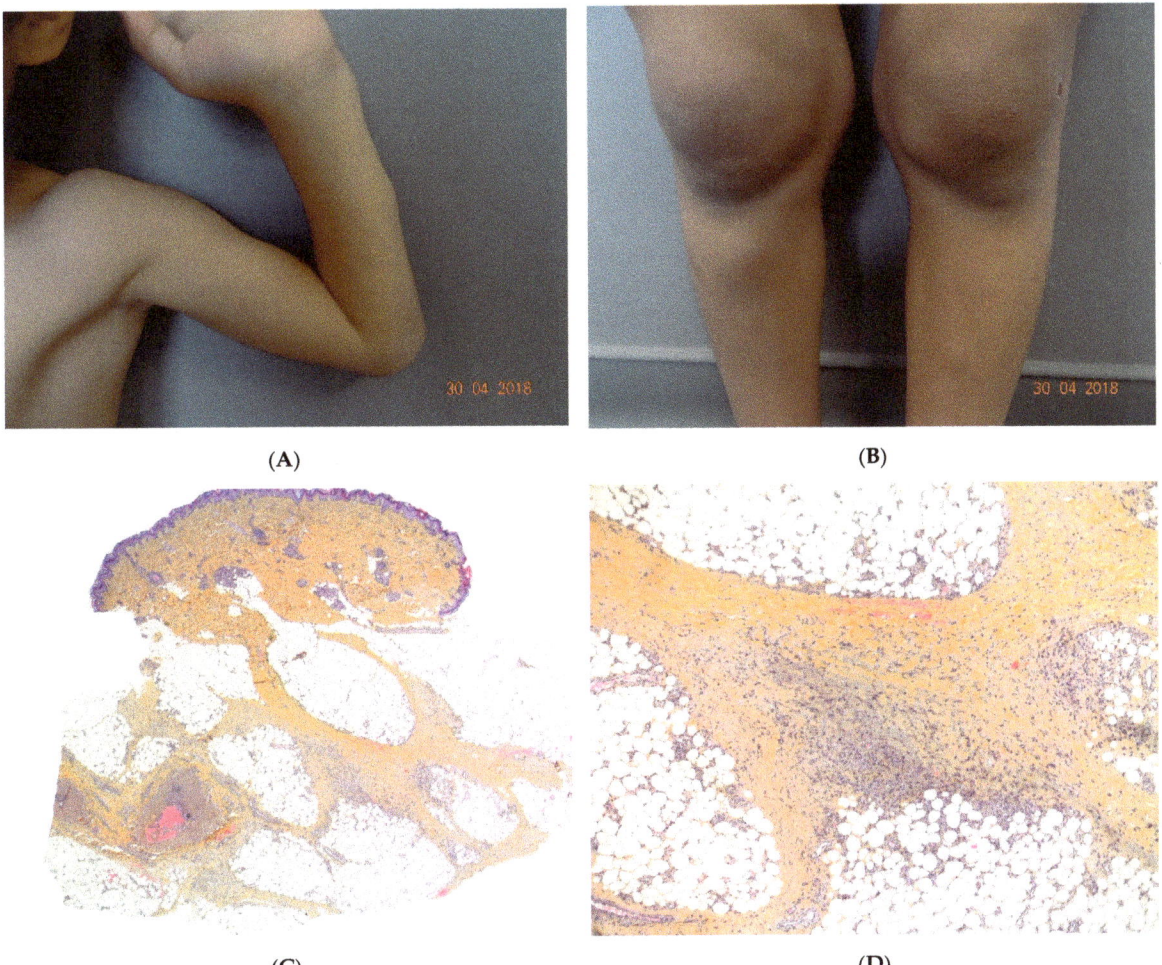

Figure 6. (**A**,**B**) Self-healing juvenile cutaneous mucinosis. Painful nodules of the limbs. *Photo Courtesy of Christine Bodemer Dermatology Department Hopital Necker Enfants Malades. Paris France.* (**C**,**D**) Chronic lobular panniculitis with features of proliferative fasciitis. (**C**) Original magnification ×20, (**D**) original magnification ×100.

Deficiency of Adenosine Deaminase 2 Deficiency

DADA2 is an autosomal recessive disorder caused by compound heterozygous missense mutations in *ADA2*. Skin manifestations may be the presenting symptoms of DADA2. They often include widespread livedo reticularis (often of the racemosa subtype) involving all the limbs and (in some cases) extending to the abdomen or trunk. Other skin manifestations include nodules, EN–like lesions, purpura, leg ulcers, and Raynaud symptoms [28,29]. Any diagnosis of polyarteritis nodosa in a child should always exclude DADA2, since early treatment with an anti-TNF may prevent a stroke.

Histopathology

A biopsy of the skin nodules may have much the same features as polyarteritis nodosa, with fibrinoid necrotising vasculitis affecting the small arteries (in acute panniculitis) and the dermal-subcutaneous junction (at the subacute or reparative stage). Other cases have been characterised by thrombosis of dermal and/or hypodermal capillaries, in the absence of vasculitis [29]. Overall, livedo racemosa with a large branching pattern, nodules or ulceration in a context of neurovascular events, recurrent fever, low immunoglobulin M levels, or paediatric onset is suggestive of DADA2.

2.5. Recurrent Lipoatrophic Panniculitis of Children

This term corresponds to a particular clinical presentation of idiopathic lobular panniculitis. It usually starts in childhood and is associated with fever, the systemic involvement of inflamed visceral fat, and (at the end of the inflammatory process) lipoatrophy. Other terms (such as "connective tissue panniculitis", "lipophagic panniculitis", and "annular lipoatrophy of the ankles") have been used to describe cases with similar features. Use of the term "connective tissue panniculitis" is unfortunate because it may lead to confusion with other typical forms of panniculitis associated with connective tissue disorders (e.g., lupus panniculitis or panniculitis of dermatomyositis. Children with recurrent lipoatrophic panniculitis have inflamed, tender, subcutaneous nodules that appear mainly on the limbs (Figure 5A). In some cases, violaceous discoloration of the overlying skin is present. New lesions appear in subsequent attacks, with fever and slight malaise. Older lesions tend to subside and leave a striking, concentric, annular lipoatrophy.

Histopathology

Recurrent lipoatrophic panniculitis of children is a lobular form with a mixed but predominantly lymphocytic infiltrate that also contains histiocytes, eosinophils, plasma cells, and neutrophils (Figure 5B,C). The degree of lipoatrophy is variable. Lipidised giant cells are usually seen in the conditions called "lipophagic panniculitis of children" and "annular lipoatrophy of the ankles". Several cases have been linked to autoimmune disorders: insulin-dependent diabetes mellitus, juvenile rheumatoid arthritis, Graves' disease, Hashimoto thyroiditis, alopecia areata, vitiligo, coeliac disease, Raynaud's phenomenon, Crohn's disease, and partial IgA deficiency [30].

2.6. Panniculitis in Self-Healing Juvenile Cutaneous Mucinosis (SHJCM)

SHJCM typically presents as an acute eruption in an otherwise healthy child. The cutaneous lesions occur suddenly 3 to 10 days after prodromal fever and spread within a few days to become subcutaneous noninflammatory nodules on the head, hands, elbows, arms, and knees (Figure 6A,B). Additional nontender ivory-white papules may arise on the hands, head, and trunk at disease onset or during disease progression. Nodules are a common clinical feature and can precede the papules. Periorbital oedema, asthenia, and joint pain may also be encountered.

Histopathology

In the absence of mucinous papules, the diagnosis of SHJCM is challenging. A histopathological assessment of the papules reveals moderate dermal mucin deposition, whereas the nodules show features of proliferative fasciitis or non-specific chronic lobular panniculitis (Figure 6C) [31].

3. Paediatric Aspects of Forms of Panniculitis That Occur Mainly in Adults
3.1. Erythema Nodosum

Although EN is the most common form of panniculitis at all ages, the incidence peaks during adolescence. There is no sex predominance [32]. In children, lesions are most frequent on the anterior aspects of the thighs, upper limbs, trunk, and face (Figure 7A). The aetiology is similar to that of adult EN, with streptococcal and gastrointestinal infections as the main causes. Idiopathic EN accounts for 40% of cases in children. A skin biopsy is not generally performed, but is advisable for patients with an atypical presentation or a protracted course of disease.

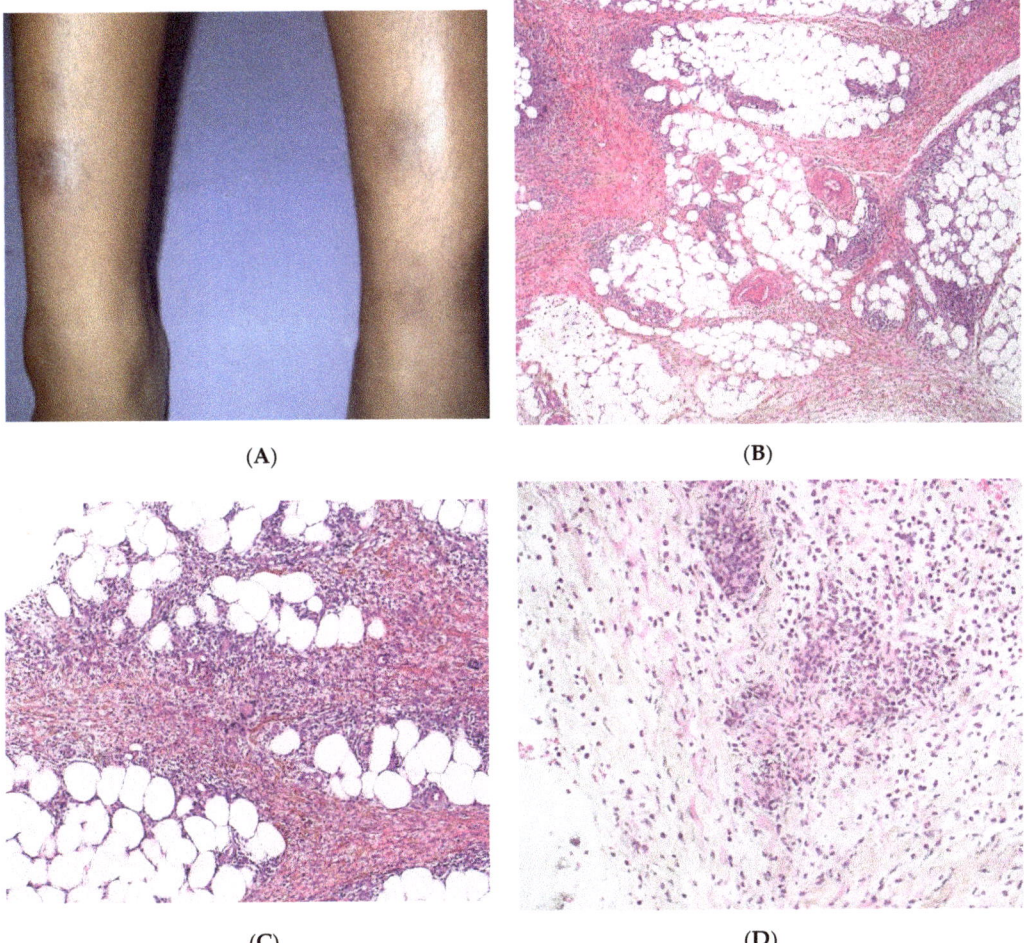

Figure 7. Erythema nodosum. (**A**) Nodules of the legs in an 8-year-old child. *Photo Dermatology Department Hopital Necker Enfants Malades. Paris France.* (**B**) Fibrosing septal pattern with involvement of the periphery of the fat lobules. The process extends into the fat lobules (original magnification ×40). (**C**) Thickened septa of subcutaneous fat with granulomatous inflammation (original magnification ×100). (**D**) Miescher granuloma consisting of small nodular aggregation of histiocytes around a central stellate-shaped cleft located near the junction of the adipocytes and the septum (original magnification ×200).

Histopathology

The aspect is similar to that of EN in adults, with mostly septal panniculitis. The septa of the subcutaneous fat are thickened, and an inflammatory cell infiltrate is present (Figure 7B,C) Neutrophils predominate in acute lesions, whereas mononuclear cells and histiocytes predominate in chronic lesions. Miescher's radial granuloma—an aggregation of histiocytes around a central stellate or "banana-shaped" cleft—is specific for EN but is not always present (Figure 7D).

3.2. Infectious Panniculitis

Infectious panniculitides are very rare and mostly occur in immunosuppressed patients. Several pathogens can infect the subcutaneous fat.

Histopathology

Infectious panniculitis is mostly lobular, with a predominance of neutrophils in the infiltrate. Necrosis and suppurative granulomas are frequent but vasculitis is rare. Microorganisms are rarely found in biopsies from non-immunocompromised patients. Bacteriological cultures may be required in immunocompromised patients.

3.3. Pancreatic Panniculitis

Pancreatic panniculitis is very rare in children. The aetiology of pancreatitis in children differs from that seen in adults; it arises in a systemic disease setting that often involves a genetic disorder [33,34]. The histopathological features and management are much the same as for the adult disease; lobular panniculitis exhibits mixed inflammation, with coagulative necrosis of adipocytes and ghost cells. Calcification is common.

3.4. Panniculitis during Vemurafenib Treatment

Panniculitis has been reported in children treated with vemurafenib for neural tumours of the central nervous system or for Langerhans cell histiocytosis [35,36]. The paediatric cases correspond to the adult phenotype with cutaneous nodules appearing soon after vemurafenib initiation. Vemurafenib panniculitis may be accompanied by fever, which (along with the presence of polymorphonuclear cells in a histological assessment) might prompt the physician to suspect an infectious cause in immunocompromised patients with new skin nodules. The lesions may or may not resolve spontaneously in patients who continue treatment with vemurafenib.

Histopathology

Vemurafenib panniculitis is a mostly lobular neutrophilic form, and lesion cultures for microorganisms are negative.

3.5. Factitial and Iatrogenic Panniculitis

Factitial panniculitis (the iatrogenic consequence of certain drug injections) is rare in children. The clinical features of factitial panniculitis are quite variable and depend on the causative agent [37]. In young children, factitial lesions should prompt the clinician to consider a diagnosis of Munchausen syndrome [38]. Subcutaneous aluminium granuloma can develop at the injection site weeks, months, or even years (median: 3 months) after the administration of aluminium-absorbed vaccines (diphtheria/tetanus/pertussis, hepatitis A, hepatitis B, and human papillomavirus vaccines). Factitial panniculitis presents as single or multiple itching subcutaneous nodules and resolves spontaneously.

Histopathology

Biopsies are not usually performed in cases of factitial panniculitis but they usually reveal an acute, lobular form of panniculitis associated with fat necrosis and an abundant, predominantly neutrophilic inflammatory infiltrate. Post-vaccination subcutaneous aluminium granuloma shows a dense, deep dermal and subcutaneous nodular mixed infiltrate of lymphocytes, histiocytes, and eosinophils, with germinal centre formation in some cases [39,40]. The bluish, amphophilic granular cytoplasm observed in most of the histiocytes is a characteristic feature of "aluminium granulomas". Moreover, the granules stain positive for aluminium (Morin reagent) (Figure 8).

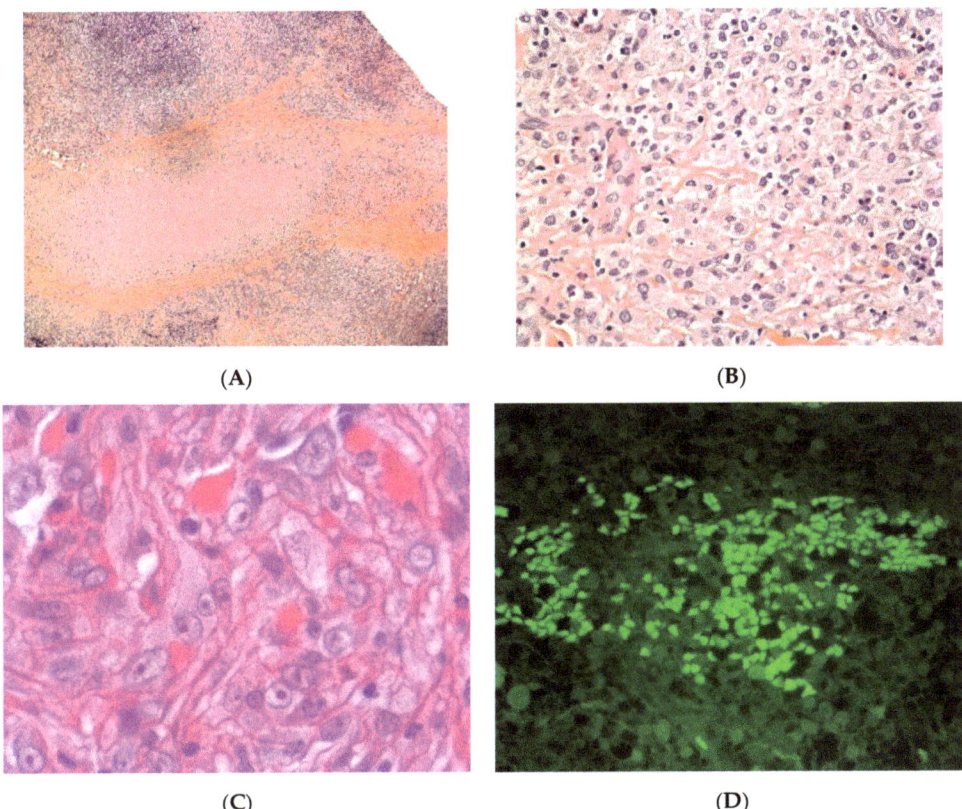

Figure 8. Subcutaneous aluminium granuloma. (**A**) Dense, deep dermal and subcutaneous nodular infiltrate surrounding areas of necrosis (original magnification ×80). (**B**) Mixed infiltrate of lymphocytes, histiocytes, and eosinophils (original magnification ×250). (**C**) Histiocytes containing violaceous granular within their cytoplasm (original magnification ×400). (**D**) The granules stain positive with aluminon staining (Morin, (original magnification ×200)), which reveals the existence of aluminium.

3.6. Alpha-1-Antitrypsin Deficiency

Panniculitis caused by alpha-1-antitrypsin is a rare autosomal recessive disorder in adults and is even rarer in children. Panniculitis occurs most commonly in individuals who are homozygous for the Z allele of the *SERPINA1* alpha-antitrypsin gene [41]. In most paediatric cases, lesions develop on trauma-damaged areas. Zones of erythema and induration are observed and often mimic cellulitis. The zones rapidly progress to deep nodules with ulceration and exudation of an oily substance produced by adipocyte necrosis. The lesions relapse and heal with atrophic scarring. A paediatric disease onset does not mean that the prognosis is more favourable, because lesions can continue to appear into adulthood. The panniculitis may precede (sometimes by several years) emphysema and other manifestations of an antitrypsin deficiency or may be the only clinical sign [42].

Histopathology

The combination of extensive liquefactive necrosis of the dermis, neutrophilic inflammation, and destructive changes in the fibrous septa of the subcutis (resulting in separation of the subcutis' lobules) is pathognomonic for alpha 1-antitrypsin deficiency [43].

3.7. H Syndrome (OMIM #612391)

H syndrome (OMIM #612391) is a recently described autosomal recessive genodermatosis, the systemic manifestations of which are linked to mutations in the *SLC29A3* gene (coding for a nucleoside transporter). The disease is characterised by the progressive, sclerodermatous thickening of the skin with overlying hyperpigmentation and hypertrichosis located mainly on the upper inner thighs. The involvement of the genitalia, lower trunk, and limbs is variable. The additional systemic manifestations that gave the syndrome its "H" name included hepatosplenomegaly, hearing loss, heart anomalies, hypogonadism, low height, hallux valgus with fixed flexion contractures of the toe joints and proximal interphalangeal joints of the hands, and (occasionally) hyperglycaemia/diabetes mellitus. Induration of the skin is often observed.

Histopathology

The dermis and hypodermis contain interstitial chronic inflammatory infiltrates mainly consisting of monocyte-derived cells (small CD68+, large CD68+, CD163+, S100+, CD1a- histiocytes with emperipolesis, and CD34+ and FXIIIa+ dendrocytes) and plasma cells. This inflammatory component is associated with striking fibrosis of the subcutis and moderate fibrosis of the dermis [44].

3.8. Panniculitis Associated with Connective Tissue Diseases and Vasculitis
3.8.1. Lupus Erythematosus Panniculitis (LEP)

Lupus erythematosus panniculitis is very rare in children and is often found as an isolated phenomenon with no systemic or other cutaneous findings. However, LEP can be observed in patients with discoid lupus erythematosus [45], systemic lupus erythematosus [46], or (very rarely) neonatal lupus [47].

Clinically, LEP manifests itself as tender nodules or plaques, with female predominance. In children, the most common lesion sites are the face, upper arms, and shoulders [48]. The lesions often heal with scarring and lipoatrophy.

Histopathology

LEP is a lobular panniculitis with a prominent lymphocytic infiltrate (lymphocytic lobular panniculitis) (Figure 9). Concomitant septal involvement is often present, with sclerosing and thickening of the septa. Myxoid and hyaline changes may be found in the connective tissue septa and the lower dermis. Lymphocytic vasculitis with lymphocytic nuclear dust is sometimes present. A characteristic feature includes fat necrosis and the presence of lymphoid follicles (sometimes with germinal centres) adjacent to the fibrous septa. Plasma cells are present in many cases. Epidermal and dermal changes (particularly basal vacuolar changes) may be present [49].

3.8.2. Panniculitis and Dermatomyositis (DM)

Panniculitis is a rare clinical finding in juvenile DM and may be the disease's only cutaneous manifestation. The typical clinical picture involves erythematous, painful subcutaneous nodules or plaques that typically occur on the buttocks, thighs, and arms and are often attributed to a flare of DM [50]. Migratory subcutaneous nodules have also been described.

Histopathology

Panniculitis in DM is very similar to lupus panniculitis. It is mostly lobular, with lymphocytes and plasma cells found among the adipocytes. The collagen bundles of the septa show hyaline sclerosis, and the fat is progressively replaced by fibrous tissue [50]. In DM, panniculitis associated with calcification of muscle and deep tissue is more common than isolated panniculitis. In cases with calcification, the fat lobules show lipophagic granuloma and various degrees of acute and/or chronic inflammation [50].

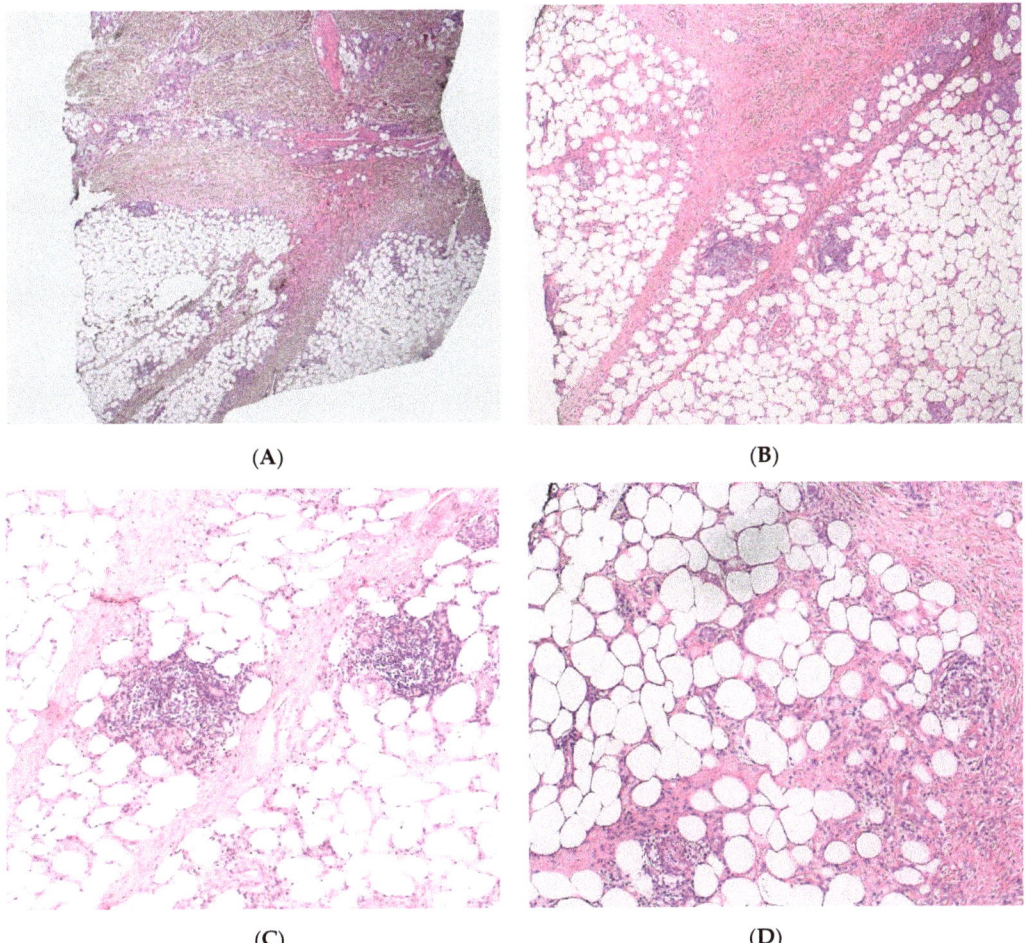

Figure 9. Lupus panniculitis. (**A**) Dense dermal infiltrate with extension into subcutaneous fat (original magnification ×30). (**B**) Septae appear fibrotic (original magnification ×100). (**C**) Lymphoid follicles (original magnification ×120). (**D**) Necrosis of adipocytes with hyalinisation of the fat lobular panniculitis with lymphocytes among necrotic adipocytes (original magnification ×120).

3.9. Cytotoxic T-Cell Clonal Panniculitis

Subcutaneous panniculitis-like cytotoxic T-cell clonal proliferation arises mainly in adults and is very rare in children. The prognosis in children is usually excellent, and thus, the term "cytotoxic T-cell clonal panniculitis" is more appropriate than "subcutaneous panniculitis-like cytotoxic T-cell lymphoma" [51]. This T-cell clonal proliferation is frequently associated with an autoimmune disease, and thus, a thorough diagnostic work-up is required. The condition can appear after an infection like toxoplasmosis, chicken pox, and viral nasopharyngitis. Cytotoxic T-cell clonal panniculitis might result from a dysregulation of T cell responses after recognition of an autoantigen or an antigen from a pathogen [52]. Cases with a severe haemophagocytic syndrome are significantly linked with germline mutations in *HAVCR2* gene encoding T-cell immunoglobulin mucin-3 (TIM-3), an inhibitory receptor expressed on T-cells and innate immune cells. *HAVCR2* mutations are found in 60–85% of cases of cytotoxic T-cell clonal panniculitis and are associated with younger age at onset and a more frequent association with haemophagocytic lymphohistiocytosis [53].

Detection of a TIM-3 deficiency provides a rationale for treatment with anti-inflammatory agent (steroids or interferon) rather than polychemotherapy.

Clinically, patients present with solitary or multiple nodules and erythematous subcutaneous plaques, which are predominantly located on the limbs and trunk. The lesions have overlying erythema, are usually painless, and range in size from 0.5–2.0 cm. Lesions at different stages of healing may be observed, which suggests a relapsing-remitting clinical course. Lipoatrophy or persistent facial swelling may be associated with these cutaneous manifestations. A haemophagocytic syndrome is sometimes also present, albeit far less frequently in children than in adults. The syndrome's features including fever, chills, malaise, weight loss, pancytopenia, lymphadenopathy, hepatosplenomegaly, abnormal liver enzyme levels, and coagulation disorders [54].

Histopathology

Cytotoxic T-cell clonal panniculitis is a lobular panniculitis with a dense, nodular or diffuse infiltrate of small to medium pleomorphic lymphocytes in the subcutaneous fat (Figure 10). The cells are arranged around the adipocytes—the so-called "rimming of the adipocytes". Necrosis is often a prominent feature and may mask specific histopathological features. The pathologist can search for small aggregates of atypical lymphocytes within the necrotic region, together with ghost cells (necrotic lymphocytes). Apoptosis with karyorrhectic debris is frequently associated with the presence of haemophagocytic cells. Paediatric lesions often contain plasma cells. In some cases, the specific features are confined to a small portion of the subcutaneous fat; a thorough examination of the biopsy specimen and multiple serial sections of the skin biopsy are needed for a firm diagnosis. Immunohistochemical studies show that the lymphocytes are mostly cytotoxic CD8+ cells expressing the cytotoxic proteins TIA1, granzyme B, and perforin, but not CD56. In situ hybridisation (to detect the EBER-1 small RNA from the Epstein-Barr virus) is usually negative [55].

T-cell clonality can be demonstrated by identifying $\alpha\beta$ T-cell receptor rearrangements using polymerase chain reactions or high-throughput sequencing.

In most cases, the prognosis is excellent, and conservative treatment with an immunosuppressant is recommended [56]. Some cases may even regress spontaneously. In patients with an immunodeficiency (particularly TIM3 deficiency), bone marrow transplantation is curative. Patients with cytotoxic T-cell clonal panniculitis and haemophagocytic syndrome should always be screened for an immunodeficiency.

The term "cytophagic histiocytic panniculitis" has been used to describe subcutaneous nodules or plaques that show (in a histological examination) macrophage infiltrates also containing erythrocytes, lymphocytes, and/or karyorrhectic debris (i.e., haematophagocytosis). With the advent of immunophenotyping and genetic techniques, it has become apparent that the vast majority of patients have lymphoma, with atypical lymphoid cells also present in the panniculus; hence, the term "cytophagic histiocytic panniculitis" is no longer used.

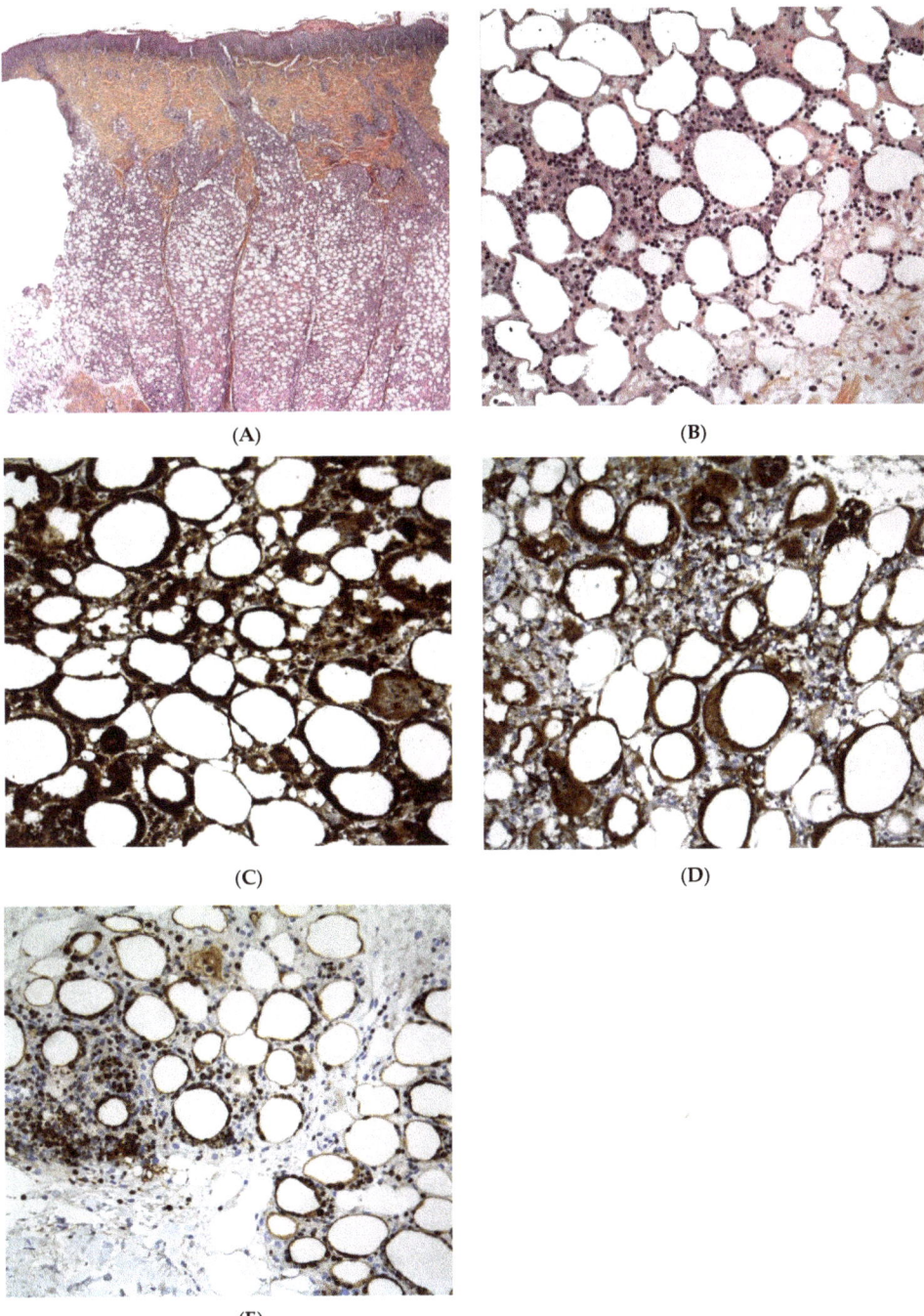

Figure 10. Cytotoxic T clonal panniculitis. (**A**) Lobular panniculitis with lymphoid cell infiltration (original magnification ×30). (**B**) Atypical lymphoid cells with adipocyte rimming and adipocyte necrosis showing infiltration by cells expressing (**C**) CD3, (**D**) Tia1, and (**E**) granzyme (original magnification ×400).

4. Conclusions

Panniculitis in children is rare but can have many possible causes. Certain types are specific for childhood, whereas others are rare at a young age. A biopsy is not always necessary but is often useful if sufficient tissue is available; clinicians must, therefore, choose the best time and best site for sampling. Patients with panniculitis but who lack an aetiological diagnosis should be monitored for immunodeficiency and autoinflammatory diseases.

Author Contributions: Conceptualization I.M., S.F.; Validation, I.M., S.F.; Writing—original draft preparation, I.M.; Writing—review and editing, I.M., S.F.; Visualization, supervision, I.M., S.F.; project administration, I.M., S.F. All authors have read and agreed to the published version of the manuscript.

Funding: This research received no external funding.

Institutional Review Board Statement: Not applicable.

Informed Consent Statement: Not applicable.

Conflicts of Interest: The authors declare no conflict of interest.

References

1. Bodemer, C. *Panniculitis in Harper's Textbook of Pediatric Dermatology*, 4th ed.; Wiley-Blackwell: Oxford, UK, 5 December 2019; pp. 1207–1220. (In English)
2. Torrelo, A.; Hernández, A. Panniculitis in children. *Dermatol. Clin.* **2008**, *26*, 491–500. [CrossRef] [PubMed]
3. Polcari, I.C.; Stein, S.L. Panniculitis in childhood. *Dermatol. Ther.* **2010**, *23*, 356–367. [CrossRef]
4. Requena, L.; Yus, E.S. Panniculitis. Part I. Mostly septal panniculitis. *J. Am. Acad. Dermatol.* **2001**, *45*, 163–183. [CrossRef] [PubMed]
5. Requena, L.; Yus, E.S. Panniculitis. Part II. Mostly lobular panniculitis. *J. Am. Acad. Dermatol.* **2001**, *45*, 325–364. [CrossRef] [PubMed]
6. Del Pozzo-Magaña, B.R.; Ho, N. Subcutaneous Fat Necrosis of the Newborn: A 20-Year Retrospective Study. *Pediatr. Dermatol.* **2016**, *33*, e353–e355. [CrossRef] [PubMed]
7. Lara, L.G.; Villa, A.V.; Rivas, M.M.; Capella, M.S.; Prada, F.; Enseñat, M.A.G. Subcutaneous Fat Necrosis of the Newborn: Report of Five Cases. *Pediatr. Neonatol.* **2017**, *58*, 85–88. [CrossRef]
8. Stefanko, N.S.; Drolet, B.A. Subcutaneous fat necrosis of the newborn and associated hypercalcemia: A systematic review of the literature. *Pediatr. Dermatol.* **2019**, *36*, 24–30. [CrossRef]
9. Ricardo-Gonzalez, R.R.; Lin, J.R.; Mathes, E.F.; McCalmont, T.H.; Pincus, L.B. Neutrophil-rich subcutaneous fat necrosis of the newborn: A potential mimic of infection. *J. Am. Acad. Dermatol.* **2016**, *75*, 177–185. [CrossRef]
10. Zeb, A.; Darmstadt, G.L. Sclerema neonatorum: A review of nomenclature, clinical presentation, histological features, differential diagnoses and management. *J. Perinatol.* **2008**, *28*, 453–460. [CrossRef]
11. Silverman, R.A.; Newman, A.J.; LeVine, M.J.; Kaplan, B. Poststeroid panniculitis: A case report. *Pediatr. Dermatol.* **1988**, *5*, 92–93. [CrossRef]
12. Malia, L.; Wang, A.; Scheiner, L.; Laurich, V.M. Cold Panniculitis After Ice Therapy for Supraventricular Tachycardia. *Pediatr. Emerg. Care* **2019**, *35*, e174–e176. [CrossRef] [PubMed]
13. Bader-Meunier, B.; Rieux-Laucat, F.; Touzot, F.; Frémond, M.L.; André-Schmutz, I.; Fraitag, S.; Bodemer, C. Inherited Immunodeficiency: A New Association with Early-Onset Childhood Panniculitis. *Pediatrics* **2018**, *141* (Suppl. 5), S496–S500. [CrossRef]
14. Escudier, A.; Mauvais, F.X.; Bastard, P.; Boussard, C.; Jaoui, A.; Koskas, V.; Lecoq, E.; Michel, A.; Orcel, M.C.; Truelle, P.E.; et al. Peau et fièvres récurrentes auto-inflammatoires [Dermatological features of auto-inflammatory recurrent fevers]. *Arch. Pediatr.* **2018**, *25*, 150–162. (In French) [CrossRef] [PubMed]
15. Torrelo, A.; Patel, S.; Colmenero, I.; Gurbindo, D.; Lendínez, F.; Hernández, A.; López-Robledillo, J.C.; Dadban, A.; Requena, L.; Paller, A.S. Chronic atypical neutrophilic dermatosis with lipodystrophy and elevated temperature (CANDLE) syndrome. *J. Am. Acad. Dermatol.* **2010**, *62*, 489–495. [CrossRef]
16. Ohmura, K. Nakajo-Nishimura syndrome and related proteasome-associated autoinflammatory syndromes. *J. Inflamm. Res.* **2019**, *12*, 259–265. [CrossRef] [PubMed]
17. Volpi, S.; Picco, P.; Caorsi, R.; Candotti, F.; Gattorno, M. Type I interferonopathies in pediatric rheumatology. *Pediatr. Rheumatol. Online J.* **2016**, *14*, 35. [CrossRef]
18. Torrelo, A.; Colmenero, I.; Requena, L.; Paller, A.S.; Ramot, Y.; Richard Lee, C.C.; Vera, A.; Zlotogorski, A.; Goldbach-Mansky, R.; Kutzner, H. Histologic and Immunohistochemical Features of the Skin Lesions in CANDLE Syndrome. *Am. J. Dermatopathol.* **2015**, *37*, 517–522. [CrossRef]
19. Figueras-Nart, I.; Mascaró, J.M., Jr.; Solanich, X.; Hernández-Rodríguez, J. Dermatologic and Dermatopathologic Features of Monogenic Autoinflammatory Diseases. *Front. Immunol.* **2019**, *10*, 2448. [CrossRef]

20. Leiva-Salinas, M.; Betlloch, I.; Arribas, M.P.; Francés, L.; Pascual, J.C. Neutrophilic lobular panniculitis as an expression of a widened spectrum of familial mediterranean fever. *JAMA Dermatol.* **2014**, *150*, 213–214. [CrossRef]
21. Zhou, Q.; Yu, X.; Demirkaya, E.; Deuitch, N.; Stone, D.; Tsai, W.L.; Kuehn, H.S.; Wang, H.; Yang, D.; Park, Y.H.; et al. Biallelic hypomorphic mutations in a linear deubiquitinase define otulipenia, an early-onset autoinflammatory disease. *Proc. Natl. Acad. Sci. USA* **2016**, *113*, 10127–10132. [CrossRef]
22. Poline, J.; Fogel, O.; Pajot, C.; Miceli-Richard, C.; Rybojad, M.; Galeotti, C.; Grouteau, E.; Hachulla, E.; Brissaud, P.; Cantagrel, A.; et al. Early-onset granulomatous arthritis, uveitis and skin rash: Characterization of skin involvement in Blau syndrome. *J. Eur. Acad. Dermatol. Venereol.* **2020**, *34*, 340–348. [CrossRef]
23. Wouters, C.H.; Martin, T.M.; Stichweh, D.; Punaro, M.; Doyle, T.M.; Lewis, J.A.; Quartier, P.; Rose, C.D. Infantile onset panniculitis with uveitis and systemic granulomatosis: A new clinicopathologic entity. *J. Pediatr.* **2007**, *151*, 707–709. [CrossRef] [PubMed]
24. Toro, J.R.; Aksentijevich, I.; Hull, K.; Dean, J.; Kastner, D.L. Tumor necrosis factor receptor-associated periodic syndrome: A novel syndrome with cutaneous manifestations. *Arch. Dermatol.* **2000**, *136*, 1487–1494. [CrossRef] [PubMed]
25. Cattalini, M.; Meini, A.; Monari, P.; Gualdi, G.; Arisi, M.; Pelucchi, F.; Bolognini, S.; Gattorno, M.; Calzavara-Pinton, P.G.; Plebani, A. Recurrent migratory angioedema as cutaneous manifestation in a familiar case of TRAPS: Dramatic response to Anakinra. *Dermatol. Online J.* **2013**, *19*, 20405. [CrossRef] [PubMed]
26. Polat, A.; Dinulescu, M.; Fraitag, S.; Nimubona, S.; Toutain, F.; Jouneau, S.; Poullot, E.; Droitcourt, C.; Dupuy, A. Skin manifestations among GATA2-deficient patients. *Br. J. Dermatol.* **2018**, *178*, 781–785. [CrossRef]
27. Spinner, M.A.; Sanchez, L.A.; Hsu, A.P.; Shaw, P.A.; Zerbe, C.S.; Calvo, K.R.; Arthur, D.C.; Gu, W.; Gould, C.M.; Brewer, C.C.; et al. GATA2 deficiency: A protean disorder of hematopoiesis, lymphatics, and immunity. *Blood* **2014**, *123*, 809–821. [CrossRef]
28. Chasset, F.; Fayand, A.; Moguelet, P.; Kouby, F.; Bonhomme, A.; Franck, N.; Goldman-Lévy, G.; Fraitag, S.; Barbaud, A.; Queyrel, V.; et al. Clinical and pathological dermatological features of deficiency of adenosine deaminase 2: A multicenter, retrospective, observational study. *J. Am. Acad. Dermatol.* **2020**, *83*, 1794–1798. [CrossRef]
29. Shwin, K.W.; Lee, C.R.; Goldbach-Mansky, R. Dermatologic Manifestations of Monogenic Autoinflammatory Diseases. *Dermatol. Clin.* **2017**, *35*, 21–38. [CrossRef]
30. Torrelo, A.; Noguera-Morel, L.; Hernández-Martín, A.; Clemente, D.; Barja, J.M.; Buzón, L.; Azorín, D.; de Jesús, A.A.; López-Robledillo, J.C.; Colmenero, I.; et al. Recurrent lipoatrophic panniculitis of children. *J. Eur. Acad. Dermatol. Venereol.* **2017**, *31*, 536–543. [CrossRef]
31. Luchsinger, I.; Coulombe, J.; Rongioletti, F.; Haspeslagh, M.; Dompmartin, A.; Melki, I.; Dagher, R.; Bader-Meunier, B.; Fraitag, S.; Bodemer, C. Self-healing juvenile cutaneous mucinosis: Clinical and histopathologic findings of 9 patients: The relevance of long-term follow-up. *J. Am. Acad. Dermatol.* **2018**, *78*, 1164–1170. [CrossRef]
32. Moraes, A.J.; Soares, P.M.; Zapata, A.L.; Lotito, A.P.; Sallum, A.M.; Silva, C.A. Panniculitis in childhood and adolescence. *Pediatr. Int.* **2006**, *48*, 48–53. [CrossRef] [PubMed]
33. Boyd, A.S.; Wester, A.C. Pancreatic fat necrosis in a 10-year-old girl: A case report and review of the literature. *Pediatr. Dermatol.* **2019**, *36*, 982–983. [CrossRef]
34. Holstein, T.; Horneff, G.; Wawer, A.; Gaber, G.; Burdach, S. Panniculitis, pancreatitis and very severe aplastic anemia in childhood: A challenge to treat. *Ann. Hematol.* **2000**, *79*, 631–634. [CrossRef] [PubMed]
35. Boull, C.L.; Gardeen, S.; Abdali, T.; Li, E.; Potts, J.; Rubin, N.; Carlberg, V.M.; Gupta, D.; Hunt, R.; Luu, M.; et al. Cutaneous Reactions in Children Treated with MEK Inhibitors, BRAF Inhibitors, or Combination Therapy: A Multi-Center Study. *J. Am. Acad. Dermatol.* **2020**, *16*, 1554–1561. [CrossRef]
36. Finelt, N.; Lulla, R.R.; Melin-Aldana, H.; Ruth, J.S.; Lin, F.Y.; Su, J.M.; Pourciau, C.Y.; Hunt, R.D.; Kenner-Bell, B.M. Bumps in the Road: Panniculitis in Children and Adolescents Treated with Vemurafenib. *Pediatr. Dermatol.* **2017**, *34*, 337–341. [CrossRef]
37. Sanmartín, O.; Requena, C.; Requena, L. Factitial panniculitis. *Dermatol. Clin.* **2008**, *26*, 519–527. [CrossRef] [PubMed]
38. Boyd, A.S.; Ritchie, C.; Likhari, S. Munchausen syndrome and Munchausen syndrome by proxy in dermatology. *J. Am. Acad. Dermatol.* **2014**, *71*, 376–381. [CrossRef]
39. Chong, H.; Brady, K.; Metze, D.; Calonje, E. Persistent nodules at injection sites (aluminium granuloma)—Clinicopathological study of 14 cases with a diverse range of histological reaction patterns. *Histopathology* **2006**, *48*, 182–188. [CrossRef]
40. Haag, C.K.; Dacey, E.; Hamilton, N.; White, K.P. Aluminum granuloma in a child secondary to DTaP-IPV vaccination: A case report. *Pediatr. Dermatol.* **2019**, *36*, e17–e19. [CrossRef]
41. Torres-Durán, M.; Lopez-Campos, J.L.; Barrecheguren, M.; Miravitlles, M.; Martinez-Delgado, B.; Castillo, S.; Escribano, A.; Baloira, A.; Navarro-Garcia, M.M.; Pellicer, D.; et al. Alpha-1 antitrypsin deficiency: Outstanding questions and future directions. *Orphanet J. Rare Dis.* **2018**, *13*, 114. [CrossRef]
42. Hendrick, S.J.; Silverman, A.K.; Solomon, A.R.; Headington, J.T. Alpha 1-antitrypsin deficiency associated with panniculitis. *J. Am. Acad. Dermatol.* **1988**, *18*, 684–692. [CrossRef]
43. Blanco, I.; Lipsker, D.; Lara, B.; Janciauskiene, S. Neutrophilic panniculitis associated with alpha-1-antitrypsin deficiency: An update. *Br. J. Dermatol.* **2016**, *174*, 753–762. [CrossRef] [PubMed]
44. Doviner, V.; Maly, A.; Ne'eman, Z.; Qawasmi, R.; Aamar, S.; Sultan, M.; Spiegel, M.; Molho-Pessach, V.; Zlotogorski, A. H syndrome: Recently defined genodermatosis with distinct histologic features. A morphological, histochemical, immunohistochemical, and ultrastructural study of 10 cases. *Am. J. Dermatopathol.* **2010**, *32*, 118–128. [CrossRef]

45. Wimmershoff, M.B.; Hohenleutner, U.; Landthaler, M. Discoid lupus erythematosus and lupus profundus in childhood: A report of two cases. *Pediatr. Dermatol.* **2003**, *20*, 140–145. [CrossRef] [PubMed]
46. Zhang, R.; Dang, X.; Shuai, L.; He, Q.; He, X.; Yi, Z. Lupus erythematosus panniculitis in a 10-year-old female child with severe systemic lupus erythematosus: A case report. *Medicine* **2018**, *97*, e9571. [CrossRef] [PubMed]
47. Nitta, Y. Lupus erythematosus profundus associated with neonatal lupus erythematosus. *Br. J. Dermatol.* **1997**, *136*, 112–114. [CrossRef]
48. Weingartner, J.S.; Zedek, D.C.; Burkhart, C.N.; Morrell, D.S. Lupus erythematosus panniculitis in children: Report of three cases and review of previously reported cases. *Pediatr. Dermatol.* **2012**, *29*, 169–176. [CrossRef]
49. Park, H.S.; Choi, J.W.; Kim, B.K.; Cho, K.H. Lupus erythematosus panniculitis: Clinicopathological, immunophenotypic, and molecular studies. *Am. J. Dermatopathol.* **2010**, *32*, 24–30. [CrossRef] [PubMed]
50. Neidenbach, P.J.; Sahn, E.E.; Helton, J. Panniculitis in juvenile dermatomyositis. *J. Am. Acad. Dermatol.* **1995**, *33*, 305–307. [CrossRef]
51. Bader-Meunier, B.; Fraitag, S.; Janssen, C.; Brochard, K.; Lamant, L.; Wouters, C.; Bodemer, C. Clonal cytophagic histiocytic panniculitis in children may be cured by cyclosporine A. *Pediatrics* **2013**, *132*, e545–e549. [CrossRef] [PubMed]
52. Michonneau, D.; Petrella, T.; Ortonne, N.; Ingen-Housz-Oro, S.; Franck, N.; Barete, S.; Battistella, M.; Beylot-Barry, M.; Vergier, B.; Maynadié, M.; et al. Subcutaneous Panniculitis-like T-cell Lymphoma: Immunosuppressive Drugs Induce Better Response than Polychemotherapy. *Acta. Derm. Venereol.* **2017**, *97*, 358–364. [CrossRef]
53. Gayden, T.; Sepulveda, F.E.; Khuong-Quang, D.A.; Pratt, J.; Valera, E.T.; Garrigue, A.; Kelso, S.; Sicheri, F.; Mikael, L.G.; Hamel, N.; et al. Germline HAVCR2 mutations altering TIM-3 characterize subcutaneous panniculitis-like T cell lymphomas with hemophagocytic lymphohistiocytic syndrome. *Nat. Genet.* **2018**, *50*, 1650–1657. [CrossRef] [PubMed]
54. Chaweephisal, P.; Sosothikul, D.; Polprasert, C.; Wananukul, S.; Seksarn, P. Subcutaneous Panniculitis-like T-Cell Lymphoma With Hemophagocytic Lymphohistiocytosis Syndrome in Children and Its Essential Role of HAVCR2 Gene Mutation Analysis. *J. Pediatr. Hematol. Oncol.* **2021**, *43*, e80–e84. [CrossRef] [PubMed]
55. Rutnin, S.; Porntharukcharoen, S.; Boonsakan, P. Clinicopathologic, immunophenotypic, and molecular analysis of subcutaneous panniculitis-like T-cell lymphoma: A retrospective study in a tertiary care center. *J. Cutan. Pathol.* **2019**, *46*, 44–51. [CrossRef]
56. Singh, S.; Philip, C.C.; John, M.J. Pediatric Subcutaneous Panniculitis-like T-Cell Lymphoma with Hemophagocytosis Showing Complete Resolution with the BFM90 Protocol: Case Report and Review of Literature. *J. Pediatr. Hematol. Oncol.* **2019**, *41*, 478–481. [CrossRef] [PubMed]

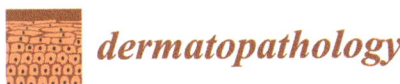

Review

Diagnostic Approach to Congenital Cystic Masses of the Neck from a Clinical and Pathological Perspective

Amanda Fanous [1,†], Guillaume Morcrette [2,†], Monique Fabre [3], Vincent Couloigner [1,4] and Louise Galmiche-Rolland [5,*]

1. Pediatric Otolaryngology-Head and Neck Surgery, AP-HP, Hôpital Universitaire Necker Enfants Malades, 75015 Paris, France; amandafanous@gmail.com (A.F.); vincent.couloigner@aphp.fr (V.C.)
2. Department of Pediatric Pathology, AP-HP, Hôpital Robert Debré, 75019 Paris, France; guillaume.morcrette@inserm.fr
3. Department of Pathology, AP-HP, Hôpital Universitaire Necker Enfants Malades, Université Paris Descartes, 75015 Paris, France; mofabre@gmail.com
4. Faculté de Médecine, Université de Paris, 75015 Paris, France
5. Department of Pathology, University Hospital of Nantes, 44000 Nantes, France
* Correspondence: louise.rolland@chu-nantes.fr
† These authors contributed equally to this work.

Abstract: Background: neck cysts are frequently encountered in pediatric medicine and can present a diagnostic dilemma for clinicians and pathologists. Several clinical items enable to subclassify neck cyst as age at presentation, anatomical location, including compartments and fascia of the neck, and radiological presentation. Summary: this review will briefly describe the clinical, imaging, pathological and management features of (I) congenital and developmental pathologies, including thyroglossal duct cyst, branchial cleft cysts, dermoid cyst, thymic cyst, and ectopic thymus; (II) vascular malformations, including lymphangioma. Key Messages: pathologists should be familiar with the diagnostic features and clinicopathologic entities of these neck lesions in order to correctly diagnose them and to provide proper clinical management.

Keywords: congenital cystic mass; pediatrics; cervical cyst; cervical malformation

1. Introduction

Congenital cystic masses of the pediatric neck can be broadly divided into medial and lateral lesions [1]. Medial lesions include thyroglossal duct cysts, dermoid cysts and bronchogenic cysts. Lateral lesions include branchial cleft cysts, lymphangiomas and thymic cysts. As most congenital lesions manifest during infancy and early childhood, the patient's age provides important diagnostic information. A painless soft or fluctuant cervical mass is the first clinical manifestation in most cases. Following physical examination, ultrasonography (US) is usually performed, defining the size and extent of the mass, demonstrating its relationship to surrounding normal structures, and confirming the cystic nature of the lesion. Computed tomography (CT) and magnetic resonance imaging (MRI) can then provide additional useful clinical information [2].

The aim of this review is to briefly describe each of the above entities in order to provide the clinician and the pathologist with the relevant clinical and pathological characteristics.

2. Details and Discussion

The range of pathology seen in the neck region is very wide and to a large extent probably mirrors the complex signaling pathways and careful orchestration of events occurring during the development of this region. As is true of pediatric pathology on general pathology, within this age group is as diverse as its adult counterpart. Cases that come across the pediatric neck surgical pathology bench are more heavily weighted toward developmental and congenital lesions.

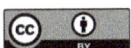

We report on the clinical presentation, diagnostic evaluation and therapeutic management of cystic lesions of the neck. Congenital cystic masses of the neck include thyroglossal duct cysts, branchial cleft cysts, lymphangioma, dermoid/epidermoid cysts, thymic and bronchogenic cysts (visceral cysts). These lesions vary in prevalence from common (thyroglossal duct cysts, branchial cleft cysts, and lymphangioma) to very rare (thymic cysts and cervical bronchogenic cysts). The vast majority of these cysts are benign in nature, unlike what is observed in adults.

The evaluation of a patient suspected of having a congenital cervical cystic mass should follow an orderly progression [3]. The clinical history and physical examination of the patient are the most important factors in the evaluation of a congenital neck mass. An appropriate knowledge of the embryology and anatomy of the cervical region frequently allows the differential diagnosis to be narrowed.

An algorithm of the decision behind cervical cysts in the pediatric population is proposed (Figure 1).

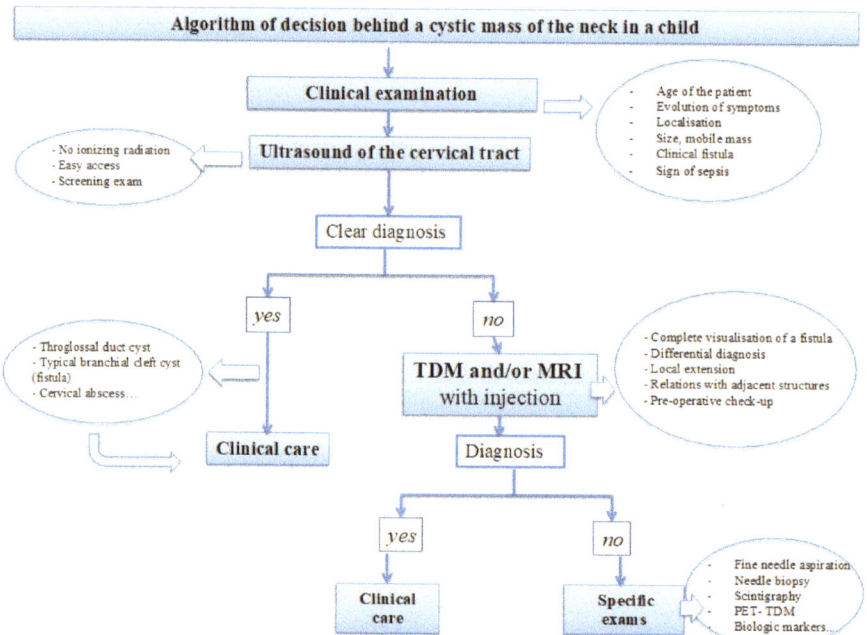

Figure 1. Diagnostic algorithm with the different steps depending on clinical examination and imaging.

The patient's age and location of the cyst provide important diagnostic information. A painless soft or fluctuant cervical mass is the first clinical manifestation in most cases. These lesions are usually slow-growing masses and typically cause symptoms due to enlargement or infection. Congenital "benign" lesions can sometimes cause significant morbidity and even mortality if they compress the airway or other vital structures.

Following physical examination, ultrasonography (US) is the most frequently used imaging modality due to its accessibility and absence of ionizing radiation. US helps to define the size and extent of the mass, demonstrates its relationship to surrounding normal structures, and confirms the cystic nature of the lesion. US may be sufficient if diagnosis is clear and in adequation with clinical presentation, typically for most thyroglossal duct cyst and branchial cleft cysts with cutaneous fistulization. Computed tomography (CT) also provides this information and is ideally suited for the evaluation of soft tissue adjacent to larger masses that cannot be entirely visualized with US. Moreover, CT is superior for detecting calcification and, when contrast material is administered, the vascularity of lesions. Magnetic resonance (mass MR) imaging, with its multiplanar capability and superior contrast resolution, demonstrates the full extent of the mass and gives important additional information for accurate preoperative planning. This can be especially relevant in cases of extension into the mediastinum or deep spaces of the neck. Furthermore, MR imaging offers superior resolution for evaluating masses located in anatomically complex areas, such as the floor of the mouth [2].

Malignant neoplastic lesions originating from these cervical cysts are very rare and arise in association with a heterotopic tissue. However, despite the rarity of malignant cystic cervical masses in children, it remains crucial to remain very careful with differential diagnosis. One should always suspect malignancy behind heterogeneous mass with solid and cystic components or equivocal clinical and radiological presentation [4].

The purpose of this review is to present the clinical, pathological, and radiological features of the most common congenital cystic lesions of the neck, emphasizing their embryologic origin, and the differential diagnosis.

We will discuss the details of the different congenital cystic lesions of the neck, emphasizing their embryologic origin, the clinical and radiologic findings, the gross and histopathologic features, the differential diagnosis, and their management. All these items are summed up in Tables 1 and 2.

2.1. Thyroglossal Duct Cyst

In the embryo, the primitive thyroid gland begins as a ventral diverticulum arising in the floor of the embryologic pharynx, between the tuberculum impar and the copula, which later forms the foramen cecum located at the base of the tongue. The thyroid then descends caudally in close relation to the hyoid bone before reaching its final position in the midline of the neck below the level of the cricoid cartilage. The resulting thyroglossal duct tract normally atrophies by the 10th week of gestation. Thyroglossal duct cysts result from failure of the complete obliteration of the thyroglossal duct tract, and can be located anywhere along the descent of the thyroid gland.

2.1.1. Clinical Findings

A thyroglossal duct cyst is the most common congenital neck mass and the second most common of all childhood cervical neck masses. Most are diagnosed at or before 10 years of age. They can occur anywhere along the thyroglossal duct tract but are most commonly found below the hyoid bone, displaying upwards displacement with tongue protrusion and swallowing. The cysts are usually a few centimeters in diameter and are round and smooth on palpation (Figure 2A).

Table 1. Congenital cystic masses (CCM) of the neck: frequency, location, clinical and radiologic presentation, associated syndromes and treatment.

Types of Cyst	Frequency	Usual Location	Most Common Clinical Features	Imaging Presentation	Associated Syndromes	Treatment
First branchial cleft	Second most common branchial cleft anomaly (4 to 10% of branchial cysts)	Type I, periauricular Type II, periparotid or submandibular area	Otalgia, otorrhea, parotidis, recurrent abscess at the angle of the mandible or submandibular area	CT and MRI: - superficial/deep to the parotid gland cyst - with/without EAC communication	None	Complete surgical excision
Second branchial cleft	Most common branchial cleft anomaly (80 to 95% of branchial cysts)	Lateral neck anterior to sternocleido-mastoid	Fluctuant neck mass +/− pain (when upper respiratory tract infection occurs)	Unilocular cyst, well circumscribed, homogeneous	- Branchio-oto-renal - Branchio-oculo-facial	Complete surgical excision
Third/Fourth branchial cleft	Rare (1 to 8% of branchial cysts)	Left sided predominance (97%), lower anterior neck, can be in close association to thyroid gland	Slight female preponderance Lower neck lateral cyst May present as thyroiditis	Unilocular cyst	None	Complete surgical excision
Thyroglossal duct	First common midline cyst (70% of midline CCM)	Midline fluctuant neck mass, in close relation to the hyoid bone	Asymptomatic palpable midline neck mass with movement during swallowing or tongue protrusion Pain if infected, dyspnea and/or dysphagia if large	Juxta/infrahyoid cyst that may cross the hyoid bone	Cowden	Sistrunk procedure
Dermoid	Second common midline neck cyst (25% of midline CCM)	Involving the neck: midline neck mass Involving the face: nasal or palpebral region	Midline neck mass, may be associated with a tuft of hair	MRI: variable signal intensity based on their protein/lipid/keratin content	Gardner	Complete surgical excision
Thymic	Rare 2 to 13y (1% of CCM) More common in males	Left neck, anterio-lateral with/without extension into the mediastinum	- Asymptomatic or - Upper respiratory infection, hoarseness, wheezing, coughing, dysphagia, and even respiratory distress	- Elongated, unilocular cyst - MRI > CT scan	- Branchio-oculo-facial	Complete surgical excision

Table 1. Cont.

Types of Cyst	Frequency	Usual Location	Most Common Clinical Features	Imaging Presentation	Associated Syndromes	Treatment
Broncho-genic	Very rare. More common in males	Suprasternal notch or supraclavicular area	Asymptomatic swelling	- Tubular pattern anterior to the trachea - Air within the lesion if infected	None	Complete surgical excision
Lymphatic mal-formation	Very common (20% of pediatric cervical masses)	Commonly in the posterior triangle or in the submandibular space	- Soft, painless and compressible mass, - Growing slowly, quickly if secondary to hemorrhage or infection	- Multilocular predominantly cystic mass - With septa of variable thickness	- Turner - Noonan - Trisomy 13, 18, 21 - Cowchock Wapner Kurtz	- Steroids, antibiotics - Laser, sclero-therapy, radio-frequency ablation - Surgical excision

EAC, external auditory canal; y, years; CCM, congenital cystic mass.

Table 2. Congenital cystic masses of the neck: gross, histologic examination and differential diagnoses.

Types of Cyst	Histologic Examination	Differential Diagnosis
First branchial cleft	- Type 1, lined by squamous epithelium - Type 2, containing skin adnexa and cartilage - Lymphoid tissue absent, unless inflammation or infection	- Dermoid cyst - Epidermic cyst - Teratoma
Second branchial cleft	- Lined by squamous epithelium (90%) or ciliated columnar epithelium (8%) and rarely by both types of epithelium (2%) - Occasionally present: salivary tissue, sebaceous glands, and cholesterol clefts with a foreign body reaction - Nodular or diffuse lymphoid tissue.	- Epidermic cyst - Dermoid cyst - Teratoma - Bronchogenic cyst
Third/Fourth branchial cleft	- Lined by squamous epithelium or ciliated columnar epithelium and rarely by both types of epithelium - Lymphoid infiltrate - Thymic tissue - Parathyroid and thyroid gland	- Lymphoepithelial cyst - Lymphadenitis - Lymphoma

Table 2. Cont.

Types of Cyst	Histologic Examination	Differential Diagnosis
Thyro-glossal duct	- Unilocular/multilocular - Lined by stratified squamous epithelium at upper part; ciliated pseudostratified columnar epithelium at lower part; Stratified cuboidal epithelium at level of hyoid bone. - Mucous glands (salivary-type). - Ectopic thyroid follicles along the course of the duct in up to 62% of cases, ectopic parathyroid; adnexal skin structures, cartilage. - Denuded epithelium and secondary inflammation (lymphocytes, neutrophils, granulation tissue, cholesterol granuloma and fibrosis).	- Epidermic cyst - Dermoid cyst - Ectopic thyroid - Teratoma - Branchial cleft cyst - Bronchogenic cyst - Lymphoepithelial cyst - Lymph node metastasis of papillary thyroid carcinoma with cystic degeneration
Dermoid	- Unilocular - Lined by keratinized squamous epithelium with a granular layer, filled with lamellate keratin. - In case of dermoid cyst, hair follicles and sebaceous glands, eccrine sweat glands in 35%, apocrine glands in 15%, occasionally smooth muscle	Sebaceous cyst Dermoid teratoma Follicular cyst Steatocystoma Vellus hair cyst
Thymic	- Unilocular - Thin wall with a few layers of bland squamoid or cuboidal cells - Thymic tissue in wall	- Acquired thymic cyst (Sjögren) - Lymphatic vascular malformation - Thyroid tumors
Broncho-genic	- Unilocular or multilocular - Lined by columnar, ciliated, pseudostratified epithelial. Squamous metaplasia in previously infected cyst - Blood vessels, hyaline cartilage, smooth muscles, sero-mucinous glands, and elastic fibers in the cyst wall.	- Branchial cysts - Thyroglossal duct cyst - Teratoma - Tracheal diverticulum

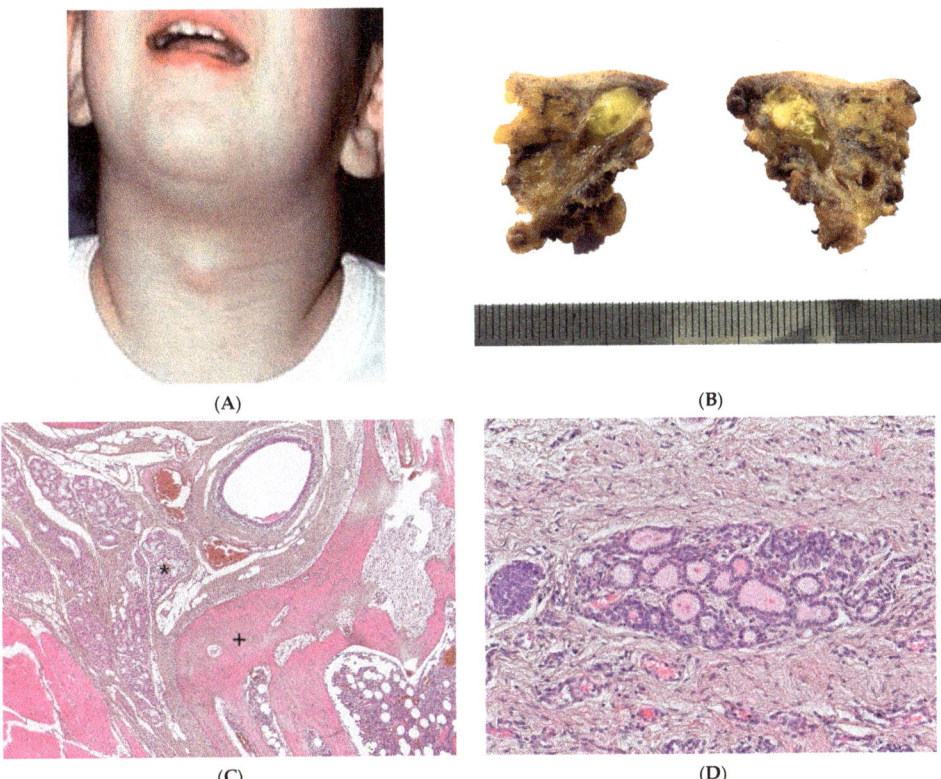

Figure 2. Thyroglossal duct cyst. (**A**) Clinical examination: typical picture of a non-infected thyroglossal duct cyst presenting as a midline neck mass. (**B**) Gross examination: cystic lumen filled with gelatinous and inflammatory material. (**C**) (H.E.S). Small cystic structure lined by ciliated pseudostratified columnar epithelium; mucous glands (*) on the left; hyoid bone (+) on the right, in close relation to the cyst. (**D**) (H.E.S), ectopic thyroid follicles in the cystic wall.

Thyroglossal duct cysts are often asymptomatic. If very large, dysphagia may be present. Infection may occur, often in conjunction with upper respiratory tract infections, and can cause painful cystic enlargement, abscess development or rupture with cutaneous sinus formation.

The main clinical differential diagnosis includes dermoid cyst, ectopic or lingual thyroid and lymphadenopathy. Ultrasonography is the first line radiological assessment tool, followed by magnetic resonance imaging (MRI).

Heterotopia-associated thyroid carcinoma, most often papillary thyroid carcinoma, may extremely rarely arise in thyroglossal duct cysts, with 27 case reports at a mean age of 12 years of age. The prognosis remains excellent. All carcinomas have been discovered after surgical excision.

2.1.2. Gross and Histopathological Features

A thyroglossal duct cyst usually corresponds to a single cyst, typically less than 2 cm in size, filled with mucoid, squamous or purulent material (Figure 2B). It may also be composed of several smaller cysts that are sometimes difficult to identify macroscopically. Occasionally, when inflammatory processes are prominent, no residual cystic space may be clearly identified.

In non-inflamed cysts, the cyst lining is ciliated pseudostratified columnar and/or squamous epithelium. Small cystic structures might only be noted in close relation to the hyoid bone, which must be sampled (Figure 2C). Ectopic normal thyroid tissue in the cyst wall can be found in 50 to 70% of cases, varying with sampling by the pathologist (Figure 2D). Inflammation and foreign body giant cell reaction are commonly noted. Mucous glands may also be present. C-cells are not present in thyroglossal duct cysts due to the different embryologic origin [5–7].

2.1.3. Brief Account of Patient Management

The recommended treatment for thyroglossal duct cysts is a Sistrunk procedure, which entails complete resection of the cyst, the entire remnant thyroglossal tract stalk, and the body of the hyoid bone. Occasionally, an extension to the tongue base requiring a concomitant intra-oral surgical approach is present. This is the only accepted surgical procedure to limit complications (1%) and recurrence (3%).

2.2. Branchial Cleft Cysts

Branchial cleft cysts are the second most common congenital neck masses in the pediatric population. Branchial cleft anomalies are congenital malformations related to embryological developmental alterations of the branchial apparatus resulting in cysts (no opening), sinuses (single opening to skin or digestive tract) or fistulas (opening to both skin and digestive tract) [8].

The branchial apparatus first appears in the developing embryo at 4 weeks. It consists of six paired mesodermal arches, separated internally by endoderm making up the four pharyngeal pouches, and externally by ectoderm making up the four branchial clefts. The first four arches proliferate, and the last two become rudimentary. Each arch and cleft give rise to its own cartilaginous, muscular, vascular, glandular, and neural components [9].

Branchial cleft cysts are clinically divided into first, second, third or fourth branchial cleft cysts, depending on the anatomical location of the lesion. This stratification corresponds to the arch involved in pathogenesis. These cysts are closed structures lined by squamous epithelium.

The first branchial apparatus normally gives rise to the eustachian tube, the tympanic cavity, the mastoid antrum, a portion of the tympanic membrane, the external auditory canal (EAC), the mandible, the maxilla, and the mall eus and incus. For this reason, first branchial cleft cysts, which represent the second most common branchial cleft anomaly accounting for less than 10% of all branchial cleft defects, can arise anywhere from the external auditory canal through the parotid gland to the submandibular triangle [10].

Two types of first branchial cleft cysts have been described: type I (Figure 3A), periauricular, of ectodermal origin, corresponding to a duplicated EAC and type II (Figure 3B), periparotid, of both ectodermal and mesodermal origin, containing skin and cartilage. An important anatomical difference of clinical and surgical importance is that the cystic tract of type I cysts passes lateral (superior) to the seventh cranial nerve, whereas in type II cysts the tract passes medial (inferior) to the seventh cranial nerve.

Lesions of the second branchial arch are by far the most common branchial anomaly, accounting for 67–93% of cases. Clinically, these cysts are present in the lateral neck, along the anterior border of the sternocleidomastoid muscle. The fistula pathway begins in the lateral neck, runs in between the external and internal carotid arteries, deep to cranial nerve 7 and superficial to cranial nerves 9 and 12, with an internal opening at the level of the oropharynx [11].

Third/fourth branchial cleft anomalies are excessively rare, rendering distinction between these two identities challenging. Anomalies usually manifest themselves as a sinus tract rather than a cyst or fistula. The cysts appear in the lower neck, predominantly left-sided due to the asymmetric development of the vascular structures (on the left, the aortic arch, and on the right, the proximal subclavian artery). Sinuses and fistulas have an internal opening at the level of the piriform sinus [12,13].

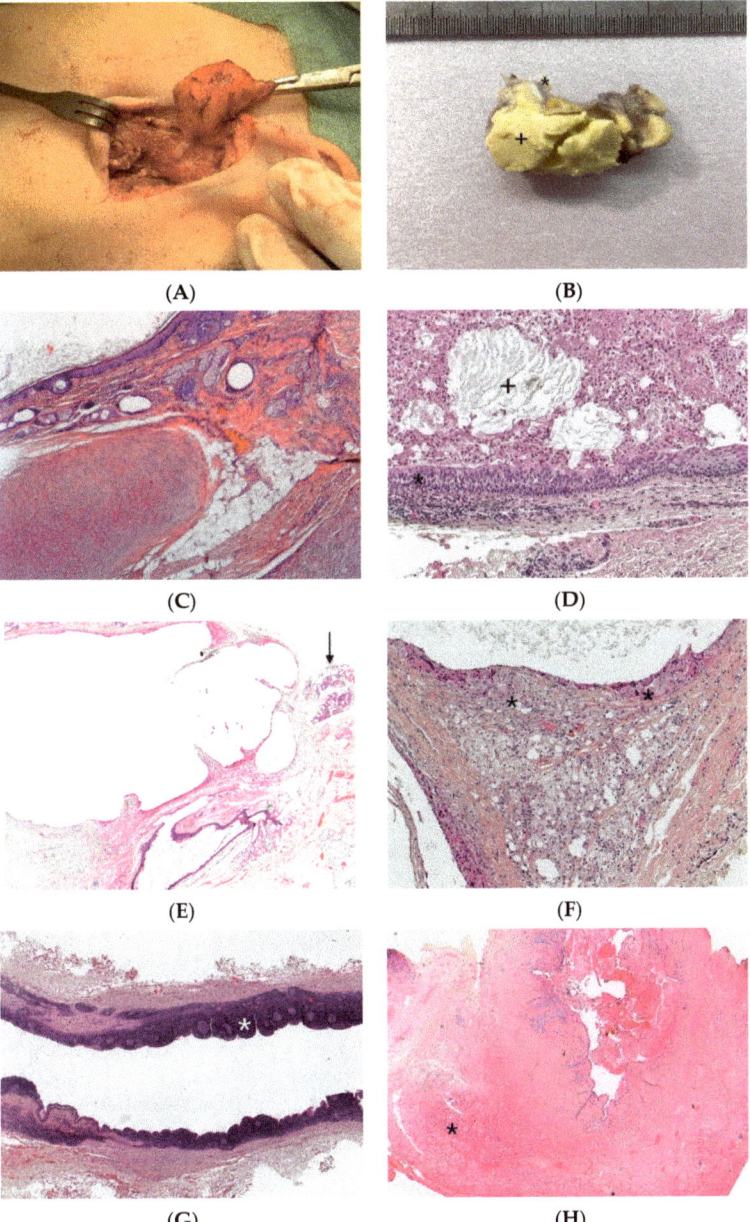

Figure 3. Branchial cleft cysts. First branchial cleft cyst (**A**), operating view. Periauricular type I cyst (**B**), gross examination. Cartilage (*) and necrosis (+) are visible. Periparotid type II with inflammatory changes (**C**) (H.E.S). lined by squamous epithelium and containing cartilage (**D**) (H.E.S). Lined by squamous epithelium and ciliated columnar epithelium (*). The lumen contains macrophages and squamous debris (+) (**E**) (H.E.S), located within the parotid gland (at the upper part, arrow), mainly denuded due to inflammatory changes (**F**) (H.E.S). The epithelial border is mainly replaced by foreign body giant cells (*). Lipid-laden macrophages are observed in the cyst wall and squamous debris within the cyst lumen. Second branchial fistula (**G**) (H.E.S), lined by respiratory epithelium and confluent lymphoid follicles (*). Fourth branchial fistula (**H**) (H.E.S). The wall of the fistula contains thyroid tissue (*).

2.2.1. Clinical Findings

Classical branchial anomalies are usually isolated. Cysts present as nontender, fluctuant masses, which may become infected and lead to abscess formation. Sinuses and fistulas may be associated with discharge of mucoid and/or purulent secretions from the internal and/or external tract opening.

Differential diagnosis may be challenging between infected branchial cyst and a cervical lymphadenopathy. Anatomical localization should be carefully detailed. Moreover, recurrent or persistent cervical "nodal" mass should raise the question of an underneath branchial cleft cyst and US is usually helpful to clarify the diagnosis.

Precise topographic anatomical assessment allows to define which branchial arch is involved and therefore to diagnose the cyst type. As previously mentioned, first branchial cleft cysts are present in the preauricular or submandibular region, second branchial cleft cysts along the anterior border of the sternocleidomastoid muscle, and third/fourth branchial cleft cysts in the lower neck. Given the close association between third/fourth branchial cleft anomalies and the thyroid gland, an infection can present itself as acute suppurative thyroiditis.

In terms of imaging, US is the initial investigation of choice. CT scan and MRI scan can also aid in diagnosis and precise surgical mapping. When uncomplicated, they are typically visualized as well delineated cystic structures appearing centrally hypoechoic on US with posterior acoustic enhancement. Their US appearances can vary, however, sometimes appearing multilocular with septations, inhomogeneous or even solid. They are uniformly hypodense on CT and can demonstrate the 'notch' or 'beak sign' between the internal and external carotid arteries. MRI can help in determining the presence and path of sinus formation and presence of inflammatory changes within the adjacent soft tissues. Bilaterality is rare (only 2% to 3%) and often associated with familial predisposition [14].

Branchio-oto-renal syndrome (BOR) may be suspected based on family history, or when second branchial arch anomalies are clinically associated with deafness, pre-auricular pits, auricular malformation and/or renal anomalies (malformations or hypoplasia). If suspected, audiology workup and renal US should be performed. BOR syndrome is inherited in an autosomal dominant pattern, with a prevalence of 1/40,000 in Western countries and results from a mutation in the *EYA1* gene [15,16].

2.2.2. Histopathological Features

Branchial cleft cysts are usually lined by squamous epithelium (90%) or ciliated columnar epithelium (8%) and rarely by both types of epithelia (2%) (Figure 3C,D). Occasionally, the cyst is denudated (Figure 3E) or lined by cholesterol clefts with a foreign body reaction (Figure 3F) due to inflammatory changes. Lymphoid tissue is generally identified (Figure 3G). Salivary tissue, sebaceous glands as well as thyroid tissue may be present (Figure 3H). An ectopic or undescended parathyroid gland may be associated with third/fourth branchial cleft anomalies, since parathyroid glands embryologically arise from these branchial arches. Parathyroid adenomas have also been reported in association with branchial cleft cysts.

2.2.3. Brief Account of Patient Management

Complete surgical excision is undertaken in order to avoid infection and prevent recurrence. This includes a complete excision of the cyst as well as any sinuses or fistulous tracts. Given the various communication patterns of these anomalies, a combined approach is commonly used including a mix of endaural, trans-cervical, trans-parotid and intra-oral/intra-laryngeal (endoscopic) routes.

2.3. Lymphatic Malformations

Lymphatic malformations are thought to arise from the early sequestration of embryonic lymphatic channels. There are three main types of lymphatic malformations: microcystic (<2 mL, occurring mostly above the level of the mylohyoid muscle, commonly involving the oral cavity), macrocystic (≥1 cyst, ≥2 mL in size, occurring below the level of the mylohyoid muscle) and mixed (by far the most common, also referred to as lymphangioma, formerly called cystic hygroma). Lymphatic malformations constitute about 5% of all benign tumors of infancy and childhood. The sequestration of lymphatic channels occurs more commonly in the developing jugular lymph sac pair than in the other four embryonic sites of lymphatic system development. From this location, the sequestered site follows the path of the surrounding mesenchyme destined for either the neck or the developing mediastinum. Therefore, these lesions tend to occur in the neck, axilla, and upper mediastinum.

2.3.1. Clinical Findings

The overwhelming majority (about 80–90%) are diagnosed by the time the patient turns 2 years old, the age of greatest lymphatic growth. No gender predilection is reported. Approximately 75–80% of lymphatic malformations involve the neck and the lower third of the face. In children, the most common location is the posterior cervical space, followed by the oral cavity.

These lesions are characteristically infiltrative in nature. Consequently, they may extend inferiorly from the posterior cervical triangle into the axilla and mediastinum or anteriorly into the floor of the mouth and the tongue. If the mass is very large, it may extend across the midline. Only 3–10% of cervical lymphatic malformations are associated with extension into the mediastinum.

Most patients are clinically asymptomatic. The lesion presents itself as a soft, painless and compressible mass in the neck. Size is extremely variable. Very large masses may cause dysphagia or dyspnea by extrinsic compression. The lesion may become painful or enlarge rapidly from acute spontaneous hemorrhage or infection. Disfigurement may also be a significant concern.

They may be associated with chromosomal defects, such as Turner's syndrome, Trisomy 13, 18 and 21 as well as Noonan syndrome. Additional investigations by means of amniocentesis are therefore indicated when detected on antenatal US.

2.3.2. Histopathological Features

Lymphatic malformations are composed of multiple dilated cystic spaces separated by minimal intervening stroma (Figure 4A). The cysts vary in diameter from a few millimeters to more than 10 cm, and most contain chylous fluid, a variable number of lymphocytes and/or macrophages, and occasional erythrocytes. These thin-walled spaces are lined by endothelial cells and supporting connective tissue stroma. Focally disorganized smooth muscle is present in the wall of larger channels. Lesions may extend into adjacent soft tissues, invade into muscle, and surround vascular structures.

The macrocystic type is defined by collections of large interconnected lymphatic cisterns; some vessels may have a relatively thick but incomplete smooth muscular lining. Mural lymphoid aggregates are commonly present and help distinguish these lesions from venous malformations.

The microcystic type is comprised of smaller lymphatic channels that may interdigitate between local tissue elements. In superficial lesions, these often protrude into and expand dermal or mucosal papillae, forming lymph-filled vesicles.

An immunohistochemical panel consisting of D2-40 (more consistent staining of small versus large lymphatic channels), Prospero-related homeobox gene-1 (*Prox-1*), vascular endothelial growth factor receptor 3 (VEGFR3), CD31, and CD34 antibodies allows the differentiation of lymphatic malformations from venous ones in pathologic practice (Figure 4B,C) [17,18].

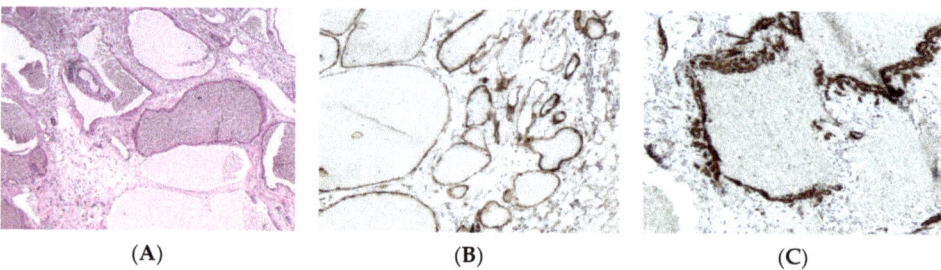

Figure 4. Lymphatic malformation. (**A**), (H.E.S). Collection of large interconnected lymphatic cisterns. Small lymphoid aggregates are also present (at the upper left quarter). (**B**), (D2-40). Positive cytoplasmic immunostaining of endothelial cells. (**C**), (smooth muscle actin). Positive cytoplasmic immunostaining of disorganized smooth muscle in the wall of larger channels.

2.3.3. Brief Account of Patient Management

MRI is the diagnostic investigation of choice. If the lesion is asymptomatic, watchful waiting for spontaneous regression may be considered. Medical treatment includes antibiotics if the cyst is superinfected and corticosteroids as needed. Non-surgical treatment remedies include sclerotherapy (with either alcohol, bleomycin or picibanil), radiofrequency ablation or laser therapy. Surgical resection may be considered as a last resort for macrocystic lesions but may be the only viable option for microcystic lesions given that the cysts are too small for sclerotherapy. PIK3CA is known to play a role in regulating cell growth by signaling through the PI3K/mTOR pathway. Medical therapy with the drugs sirolimus or sildenafil can be used to treat both localized and diffuse lymphatic malformations [19].

2.4. Dermoid Cyst

Dermoid cysts are congenital masses that result from the sequestration of cutaneous tissues along embryonal fusion lines. They are composed of ectodermal and mesodermal elements only, including epidermal appendages such as hair follicles and sebaceous glands. This is in contrast to teratoid cyst, which are composed of all three embryonic layers (endodermal derivatives, e.g., gastrointestinal or respiratory mucosa or smooth muscle), and epidermoid cysts, composed of ectodermal elements only (without epidermal appendages).

2.4.1. Clinical Findings

Dermoid cysts are present at birth and may grow slowly thereafter or remain stable in size. Most cysts are subcutaneous and recognized in children younger than 5 years old. Dermoid cysts may occur anywhere in the body, with 50% presenting in the head and neck area (30% face and 20% neck). Nasal and palpebral sites are most common in the face. In the neck, the midline location is very characteristic of the diagnosis and may be associated with a tuft of hair. Diagnosis is made by excisional biopsy.

Given the midline location, differential diagnosis includes thyroglossal duct cyst. In contrast to thyroglossal duct cysts, dermoid cysts are smaller in size, perfectly round, more superficial (subcutaneous, superficial to strap muscles) and do not move with swallowing. Submental localization raises specific differential diagnosis: ranula is usually developed on the buccal floor but can expand to posterior part of mylohyoid muscle. Anatomical localization and extension of the cyst should be finely analyzed in order not to ignore such lesion due to salivary retention [20].

2.4.2. Histopathological Features

At gross examination, the cyst has yellowish-white keratinous material and might reach 12 cm in size. They are lined by stratified squamous epithelium with associated small hair follicles and sebaceous glands (Figure 5A,B). Eccrine sweat glands and apocrine glands are less commonly present. The cavity contains laminated keratin and numerous vellus hairs oriented haphazardly (Figure 5C). Acute inflammation may result in the subsequent disruption of the cyst wall, with the development of an intense foreign body giant cell reaction (Figure 5D).

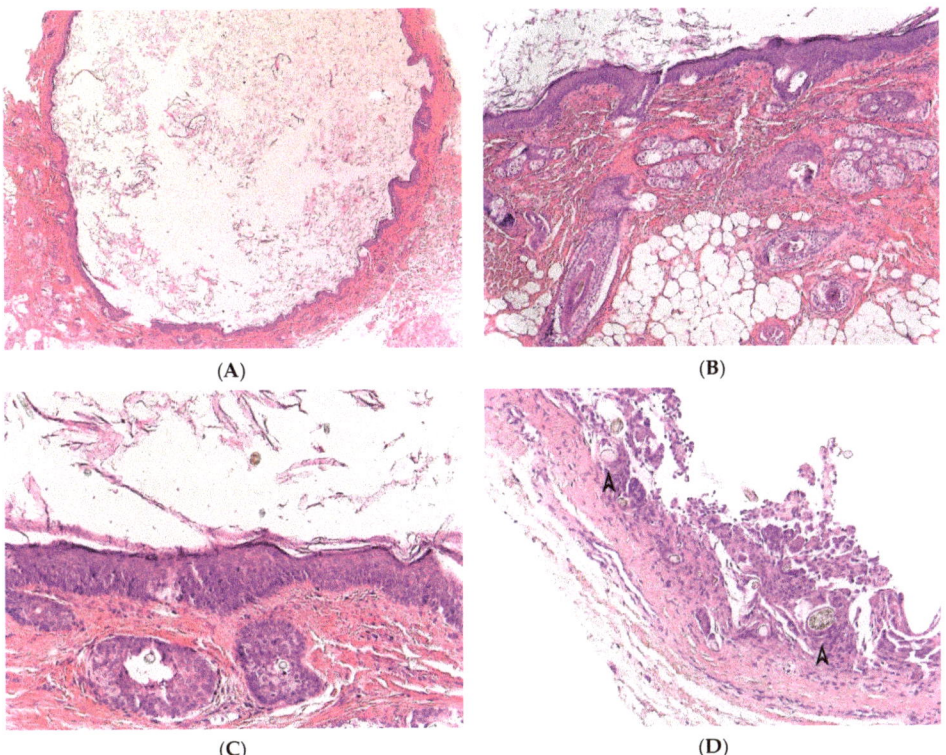

Figure 5. Dermoid cyst. (**A**) (H.E.S). The cyst is lined by keratinizing stratified squamous epithelium. (**B**) (H.E.S). The cyst is deeply located in the subcutis. Small hair follicles and sebaceous glands are attached to the epithelium. (**C**) (H.E.S). The lumen contains numerous vellus hair shafts and lamellated keratin, and the epithelium has a granular layer. (**D**), (H.E.S). Several vellus hairs (arrowheads) are observed within the granuloma.

2.4.3. Brief Account of Patient Management

The treatment of neck dermoid cysts involves complete surgical excision of the lesion [21,22].

2.5. *Thymic Cyst*

Cervical thymic cysts and ectopic thymus are extremely rare entities, with only about 100 cases reported in the literature [23]. However, the presence of asymptomatic thymic tissue in the neck is much more common, with a reported incidence of 30% in children at autopsy. They therefore represent less than 1% of cystic cervical masses. They are thought to arise due to the persistence of the embryonic thymopharyngeal ducts, derived from the ventral surface of the third pharyngeal pouch during the sixth week of intrauterine life. Failure of these ducts to regress during the eighth week of development can cause cervical thymic cysts to form.

They can arise anywhere along the descent of the thymic primordia from the mandible to the mediastinum [24]. They are most commonly found in the left neck, anterior to the sternocleidomastoid muscle, with approximately 50% showing extension into the superior mediastinum. They are most commonly present during the first decade of life, with a slight preponderance towards males.

2.5.1. Clinical Findings

Cervical thymic cysts are painless neck masses that can present suddenly in children, or in association with cutaneous pharyngeal defects and ocular and facial anomalies as in branchio-oculo-facial syndrome (BOFS), an autosomal-dominant transmitted disorder with mutations in the *TFAP2A* gene. The presence of an ectopic thymus (dermal) can justify a BOFS diagnosis [25].

2.5.2. Histopathological Features

The cystic fluid may be clear, yellow, brown, green, or even purulent. The diagnosis is established by histologic demonstration of residual thymic tissue showing Hassall's corpuscles and cortico-medullary differentiation (Figure 6A). The cyst wall lining may be spindle, cuboidal, or columnar, stratified or pseudostratified, ciliated or non-ciliated (Figure 6B). Cholesterol crystals, giant cells, histiocytes, inflammatory cells, and hemosiderin have also been described.

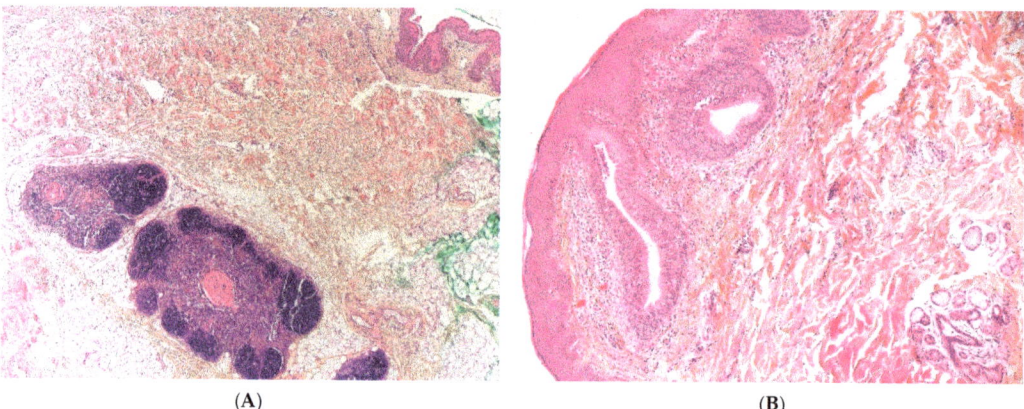

Figure 6. Thymic cyst. (**A**), (H.E.S). Mature thymic tissue showing Hassall's corpuscles (arrow) and cortico-medullary differentiation and arranged in lobules at the hypodermis. The overlying dermis is devoid of adnexa and replaced by scar-like fibrous tissue. (**B**), (H.E.S). Ductal-like structures (arrow) opening at the surface of the skin, lined by a columnar, pseudostratified epithelium (at the left, half part).

Congenital thymic cysts should be differentiated from multilocular thymic cyst, as the latter represents an acquired, multilocular, inflammatory lesion arising from cystic dilatation of the medullary duct and associated with autoimmune diseases, such as Sjogren's syndrome and aplastic anemia. These acquired thymic cysts are lined by squamoid, cuboidal, columnar, micropapillary or mixed glandular epithelium, and can present with pseudo-epitheliomatous hyperplasia. Secondary inflammation is commonly found but no cartilage or smooth muscle can be identified [26].

2.5.3. Brief Account of Patient Management

Complete surgical excision, even with asymptomatic lesions, is used for diagnosis and treatment. Confirmation of the presence of mediastinal thymic tissue should be performed prior to the removal of thymic cysts or ectopic thymic tissue to prevent immunocompromise.

2.6. Bronchogenic Cyst

Bronchogenic cysts correspond to embryonic foregut abnormalities arising from aberrant budding of the tracheobronchial tree. These cysts predominantly appear in the mediastinum, especially the hilar or middle-mediastinal area. The anatomical presentation may vary, from the midline subcutaneous region of the suprasternal area to beneath the diaphragm. Cutaneous bronchogenic cysts are often supra-sternal.

2.6.1. Clinical Findings

Bronchogenic cysts are often incidentally found in children and later in life. The volume usually increases with age, with the diameter ranging from 1 to 4 cm in infants. Bronchogenic cysts are usually sporadic. They are encountered predominantly within the mediastinum or the lung parenchyma and, in few instances, within the neck. Symptoms secondary to infection may occur, such as fever, hemorrhage or perforation. Bronchogenic cysts may be compressive in infants and responsible for respiratory distress. They are, however, not connected to the respiratory tract. Clinical differential diagnosis includes esophageal and enteric duplication cysts and pericardial cysts [27,28]. Diagnosis is often performed with histological analysis because of poorly specific clinical presentation: midline cyst also raise differential diagnosis as thyroglossal duct cyst, dermoid cyst, vascular malformation or thymic cervical cyst.

2.6.2. Histopathological Features

The bronchogenic cyst presents itself as an extrapulmonary unilocular cyst. The lumen contains fluid, turbid, mucinous or purulent material. Its wall is lined by respiratory epithelium overlying fibromuscular connective tissue containing seromucinous glands and cartilage plates (Figure 7A,B). Squamous metaplasia may occur. The presence of cartilage tissue is important for establishing the final diagnosis and differentiating between bronchogenic cysts and other cysts of the neck [27,29].

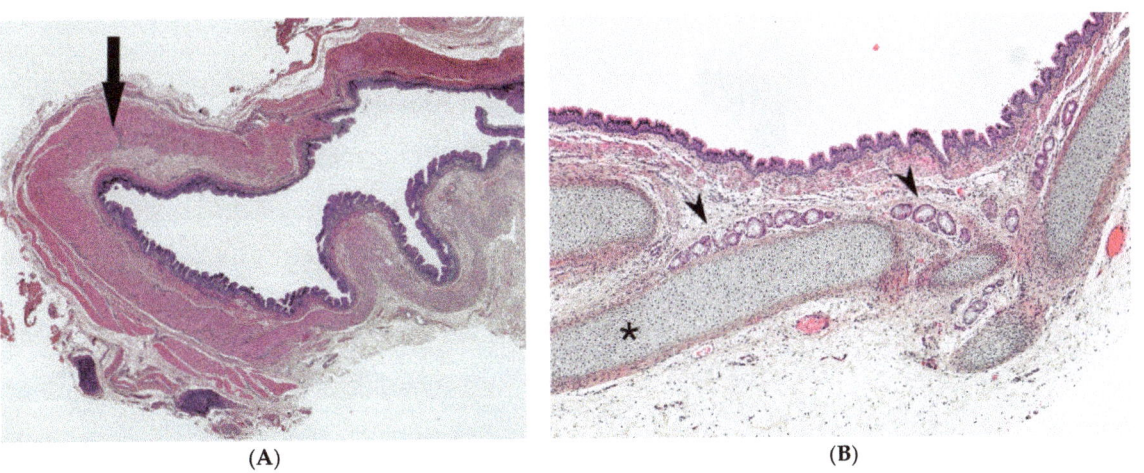

Figure 7. Bronchogenic cyst. (**A**), (H.E.S). unilocular cyst lined by respiratory epithelium overlying circular muscular tunic (arrow). (**B**), (H.E.S.). In the wall, seromucous glands (arrowheads) and cartilage plates (*).

2.6.3. Brief Account of Patient Management

Surgical excision is usually necessary to confirm the diagnosis and avoid infection or hemorrhage. Bronchogenic cysts have no malignant potential.

2.7. Risk of Malignancy

Rare cases of malignant transformations are described at the level of congenital cystic formations. The risk of carcinomatous degeneration of the thyroglossal tract cyst is less than 1%, most often affecting the adults. Of the 180 cases reported in the literature, 21 concerned children under 18 years of age with only one case in a 6-year-old child. Most of these lesions were histologic findings following cyst removal surgery with a pathologic diagnosis of papillary carcinoma [30]. Carcinomas developed on congenital branchial cysts are also described. The reported cases concern adults and the distinction between primary carcinoma developed on an underlying congenital branchial cyst and cystic metastasis from oropharyngeal cancer remains controversial [31–33].

We would like to highlight the role of initial clinical and radiological evaluation in order not to miss malignant lesions. Radiological heterogenous aspect with even a minor solid component associated to cystic component should raise attention and lead to the realization of a biopsy. Malignant tumors may be misleading and neuroblastoma, yolk sac tumor or embryonal rhabdomyosarcoma can present with partial cystic component.

3. Conclusions

When evaluating a cystic lesion of the neck in children, understanding the morphologic embryology, anatomy, clinical features, and gross/histopathologic features is critical to diagnosis.

The diagnosis of a cervical mass in a child is usually suspected based on clinical examination data. The age of the child (infant or child) and the localization of the mass (median, lateral or parotid) are extremely important elements of orientation. The relative frequency of different types of cervical cysts has also to be considered. Branchial cleft cysts are the most frequent cervical cysts and represent approximately 20% of all cervical masses in children.

Ultrasound, an easy-to-perform, non-irradiating examination that does not require sedation, is a supplement; it clarifies the anatomical situation, differentiates cystic transsonic lesions from solid echogenic lesions. Most of the time, clinical examination and US are sufficient for clear identification and correct treatment of the cervical cyst.

Large predominance of benign cystic lesions does not rule out the possibility of any rare malignancies associated with a cystic presentation. These tumors have a solid component which must not be ignored on radiological examination. These situations account for rare indications of fine needle aspiration or needle biopsy in order to perform right treatment.

Finally, correct identification of these benign lesions may have additional interest in identifying or implementing the description of a genetic predisposing syndrome or chromosomal defect. Lymphatic vascular malformations, for example, may be associated with chromosomal defects.

Research on the molecular embryology of craniofacial development in the coming years should begin to shed light on the pathogenesis of lesions and syndromes of craniofacial development.

Author Contributions: A.F., G.M., M.F. and L.G.-R. contributed equally to the acquisition, analysis and interpretation of data for this review, participated in original draft preparation. A.F. provided the clinical findings, management data, clinical and operating views. M.F. and L.G.-R. were responsible for the histopathological results, photomicrographs, tables and discussion of differential diagnoses. G.M. and V.C. participated in original draft preparation, revising tables and conclusion. All authors have read and agreed to the published version of the manuscript.

Funding: This research received no external funding.

Institutional Review Board Statement: Not applicable.

Informed Consent Statement: Not applicable.

Acknowledgments: We thanks J. Ciaran Hutchinson (Great Ormond Street Hospital for Children, London, UK).

Conflicts of Interest: The authors declare no conflict of interest.

References

1. Curtis, W.J.; Edwards, S.P. Pediatric Neck Masses. *Atlas Oral Maxillofac. Surg. Clin.* **2015**, *23*, 15–20. [CrossRef] [PubMed]
2. Friedman, E.R.; John, S.D. Imaging of Pediatric Neck Masses. *Radiol. Clin. N. Am.* **2011**, *49*, 617–632. [CrossRef] [PubMed]
3. Shengwei, H.; Zhiyong, W.; Wei, H.; Qingang, H. The Management of Pediatric Neck Masses. *J. Craniofacial Surg.* **2015**, *26*, 399–401. [CrossRef] [PubMed]
4. Goins, M.R.; Beasley, M.S. Pediatric Neck Masses. *Oral Maxillofac. Surg. Clin. N. Am.* **2012**, *24*, 457–468. [CrossRef] [PubMed]
5. Tokarz, E.; Gupta, P.; McGrath, J.; Szymanowski, A.R.; Behar, J.; Behar, P. Proposed ultrasound algorithm to differentiate thyroglossal duct and dermoid cysts. *Int. J. Pediatr. Otorhinolaryngol.* **2021**, *142*, 110624. [CrossRef]
6. Thompson, L.; Herrera, H.B.; Lau, S.K. A Clinicopathologic Series of 685 Thyroglossal Duct Remnant Cysts. *Head Neck Pathol.* **2016**, *10*, 465–474. [CrossRef]
7. Shahin, A.; Burroughs, F.H.; Kirby, J.P.; Ali, M.S.Z. Thyroglossal duct cyst: A cytopathologic study of 26 cases. *Diagn. Cytopathol.* **2005**, *33*, 365–369. [CrossRef]
8. Achard, S.; Leroy, X.; Fayoux, P. Congenital midline cervical cleft: A retrospective case series of 8 children. *Int. J. Pediatr. Otorhinolaryngol.* **2016**, *81*, 60–64. [CrossRef]
9. Adams, A.; Mankad, K.; Offiah, C.; Childs, L. Branchial cleft anomalies: A pictorial review of embryological development and spectrum of imaging findings. *Insights Imaging* **2015**, *7*, 69–76. [CrossRef]
10. Olivas, A.D.; Sherman, J.M. First branchial cleft anomalies. *Oper. Tech. Otolaryngol. Head Neck Surg.* **2017**, *28*, 151–155. [CrossRef]
11. Grohmann, N.C.; Herrington, H.C. Second branchial cleft anomalies. *Oper. Tech. Otolaryngol. Head Neck Surg.* **2017**, *28*, 156–160. [CrossRef]
12. Lee, J.W.; Funamura, J.L. Third branchial cleft anomalies. *Oper. Tech. Otolaryngol. Head Neck Surg.* **2017**, *28*, 161–166. [CrossRef]
13. Doody, J.; Sobin, L. Fourth branchial pouch or cleft anomalies. *Oper. Tech. Otolaryngol. Head Neck Surg.* **2017**, *28*, 167–172. [CrossRef]
14. Brown, R.E.; Harave, S. Diagnostic imaging of benign and malignant neck masses in children—A pictorial review. *Quant. Imaging Med. Surg.* **2016**, *6*, 591–604. [CrossRef] [PubMed]
15. Au, P.-Y.B.; Chernos, J.E.; Thomas, M.A. Review of the recurrent 8q13.2q13.3 branchio-oto-renal related microdeletion, and report of an additional case with associated distal arthrogryposis. *Am. J. Med. Genet. Part A* **2016**, *170*, 2984–2987. [CrossRef] [PubMed]
16. Newton, S.S. Thyroglossal duct cyst: Operative technique. *Oper. Tech. Otolaryngol. Head Neck Surg.* **2017**, *28*, 173–178. [CrossRef]
17. Aboutalebi, A.; Jessup, C.J.; North, P.E.; Mihm, M.C. Histopathology of Vascular Anomalies. *Facial Plast. Surg.* **2012**, *28*, 545–553. [CrossRef]
18. Castro, E.C.C.; Galambos, C. Prox-1 and VEGFR3 antibodies are superior to D2-40 in identifying endothelial cells of lymphatic malformations—A proposal of a new immunohistochemical panel to differentiate lymphatic from other vascular malformations. *Pediatr. Dev. Pathol.* **2009**, *12*, 187–194. [CrossRef]
19. Lerat, J.; Mounayer, C.; Scomparin, A.; Orsel, S.; Bessede, J.-P.; Aubry, K. Head and neck lymphatic malformation and treatment: Clinical study of 23 cases. *Eur. Ann. Otorhinolaryngol. Head Neck Dis.* **2016**, *133*, 393–396. [CrossRef] [PubMed]
20. Chorney, S.R.; Irace, A.L.; Sobin, L. Cervical dermoid cysts. *Oper. Tech. Otolaryngol. Head Neck Surg.* **2017**, *28*, 179–182. [CrossRef]
21. Orozco-Covarrubias, L.; Lara-Carpio, R.; Saez-De-Ocariz, M.; Duran-McKinster, C.; Palacios-Lopez, C.; Ruiz-Maldonado, R. Dermoid cysts: A report of 75 pediatric patients. *Pediatr. Dermatol.* **2013**, *30*, 706–711. [CrossRef]
22. Paradis, J.; Koltai, P.J. Pediatric Teratoma and Dermoid Cysts. *Otolaryngol. Clin. N. Am.* **2015**, *48*, 121–136. [CrossRef]
23. Caluwé, D.D. Cervical thymic cysts. *Pediatr. Surg. Int.* **2002**, *18*, 477–479. [CrossRef] [PubMed]
24. Statham, M.M.; Mehta, D.; Willging, J.P. Cervical thymic remnants in children. *Int. J. Pediatr. Otorhinolaryngol.* **2008**, *72*, 1807–1813. [CrossRef] [PubMed]
25. Drut, R.; Galliani, C. Thymic tissue in the skin: A clue to the diagnosis of the branchio-oculo-facial syndrome: Report of two cases. *Int. J. Surg. Pathol.* **2003**, *11*, 25–28. [CrossRef] [PubMed]
26. Sturm, J.; Dedhia, K.; Chi, D.H. Diagnosis and Management of Cervical Thymic Cysts in Children. *Cureus* **2017**, *9*, e973. [CrossRef] [PubMed]
27. Jiang, J.-H.; Yen, S.-L.; Lee, S.-Y.; Chuang, J.-H. Differences in the distribution and presentation of bronchogenic cysts between adults and children. *J. Pediatr. Surg.* **2015**, *50*, 399–401. [CrossRef]
28. Mammadov, E.; Eliçevik, M.; Adaletli, I.; Dervişoğlu, S.; Celayir, S. Bronchogenic Cysts Located in Neck Region: An Uncommon Entity with a Common Reason for Misdiagnosis. *Ann. Pediatr. Surg.* **2010**, *6*, 167–169.
29. Lee, D.H.; Yoon, T.M.; Lee, J.K.; Lim, S.C. Bronchogenic Cyst in the Head and Neck Region. *J. Craniofacial Surg.* **2017**, *28*, e303–e305. [CrossRef]
30. Carter, Y.; Yeutter, N.; Mazeh, H. Thyroglossal duct remnant carcinoma: Beyond the Sistrunk procedure. *Surg. Oncol.* **2014**, *23*, 161–166. [CrossRef]
31. Girvigian, M.R.; Rechdouni, A.K.; Zeger, G.D.; Segall, H.; Rice, D.H.; Petrovich, Z. Squamous Cell Carcinoma Arising in a Second Branchial Cleft Cyst. *Am. J. Clin. Oncol.* **2004**, *27*, 96–100. [CrossRef] [PubMed]
32. Jablokow, V.R.; Kathuria, S.; Wang, T. Squamous cell carcinoma arising in branchiogenic cyst branchial cleft carcinoma. *J. Surg. Oncol.* **1982**, *20*, 201–204. [CrossRef] [PubMed]
33. Chauhan, A.; Tiwari, S.; Pathak, N. Primary branchiogenic carcinoma: Report of a case and a review of the literature. *J. Cancer Res. Ther.* **2013**, *9*, 135. [CrossRef] [PubMed]

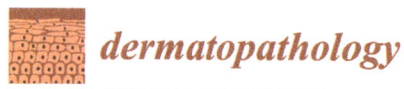

Review

Pseudomalignancies in Children: Histological Clues, and Pitfalls to Be Avoided

Sébastien Menzinger [1,2,*] and Sylvie Fraitag [3]

1 Department of Dermatology, University Hospital of Geneva, 1205 Geneva, Switzerland
2 Department of Clinical Pathology, University Hospital of Geneva, 1205 Geneva, Switzerland
3 Department of Pathology, Hôpital Necker-Enfants Malades, APHP, 75015 Paris, France; sylvie.fraitag@aphp.fr
* Correspondence: sebastien.menzinger@hcuge.ch

Abstract: The term "pseudomalignancy" covers a large, heterogenous group of diseases characterized by a benign cellular proliferation, hyperplasia, or infiltrate that resembles a true malignancy clinically or histologically. Here, we (i) provide a non-exhaustive review of several inflammatory skin diseases and benign skin proliferations that can mimic a malignant neoplasm in children, (ii) give pathologists some helpful clues to guide their diagnosis, and (iii) highlight pitfalls to be avoided. The observation of clinical–pathological correlations is often important in this situation and can sometimes be the only means (along with careful monitoring of the disease's clinical course) of reaching a firm diagnosis.

Keywords: pseudomalignancies; pediatrics; pseudolymphoma; pityriasis lichenoides; lymphomatoid papulosis; mycosis fungoides; lymphoplasmacytic plaque; acral pseudo-lymphomatous angiokeratoma of children; histiocytic infiltrate; langerhans cell histiocytosis; CD1a+ dendritic cell hyperplasia; melanocytic disorders; congenital melanocytic lesion; proliferative nodule; Spitz tumor

1. Introduction

The term "pseudomalignancy" covers a large, heterogenous group of diseases characterized by a benign cellular proliferation, hyperplasia, or infiltrate that resembles a true malignancy clinically or histologically. Several inflammatory skin diseases or benign skin proliferations in children can mimic malignant neoplasms [1]. However, when examining a child's skin biopsy, the pathologist must bear in mind that benign disorders are more frequent than malignancies.

Here, we review cellular infiltrates of the skin that can mimic neoplasms of the skin in children. The article is divided into three subsections, according to the specific type of cellular infiltrate (lymphocytic, histiocytic, and melanocytic infiltrates).

2. Lymphocytic Infiltrates

Cutaneous lymphocytic infiltrates that mimic lymphoma can be referred to cutaneous pseudo-lymphomas. This heterogenous group has been described in the literature as reactive lymphoproliferation that histopathologically and clinically imitates cutaneous lymphomas [2]. The causes are many and varied. Cutaneous lymphocytic infiltrates can be subdivided as a function of the histological pattern or the predominant immunophenotype (T or B), amongst others.

2.1. Vitiligo

Many inflammatory skin disorders can mimic mycosis fungoides (MF) clinically or histologically; this is the case for vitiligo. This acquired chronic depigmentation disorder results from the selective destruction of melanocytes; although the etiology is unknown, an auto-inflammatory or auto-immune mechanism is most strongly suspected [3].

Clinical differentiation between vitiligo and MF in children can be challenging, especially because hypopigmented MF is particularly frequent in children with a darker skin type (Fitzpatrick types IV–VI) [4] and can clinically mimic vitiligo or other pathologies with hypopigmentation or depigmentation (e.g., pityriasis alba, pityriasis versicolor, post-inflammatory hypopigmentation, progressive macular hypomelanosis, and hypopigmented pityriasis lichenoides (PL) chronica).

In the early (inflammatory) phase of vitiligo, a marked superficial perivascular lymphocytic infiltrate can be observed; it sometimes has a lichenoid pattern and can be mistaken for epidermotropism [5] (Figure 1). Moreover, the intra-epidermal lymphocytes in inflammatory vitiligo are predominantly CD8-positive [6], as in hypopigmented MF [4,6]. Furthermore, the melanocyte count can also be abnormally low in cases of hypopigmented MF [6]. On one hand, some features tend to indicate a diagnosis of hypopigmented MF: partial depigmentation, the persistence of some melanocytes, wiry fibrosis of the papillary dermis, and increased density of the dermal infiltrate. On the other hand, some features argue in favor of vitiligo: complete loss of pigmentation, the complete absence of melanocytes, and fewer lymphocytes in the papillary dermis. When observed, the loss of cell surface "pan-T" antigens (CD2, CD5, and CD7) and the presence of clonal T-cell receptor rearrangements may be of diagnostic value. In difficult cases, the observation of clinical-pathological correlations and the course of the disease should enable a definitive diagnosis.

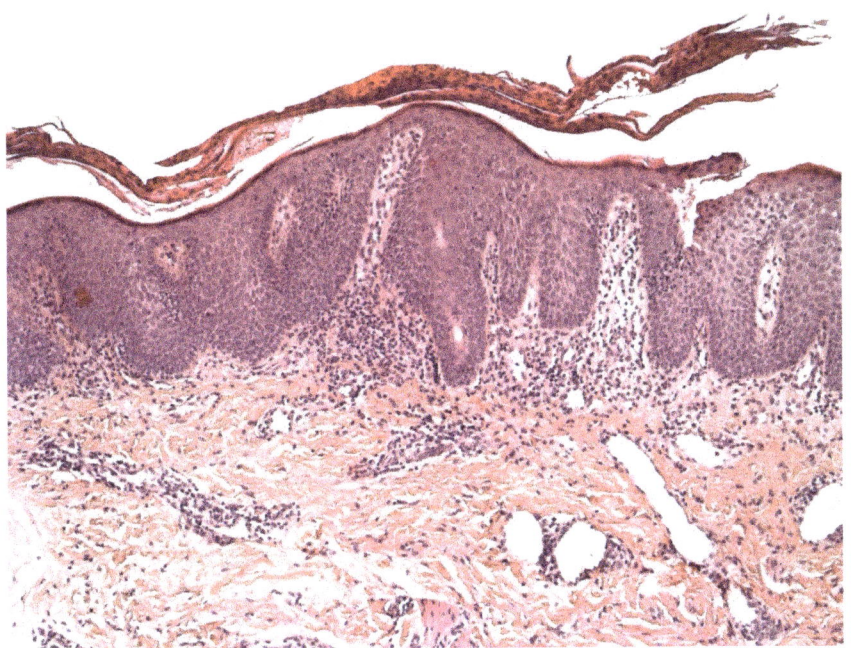

Figure 1. An example of vitiligo (inflammatory phase): parakeratosis, epidermal hyperplasia, slight spongiosis, lymphocyte exocytosis, and a discrete lymphocytic infiltrate in the superficial dermis. HE ×200.

2.2. Immunodeficiencies Rashes

A skin rash (sometimes presenting as neonatal erythroderma) is a feature of several immunodeficiencies, including severe combined immunodeficiency, Omenn syndrome, and immune dysregulation-poly-endocrinopathy-enteropathy-X-linked syndrome [7]. These histological features can mimic MF; in particular, marked lymphocytic exocytosis resembles the epidermotropism seen in MF. This epidermotropism is commonly associated with adnexotropism. To the best of our knowledge, however, neonatal MF has never been described. However, the presence of necrotic/apoptotic changes in the epidermis and adnexal epithelium in a newborn/infant skin biopsy must alert the clinician and prompt him or her to consider a diagnosis of immunodeficiency (Figure 2).

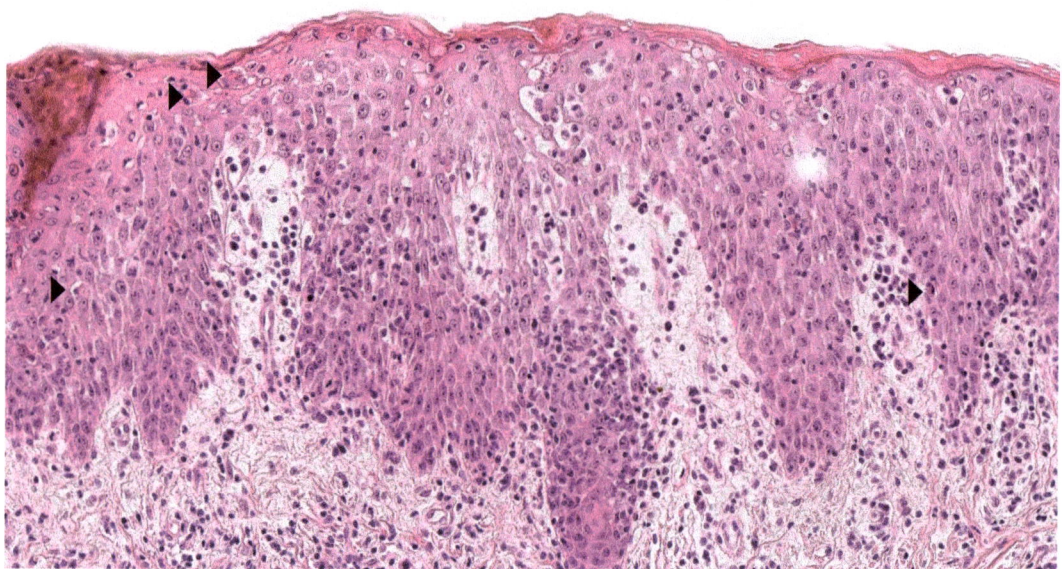

Figure 2. IPEX syndrome: Epidermal hyperplasia, marked lymphocytic exocytosis, scattered apoptotic keratinocytes (arrowhead), and a moderate lymphocytic infiltrate in the superficial dermis. HE ×400.

2.3. Pityriasis Lichenoides

Pityriasis lichenoides (PL) is an infrequent skin disorder that predominantly affects children and young adults. The clinical presentation usually differs from that of MF, although the histological picture can be very similar. Moreover, PL can be present before (or at the same time as) MF in children. The histological picture in PL usually includes parakeratosis, epidermal hyperplasia, variable numbers of necrotic keratinocytes, interface changes with prominent lymphocytic exocytosis, perivascular, and periadnexal lymphocytic infiltrates in the superficial and deep dermis, and red blood cell extravasation [8]. However, some cases present with prominent intra-epidermal lymphocytes, basal cell replacement by lymphocytes, and nuclei surrounded by a clear halo—as in MF (Figure 3). The immunohistochemical findings are not usually helpful, unless "pan-T" antigen (CD2, CD5, and CD7) loss is highlighted. Moreover, a screen for monoclonality is not very helpful because many PL cases show a clonal T-cell receptor rearrangement [9,10]. Some findings tend to indicate a diagnosis of PL: the presence of necrotic keratinocytes, superficial epidermal pallor, red blood cell extravasation (especially intra-epidermal extravasation), and the presence of deep perivascular and periadnexal lymphocytic infiltrates.

Some cases of PL are difficult to distinguish clinically from lymphomatoid papulosis (LyP); this is notably the case when the lesions are necrotic and few in number. Moreover, large CD30+ lymphoid cells can be observed in the infiltrate in the epidermis, the dermis or both in some cases of PL, which can cause confusion with LyP [11]. Furthermore, monoclonality is not very helpful for differentiating between the two entities because many PL cases show a clonal T-cell receptor rearrangement [9,10]. However, some findings tend to indicate a diagnosis of PL: an intra-epidermal lymphocytic infiltrate associated with necrotic keratinocytes, cellular monomorphism with a complete absence of eosinophils, and few or no large lymphoid cells. Furthermore, our recent study showed that the lymphocytic infiltrate is usually wedge-shaped in LyP (except for the recently described follicular variant) but is T-shaped and follows the adnexa in PL [8].

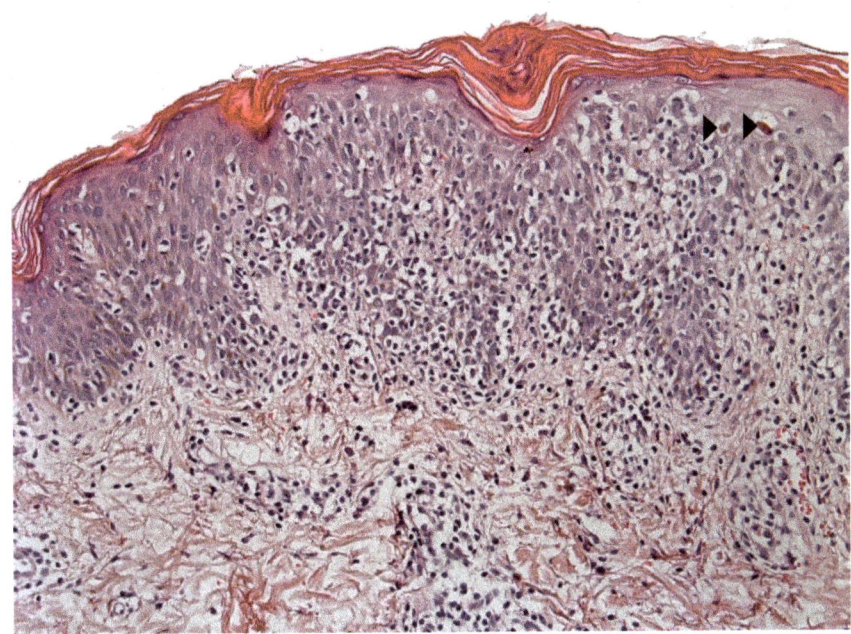

Figure 3. Mycosis fungoides-like pityriasis lichenoides. In this example there is a marked lymphocytic exocytosis, with lymphocytes displaying a clear halo. Note the few necrotic keratinocytes (arrowhead). HE ×250.

2.4. Scabies Nodules and Insect Bite Reactions

The histological features of insect bite reactions (including scabies and post-scabies nodules) may mimic those of LyP, with a dense, lymphoid, wedge-shaped infiltrate containing large numbers of eosinophils and atypical or large CD30+ lymphoid cells [12,13]. The presence of CD30+ large lymphoid cells is a feature of many infectious diseases of the skin and is considered to be a sign of lymphocyte activation [14]. CD30 is a member of the tumor necrosis factor super-family and probably has a role in the immune response to infections [15]. In LyP in children, the high eosinophil count can mask the presence of large, atypical lymphocytes. A screen for monoclonality may help in some cases. Clinical-histological correlations, and sometimes additional biopsies or response to empiric therapy, are often the only means of making a firm diagnosis [16].

2.5. Lymphoplasmacytic Plaque

Lymphoplasmacytic plaque (LPP) is a rare, recent characterized clinicopathological entity that mostly affects children. It features an asymptomatic, linear, reddish-brown, violaceous plaque, usually on the leg—hence the name "tibial" or "pretibial" LPP [17,18]. Since the initial reports, however, cases affecting other parts of the body have been described [19]. The histopathology is characterized by a dense nodular infiltrate within the upper reticular dermis or the whole dermis. This infiltrate is an admixture of plasma cells, lymphocytes, scattered histiocytes and (in some cases) epithelioid granulomas, together with vascular hyperplasia. The overlying epidermis may be hyperplastic and spongiotic [17,20] (Figure 4). This disease is closely related to another pseudo-lymphomatous disorder called "acral pseudolymphomatous angiokeratoma of children" (APACHE, see below) and may be a part of the same spectrum [20]. Importantly, the histological presentation of LP can be confused with that of cutaneous marginal zone lymphoma, a low-grade B cell lymphoma that very rarely affects children and occasionally affects teenagers [21]. Immunohistochemical analysis of the plasma cells in LPP shows a polytypic pattern of immunoglobulin light chain expression, and PCR studies do not show monoclonality [18,20,22].

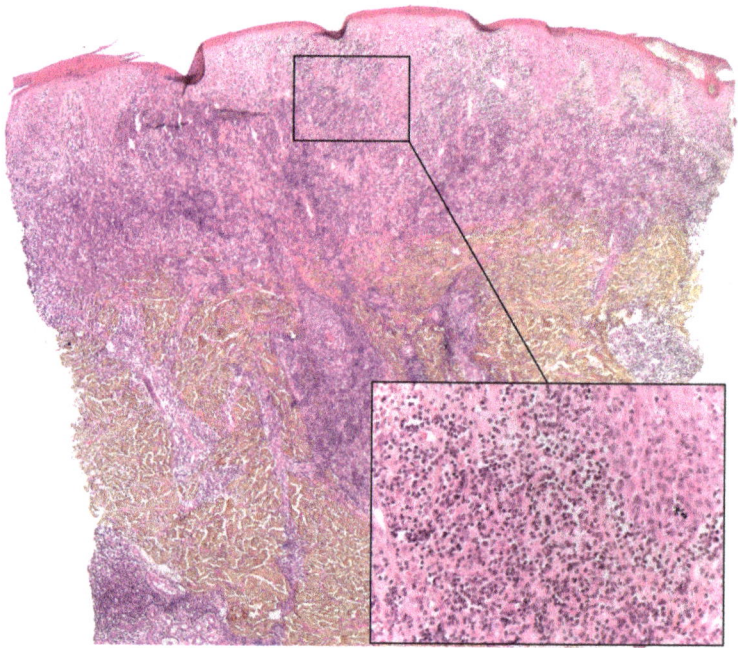

Figure 4. Lymphoplasmacytic plaque: parakeratotic scale, epidermal hyperplasia, a dense lymphoplasmacytic infiltrate in the whole dermis. Inset: note the numerous plasma cells. HE ×40 (inset: ×200).

2.6. Acral Pseudo-Lymphomatous Angiokeratoma of Children

Acral pseudo-lymphomatous angiokeratoma of children (APACHE), also named papular angiolymphoid hyperplasia, is a rare disease with female predominance [23]. It is characterized clinically by unilateral, asymptomatic, erythematous-violaceous papules and nodules with an acral distribution [24]. The histology findings are characterized by a dense superficial and deep dermal infiltrate, and a prominent vascular pattern of capillaries lined with plump endothelial cells. The infiltrate comprises lymphocytes, histiocytes, plasma cells, and eosinophils. The epidermis may also show hyperkeratosis, parakeratosis, spongiosis, and lymphocyte exocytosis [24]. Immunohistochemical studies show a slight predominance of T lymphocytes (with equal numbers of CD4+ and CD8+ cells, or slightly more CD4+ cells) and a large number of B lymphocytes. To the best of our knowledge, the presence or absence of CD30 in APACHE has not been studied immunohistochemically. A PCR analysis reveals that APACHE is a polyclonal disorder [25,26].

3. Histiocytic Infiltrates

3.1. CD1a+ Dendritic Cell Hyperplasia

CD1a+ dendritic cell hyperplasia (CD1a+ DCH) has been described in children as part of a large number of disorders including scabies, arthropod bite reactions, prurigo, warts, molluscum contagiosum, spongiotic dermatoses, psoriasis, PL, and interface dermatitis [27–29]. CD1a+ DCH can also be observed in proliferative processes, such as regressive melanocytic nevi, lymphoproliferative disorders, and the stroma of various tumors [30,31]. The CD1a+ DCH may have the typical aspect of Langerhans cell histiocytosis

(LCH), i.e., round, medium-sized histiocytes with eosinophilic cytoplasm and, in some cases, large reniform or "coffee bean" shaped nuclei. This LCH-mimicking phenomenon is often referred to as "Langerhans cell hyperplasia" and can lead to misdiagnosis. Some cases do not display these characteristic morphologic features and are only discovered after immunostaining with anti-CD1a [28,32]. The Langerhans cells are often located in the dermis around the vessels, but can also be encountered in the epidermis—mostly in spongiotic disorders, such as Langerhans cell microgranulomas and pseudo-Pautrier abscesses [32]. There are a few histological features that facilitate the differential diagnosis between CD1a+ DCH and LCH:

- The infiltrate's architecture: in CD1a+ DCH, cells are mostly located around the vessels in the dermis and do not accumulate in the papillary dermis as in LCH;
- The infiltrate's polymorphism: the CD1a+ cells are rarely predominant and are mixed with other cell types;
- Immunoreactivity: importantly, the cells are not true Langerhans cells because they do not usually express CD207 (Langerin); in fact, they are CD1a+/CD207− dendritic cells that lack Birbeck granules [27,33]. CD207 is a very sensitive, specific marker of Birbeck granules, which are located in the cytoplasm of Langerhans cells. Along with CD207, the presence of markers of MAPK pathway activation (involved in the pathogenesis of LCH [34]) can also help the pathologist to distinguish between CD1a+ DCH and LCH. In particular, cyclin D1 and pERK are expressed in all cases of LCH but are not expressed (or only weakly) in cases of "dermatitis" with CD1a+ DCH [35]. The CD1a+/CD207− dendritic cells probably come from bone marrow (as do Langerhans cells and interdigitated DCs) and might be indeterminate cells or immature Langerhans cell precursors.

Hence, immunostaining with antibodies against CD207 (and perhaps pERK and cyclin-D1) is very helpful for the differential diagnosis of CD1a+ DCH vs. LCH. In all cases, a clinical–histological correlation is always required for a firm diagnosis (Figure 5).

3.2. Juvenile Xanthogranuloma

Juvenile xanthogranuloma (JXG) is the most frequent subtype of non-Langerhans cell histiocytosis and one of the commonest skin tumors in children. This benign disorder usually affects young children and typically presents as a single erythematous to yellow papule, nodule, or plaque in the head and neck area. JXG usually regresses spontaneously and is very rarely associated with systemic disease [36]. Most JXG lesions appear during the first few years of life. There are several variants: micronodular, macronodular, giant (>5 cm), and subcutaneous JXG are observed. The giant and subcutaneous types always occur in the neonatal period. Clinically, JXG may be misleading and worrisome because of its size; it can mimic sarcoma in general and dermatofibrosarcoma protuberans in particular. Accordingly, a biopsy is essential.

These neonatal cases of JXG can also mimic malignancies histologically, since they usually display a large number of mitotic figures and have a high mitotic index (Ki67). Furthermore, early-stage JXG does not show xanthomization, and the cells tend to be monomorphous or even spindled. Early-stage JXG may also lack granulomatous inflammatory cells and, thus, can mimic spindle-cell sarcoma, round-cell sarcoma, or monoblastic leukemia. However, the cells do not show marked atypia and are commonly CD163+ and FXIIIa+—at least focally.

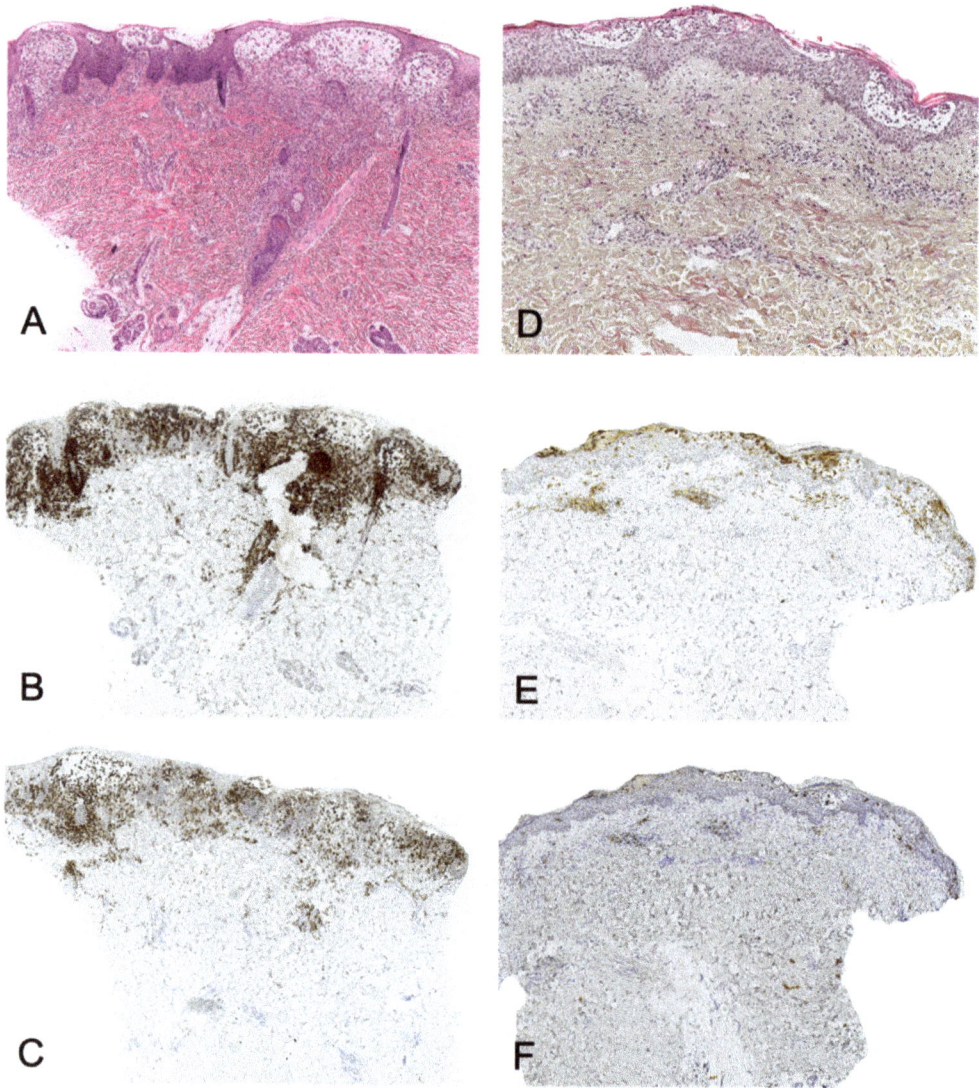

Figure 5. Left panel: Langerhans cell histiocytosis. (**A**): HE ×40. Superficial infiltrate of histiocytes with epidermotropism and edema. (**B**): CD1a immunostaining. (**C**): CD207/Langerin immunostaining. The whole infiltrate express CD207. Right panel: spongiotic dermatitis with CD1a+ dendritic cell hyperplasia. (**D**): HE ×40. (**E**): CD1a immunostaining. (**F**): CD207/Langerin immunostaining. The true Langerhans cells in the epidermal vesicles express CD207. The dermal infiltrate is almost completely negative.

4. Melanocytic Disorders

Melanoma is rare in children; it accounts for 3% of all pediatric cancers. Both sexes are affected equally. Although 2% of melanomas occur in patients under the age of 20, only 0.3% occur in prepubertal children. The most common types are Spitz melanomas in prepubescent children and "conventional" melanomas (i.e., similar to chronic sun-damage melanomas seen in adults) in postpubescent children [37]. Some melanomas are associated with a congenital nevus; this can often be large and occasionally develops even before birth. However, most pediatric melanomas develop *de novo* in the absence of a known underlying condition. A single large (≥20 cm) congenital nevus or two or more congenital nevi (regardless of the size), abnormal central nervous system MRI findings in the first months of life are factors that predispose to congenital nevi-associated melanoma. Conventional melanoma is linked to genetic factors, such as a light complexion, poor tanning ability, sun exposure, xeroderma pigmentosum, and germline mutations of the *CDKN2A* gene [38,39].

A number of common but histologically ambiguous melanocytic lesions can easily be misconstrued as melanoma; they include (i) Spitz nevus and its variants, (ii) proliferative nodules in congenital nevi, (iii) acquired melanocytic nevi on particular, "special" anatomic sites (such as the scalp, genital area, acral sites, and conjunctiva), and (iv) lesions on the blue nevus spectrum [40].

4.1. Melanocytic Lesions in Newborns

Melanoma is very rare in the neonatal period, and there are very few case reports in the literature. The tumor either arises in a giant congenital melanocytic nevus (CMN) or grows from transplacental metastases of the mother's melanoma [38,41]. The estimated risk of developing a melanoma associated with CMN is between 1% and 2% but might be as high as 10% to 15% for large and giant CMN. Early-onset (congenital, neonatal, and infantile) melanoma usually has a poor prognosis [41]. Melanocytic lesions that arise in association with a congenital melanocytic nevus will be discussed in the next subsection.

Melanocytic lesions in newborns can show worrisome histological features. The junctional component may show irregularly distributed and sometimes non cohesive nests. Pagetoid spread (a helpful criterion in the diagnosis of adult melanoma) should be interpreted with caution because it is displayed by many melanocytic lesions in newborns [40] and can, therefore, mimic superficial spreading melanoma (SSM) (Figure 6). The lesions may also be nodular and ulcerated, with many mitotic figures and a high proliferation index (Ki67/MIB); it can, therefore, mimic nodular melanoma. These lesions must be interpreted carefully so that melanoma is not erroneously diagnosed in this population. Ancillary immunochemistry or molecular biology test can be helpful (see the following section). Ideally, the clinician should seek an expert opinion before diagnosing melanoma. If doubt persists, excision of the lesion with broad margins (if possible) and long-term follow-up is recommended.

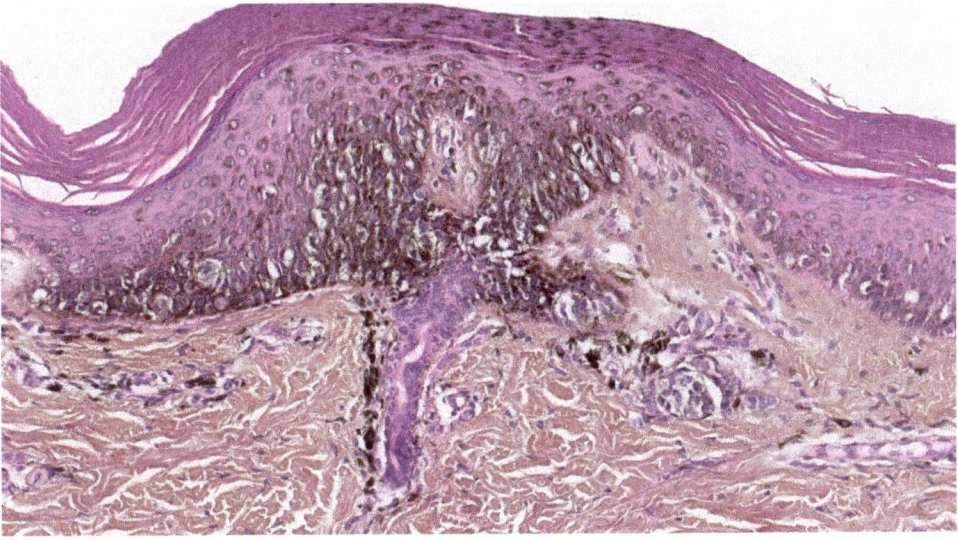

Figure 6. Junctional component of a congenital nevus in a newborn. Irregularly distributed melanocytes with pagetoid spread. HE ×250.

4.2. Melanocytic Lesions Associated with a Congenital Melanocytic Nevus

A distinct, benign, nodular proliferation arising on a congenital melanocytic nevus (CMN) and particularly on a giant CMN is referred to as a "proliferative nodule" (PN). This entity is relatively common and can mimic the clinical and histological features of melanoma [42]. The cell density is higher in the PN than in the adjacent congenital nevus. A PN can sometimes exhibit worrisome clinical features, such as rapid growth or ulceration. The typical histological characteristics of melanoma can also be seen in PN; these include a high mitotic index, sheets of large melanocytes with an epithelioid morphology, nuclear atypia, and even atypical mitoses and necrosis [43]. The features of this kind of lesion must be interpreted with caution because large/giant CMN is nevertheless the main risk factor for the development of melanoma in childhood [44,45].

Several subtypes or morphological patterns have been described, including epithelioid, Spitzoid, small round blue cell-like, blue nevus-like, nevoid melanoma-like, and complex subtypes [43]. The recent literature has provided many characteristics, features, and clues of value in distinguishing between melanoma and PN [43,46,47]. The first important observation is that PN is much more frequent than melanoma. Secondly, and in contrast to melanoma, PN presents frequently as multiple lesions. Ulceration is suggestive of melanoma, especially when extensive. Blending (i.e., a smooth transition between PN cells and nevus cells), favors PN, even when focal (Figure 7). However, this feature is not always observed, and its significance is subject to debate. A very high mitotic index, necrosis within the nodule, inflammation, pleomorphism, and high-grade atypia increase the likelihood of a diagnosis of melanoma [41].

Immunochemistry is often described as being of limited value in distinguishing between PN and melanoma [48,49]. Recently, the expression of 5-hydroxymethylcytosine (5-hmC, an intermediate product of DNA demethylation) was studied in cases of giant CMN, PN, and melanoma arising within a CMN. Strong nuclear staining for 5-hmC was observed in almost all benign giant CMNs (93%) and PNs (98%) but never in melanomas associated with a within a CMN [42]. Immunochemical screening for the trimethylated lysine residue of histone H3 (H3K27me3) is also of diagnostic value: H3K27me3 expression tends to be abnormally low most nodular melanomas associated with a giant CMN [40,50].

Furthermore, molecular assays (such as fluorescence in situ hybridization (FISH) and comparative genomic hybridization (CGH)) have been studied in PN and melanoma arising in a CMN. FISH with standard melanoma probes was not helpful in distinguishing between PN and childhood-onset melanoma in a small series of patients [49]. In contrast, CGH might be useful for distinguishing between PN and melanoma because whole-chromosome gains or losses are observed in PNs, whereas and gains or losses in melanoma are restricted to parts or fragments of chromosomes [40,51]. An in situ hybridization study of telomerase reverse transcriptase mRNA gave promising results, with signals in all melanomas arising in a giant CMN but none in PNs [52].

4.3. Juvenile Nevi

In principle, SSM does not occur in prepubertal children. However, common, acquired "juvenile-type" nevi occasionally show worrisome histological features that mimic SSM. Most of these lesions present as epithelioid Spitz nevi with a predominantly epithelioid appearance characterized by enlarged round-to-oval nuclei, often with a delicate open chromatin pattern. Some lesions are flat but some may be polypoid. These "juvenile-type" nevi may contain suprabasal intraepidermal melanocytes—especially in young children. At most, one can see features of "pagetoid Spitz nevus", with the prominent pagetoid growth of solitary units and nests of melanocytes in the stratum spinosum throughout the lesion (Figure 8). Care must be taken not to confuse a pagetoid Spitz nevus with in situ melanoma. The presence of Spitzoid cytologic features, a small lesion diameter, and sharp demarcations are important parameters for the diagnosis of a Spitz nevus rather than SSM [53].

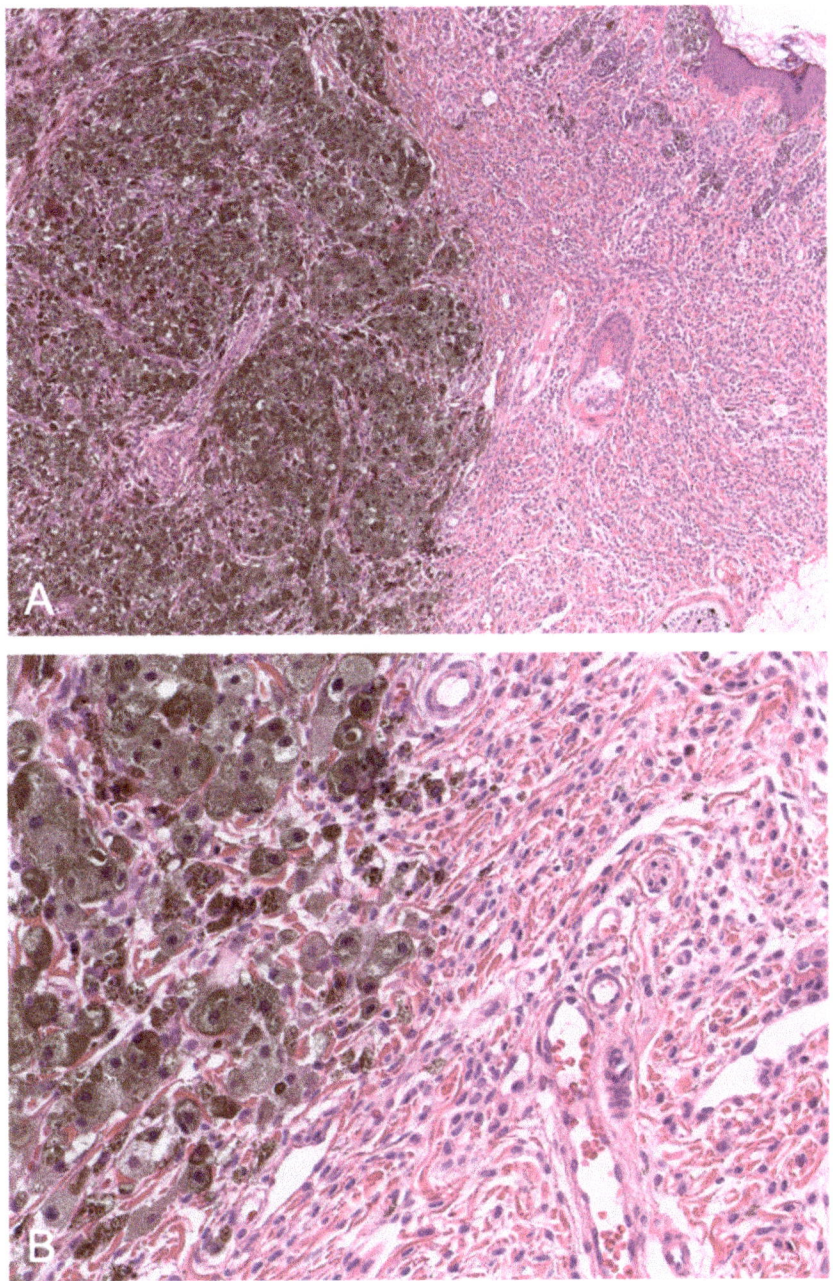

Figure 7. (**A**): (HE ×40) Proliferative nodule in a congenital melanocytic lesion. (**B**): (HE ×250) The melanocytes of the proliferative nodule are epithelioid and with a dusty cytoplasm, without nuclear atypia. Note the delicate transition (blending), which may be very focal and inconspicuous.

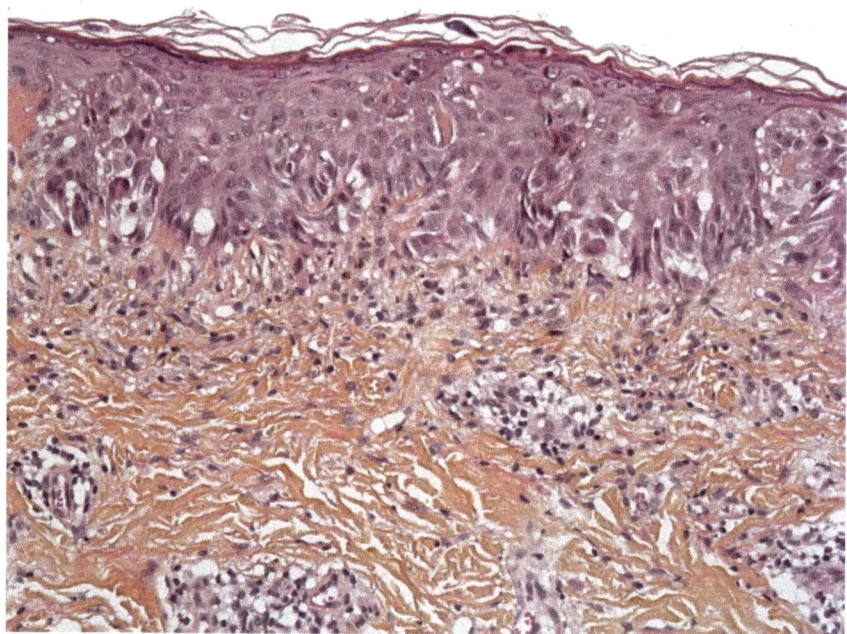

Figure 8. Pagetoid Spitz nevus (HE ×250). Epithelioid or spindle melanocytes with large nuclei and abundant "ground glass" cytoplasm, and pagetoid spread.

4.4. Spitz Nevus and Atypical Spitz Tumor

Spitz nevus and Spitzoid melanocytic lesions are part of a spectrum of melanocytic proliferations with a distinctive cellular morphology. The clinical-pathologic classification, diagnosis, and management of these lesions are among the most problematic topics in dermatopathology [54].

Histologically, Spitz nevi are mainly compound nevi and consist of epithelioid and spindle melanocytes with large nuclei and abundant "ground glass" cytoplasm. They show symmetry, sharp demarcation, uniform maturation (zonation), epidermal hyperplasia, Kamino bodies, no pleomorphism, no high-grade atypia, few mitoses, no mitoses in deep tissue, and no subcutaneous tissue involvement.

Some Spitzoid lesions present atypia and are, therefore, referred to as an "atypical Spitz nevi" or "atypical Spitz tumors". These atypia include a diameter >10 mm, asymmetry, subcutaneous fat involvement, a "pushing" deep margin, ulceration, poor demarcation, pagetoid migration, lack of maturation and zonation, few or no Kamino bodies, a high mitotic index (>2–6/mm^2), deep mitoses, a proliferation index $\geq$ 10%, and cytological atypia (e.g., a high nucleocytoplasmic ratio, hyperchromatism, and large nucleoli) [55,56]. Spitzoid lesions are discussed more exhaustively elsewhere in this issue.

5. Conclusions

Many skin conditions in children can mimic the clinical and histologic features of malignancies. The pathologist must bear in mind that a neoplasm in a young child (and especially a newborn) will frequently have a high mitosis count or mitotic index, which are usually indicative of malignancy in adults. All dermatologists and dermatopathologists are aware of the importance of clinical–pathological correlations. This is particularly true in pediatrics, and these correlations—along with careful monitoring of the disease's clinical course—sometimes constitute the only means of reaching a firm diagnosis. Except during the neonatal period, cutaneous malignancies are very rare in children; hence, the clinician is more likely to make a false-positive diagnosis than to truly miss a malignant disorder. It is also very important to ask for a second opinion from an expert center, when indicated.

Funding: The authors thank the Lions Club de Correze and Professor Nicole Brousse for financial support.

Institutional Review Board Statement: Not applicable.

Informed Consent Statement: Not applicable.

Conflicts of Interest: The authors declare no conflict of interest.

References

1. Connors, R.C.; Ackerman, A.B. Histologic pseudomalignancies of the skin. *Arch. Dermatol.* **1976**, *112*, 1767–1780. [CrossRef] [PubMed]
2. Mitteldorf, C.; Kempf, W. Cutaneous pseudolymphoma-A review on the spectrum and a proposal for a new classification. *J. Cutan. Pathol.* **2020**, *47*, 76–97. [CrossRef]
3. Ezzedine, K.; Eleftheriadou, V.; Whitton, M.; van Geel, N. Vitiligo. *Lancet Lond. Engl.* **2015**, *386*, 74–84. [CrossRef]
4. Castano, E.; Glick, S.; Wolgast, L.; Naeem, R.; Sunkara, J.; Elston, D.; Jacobson, M. Hypopigmented mycosis fungoides in childhood and adolescence: A long-term retrospective study. *J. Cutan. Pathol.* **2013**, *40*, 924–934. [CrossRef]
5. Werner, B.; Brown, S.; Ackerman, A.B. Hypopigmented Mycosis Fungoides? Is Not Always Mycosis Fungoides! *Am. J. Dermatopathol.* **2005**, *27*, 56–67. [CrossRef] [PubMed]
6. Furlan, F.C.; Pereira, B.A.D.P.; Da Silva, L.F.; Sanches, J.A. Loss of melanocytes in hypopigmented mycosis fungoides: A study of 18 patients. *J. Cutan. Pathol.* **2013**, *41*, 101–107. [CrossRef] [PubMed]
7. Leclerc-Mercier, S.; Bodemer, C.; Bourdon-Lanoy, E.; Larousserie, F.; Hovnanian, A.; Brousse, N.; Fraitag, S. Early skin biopsy is helpful for the diagnosis and management of neonatal and infantile erythrodermas. *J. Cutan. Pathol.* **2010**, *37*, 249–255. [CrossRef] [PubMed]
8. Menzinger, S.; Frassati-Biaggi, A.; Leclerc-Mercier, S.; Bodemer, C.; Molina, T.J.; Fraitag, S. Pityriasis Lichenoides: A Large Histopathological Case Series with a Focus on Adnexotropism. *Am. J. Dermatopathol.* **2020**, *42*, 1–10. [CrossRef]
9. Dereure, O.; Levi, E.; Kadin, M.E. T-Cell clonality in pityriasis lichenoides et varioliformis acuta: A heteroduplex analysis of 20 cases. *Arch. Dermatol.* **2000**, *136*, 1483–1486. [CrossRef] [PubMed]
10. Weinberg, J.M.; Kristal, L.; Chooback, L.; Honig, P.J.; Kramer, E.M.; Lessin, S.R. The Clonal Nature of Pityriasis Lichenoides. *Arch. Dermatol.* **2002**, *138*, 1063–1067. [CrossRef] [PubMed]
11. Kempf, W.; Kazakov, D.V.; Palmedo, G.; Fraitag, S.; Schaerer, L.; Kutzner, H. Pityriasis lichenoides et varioliformis acuta with numerous CD30(+) cells: A variant mimicking lymphomatoid papulosis and other cutaneous lymphomas. A clinicopathologic, immunohistochemical, and molecular biological study of 13 cases. *Am. J. Surg. Pathol.* **2012**, *36*, 1021–1029. [CrossRef] [PubMed]
12. Cepeda, L.T.; Pieretti, M.; Chapman, S.F.; Horenstein, M.G. CD30-Positive Atypical Lymphoid Cells in Common Non-Neoplastic Cutaneous Infiltrates Rich in Neutrophils and Eosinophils. *Am. J. Surg. Pathol.* **2003**, *27*, 912–918. [CrossRef]
13. Hwong, H.; Jones, D.; Prieto, V.G.; Schulz, C.; Duvic, M. Persistent Atypical Lymphocytic Hyperplasia Following Tick Bite in a Child: Report of a Case and Review of the Literature. *Pediatr. Dermatol.* **2001**, *18*, 481–484. [CrossRef] [PubMed]
14. Gallardo, F.; Barranco, C.; Toll, A.; Pujol, R.M. CD30 antigen expression in cutaneous inflammatory infiltrates of scabies: A dynamic immunophenotypic pattern that should be distinguished from lymphomatoid papulosis. *J. Cutan. Pathol.* **2002**, *29*, 368–373. [CrossRef]
15. Marín, N.D.; García, L.F. The role of CD30 and CD153 (CD30L) in the anti-mycobacterial immune response. *Tuberculosis* **2016**, *102*, 8–15. [CrossRef]
16. Miquel, J.; Fraitag, S.; Hamel-Teillac, D.; Molina, T.; Brousse, N.; De Prost, Y.; Bodemer, C. Lymphomatoid papulosis in children: A series of 25 cases. *Br. J. Dermatol.* **2014**, *171*, 1138–1146. [CrossRef] [PubMed]
17. Moulonguet, I.; Hadj-Rabia, S.; Gounod, N.; Bodemer, C.; Fraitag, S. Tibial Lymphoplasmacytic Plaque: A New, Illustrative Case of a Recently and Poorly Recognized Benign Lesion in Children. *Dermatology* **2012**, *225*, 27–30. [CrossRef]
18. Bierbrier, R.M.; Amdemichael, E.; Adam, D.N. Pretibial Lymphoplasmacytic Plaque in Children: Case Report and Review of the Literature. *Am. J. Dermatopathol.* **2019**, *41*, 300–302. [CrossRef]
19. Tsilika, K.; Montaudié, H.; Castela, E.; Cardot-Leccia, N.; Passeron, T.; Lacour, J.-P. A case of lymphoplasmacytic plaque in children. *J. Eur. Acad. Dermatol. Venereol.* **2019**, *33*, e171–e172. Available online: https://onlinelibrary.wiley.com/doi/abs/10.1111/jdv.15408 (accessed on 21 March 2021). [CrossRef] [PubMed]
20. Moulonguet, I.; Gantzer, A.; Bourdon-Lanoy, E.; Fraitag, S. A Pretibial Plaque in a Five and a Half year–Old Girl. *Am. J. Dermatopathol.* **2012**, *34*, 113–116. [CrossRef] [PubMed]
21. Kempf, W.; Kazakov, D.V.; Buechner, S.A.; Graf, M.; Zettl, A.; Zimmermann, D.R. Primary cutaneous marginal zone lymphoma in children: A report of 3 cases and review of the literature. *Am. J. Dermatopathol.* **2014**, *36*, 661–666. [CrossRef] [PubMed]
22. Fried, I.; Wiesner, T.; Cerroni, L. Pretibial Lymphoplasmacytic Plaque in Children. *Arch. Dermatol.* **2010**, *146*, 95–96. [CrossRef] [PubMed]

23. Tokuda, Y.; Arakura, F.; Murata, H.; Koga, H.; Kawachi, S.; Nakazawa, K. Acral pseudolymphomatous angiokeratoma of children: A case report with immunohistochemical study of antipodoplanin antigen. *Am. J. Dermatopathol.* **2012**, *34*, e128–e132. [CrossRef] [PubMed]
24. Lessa, P.P.; Jorge, J.C.F.; Ferreira, F.R.; Lira, M.L.D.A.; Mandelbaum, S.H. Acral pseudolymphomatous angiokeratoma: Case report and literature review. *An. Bras. Dermatol.* **2013**, *88*, 39–43. [CrossRef]
25. Hagari, Y.; Hagari, S.; Kambe, N.; Kawaguchi, T.; Nakamoto, S.; Mihara, M. Acral pseudolymphomatous angiokeratoma of children: Immunohistochemical and clonal analyses of the infiltrating cells. *J. Cutan. Pathol.* **2002**, *29*, 313–318. [CrossRef]
26. Evans, M.S.; Burkhart, C.N.; Bowers, E.V.; Culpepper, K.S.; Googe, P.B.; Magro, C.M. Solitary plaque on the leg of a child: A report of two cases and a brief review of acral pseudolymphomatous angiokeratoma of children and unilesional mycosis fungoides. *Pediatr. Dermatol.* **2018**, *36*, e1–e5. [CrossRef] [PubMed]
27. Bhattacharjee, P.; Glusac, E.J. Langerhans cell hyperplasia in scabies: A mimic of Langerhans cell histiocytosis. *J. Cutan. Pathol.* **2007**, *34*, 716–720. [CrossRef]
28. Hatter, A.D.; Zhou, X.; Honda, K.; Popkin, D.L. Langerhans Cell Hyperplasia from Molluscum Contagiosum. *Am. J. Dermatopathol.* **2015**, *37*, e93–e95. [CrossRef]
29. Kim, S.H.; Kim, D.H.; Gil Lee, K. Prominent Langerhans' cell migration in the arthropod bite reactions simulating Langerhans' cell histiocytosis. *J. Cutan. Pathol.* **2007**, *34*, 899–902. [CrossRef]
30. Jokinen, C.H.; Wolgamot, G.M.; Wood, B.L.; Olerud, J.; Argenyi, Z.B. Lymphomatoid papulosis with CD1a+ dendritic cell hyperplasia, mimicking Langerhans cell histiocytosis. *J. Cutan. Pathol.* **2007**, *34*, 584–587. [CrossRef]
31. Ezra, N.; Van Dyke, G.S.; Binder, S.W. CD30 positive anaplastic large-cell lymphoma mimicking Langerhans cell histiocytosis. *J. Cutan. Pathol.* **2009**, *37*, 787–792. [CrossRef]
32. Burkert, K.L.; Huhn, K.; Whitaker Menezes, D.; Murphy, G.F. Langerhans cell microgranulomas (pseudo-pautrier abscesses): Morphologic diversity, diagnostic implications and pathogenetic mechanisms: Langerhans cell microgranulomas. *J. Cutan. Pathol.* **2002**, *29*, 511–516. [CrossRef] [PubMed]
33. Drut, R.; Peral, C.G.; Garone, A.; Rositto, A. Langerhans cell hyperplasia of the skin mimicking Langerhans cell histiocytosis: A report of two cases in children not associated with scabies. *Fetal Pediatr. Pathol.* **2010**, *29*, 231–238. [CrossRef]
34. Tran, G.; Huynh, T.N.; Paller, A.S. Langerhans cell histiocytosis: A neoplastic disorder driven by Ras-ERK pathway mutations. *J. Am. Acad. Dermatol.* **2018**, *78*, 579–590.e4. [CrossRef]
35. Shanmugam, V.; Craig, J.W.; Hornick, J.L.; Morgan, E.A.; Pinkus, G.S.; Pozdnyakova, O. Cyclin D1 Is Expressed in Neoplastic Cells of Langerhans Cell Histiocytosis but Not Reactive Langerhans Cell Proliferations. *Am. J. Surg. Pathol.* **2017**, *41*, 1390–1396. [CrossRef] [PubMed]
36. Gianotti, F.; Caputo, R. Histiocytic syndromes: A review. *J. Am. Acad. Dermatol.* **1985**, *13*, 383–404. [CrossRef]
37. World Health Organization. ID: gnd/1007857-5. WHO Classification of Skin Tumours. In *World Health Organization Classification of Tumours*, 4th ed.; Elder, D.E., Massi, D., Scolyer, R.A., Willemze, R., Eds.; International Agency for Research on Cancer: Lyon, France, 2018; p. 470.
38. Stefanaki, C.; Chardalias, L.; Soura, E.; Katsarou, A.; Stratigos, A. Paediatric melanoma. *J. Eur. Acad. Dermatol. Venereol.* **2017**, *31*, 1604–1615. [CrossRef]
39. Wood, B.A. Paediatric melanoma. *Pathology* **2016**, *48*, 155–165. [CrossRef]
40. Busam, K.J.; Scolyer, R.A.; Gerami, P. Pathology of Melanocytic Tumors E-Book. 2018. Available online: https://nls.ldls.org.uk/welcome.html?ark:/81055/vdc_100063476428.0x000001 (accessed on 8 June 2021).
41. Masson Regnault, M.; Mazereeuw-Hautier, J.; Fraitag, S. Les mélanomes d'apparition précoce (congénitaux, néonataux, du nourrisson): Revue systématique des cas de la littérature. *Ann. Dermatol. Vénéréol.* **2020**, *147*, 729–745. [CrossRef]
42. Pavlova, O.; Fraitag, S.; Hohl, D. 5-Hydroxymethylcytosine Expression in Proliferative Nodules Arising within Congenital Nevi Allows Differentiation from Malignant Melanoma. *J. Investig. Dermatol.* **2016**, *136*, 2453–2461. [CrossRef]
43. Yélamos, O.; Arva, N.C.; Obregon, R.; Yazdan, P.; Wagner, A.; Guitart, J.; Gerami, P. A Comparative Study of Proliferative Nodules and Lethal Melanomas in Congenital Nevi from Children. *Am. J. Surg. Pathol.* **2015**, *39*, 405–415. [CrossRef] [PubMed]
44. Kinsler, V.; O'Hare, P.; Bulstrode, N.; Calonje, J.; Chong, W.; Hargrave, D.; Jacques, T.; Lomas, D.; Sebire, N.; Slater, O. Melanoma in congenital melanocytic naevi. *Br. J. Dermatol.* **2017**, *176*, 1131–1143. [CrossRef]
45. Lacoste, C.; Avril, M.-F.; Frassati-Biaggi, A.; Dupin, N.; Chrétien-Marquet, B.; Mahé, E. Malignant Melanoma Arising in Patients with a Large Congenital Melanocytic Naevus: Retrospective Study of 10 Cases with Cytogenetic Analysis. *Acta Derm. Venereol.* **2015**, *95*, 686–690. [CrossRef] [PubMed]
46. Aoyagi, S.; Akiyama, M.; Mashiko, M.; Shibaki, A.; Shimizu, H. Extensive proliferative nodules in a case of giant congenital naevus. *Clin. Exp. Dermatol.* **2007**, *33*, 125–127. [CrossRef] [PubMed]
47. Van Houten, A.H.; van Dijk, M.C.R.F.; Schuttelaar, M.-L.A. Proliferative nodules in a giant congenital melanocytic nevus-case report and review of the literature. *J. Cutan. Pathol.* **2010**, *37*, 764–776. [CrossRef] [PubMed]
48. Nguyen, T.L.T.; Theos, A.; Kelly, D.R.; Busam, K.; Andea, A.A. Mitotically active proliferative nodule arising in a giant congenital melanocytic nevus: A diagnostic pitfall. *Am. J. Dermatopathol.* **2013**, *35*, e16–e21. [CrossRef] [PubMed]
49. Vergier, B.; Laharanne, E.; Prochazkova-Carlotti, M.; De La Fouchardière, A.; Merlio, J.-P.; Kadlub, N.; Avril, M.-F.; Bodemer, C.; Lacoste, C.; Boralevi, F.; et al. Proliferative Nodules vs Melanoma Arising in Giant Congenital Melanocytic Nevi During Childhood. *JAMA Dermatol.* **2016**, *152*, 1147–1151. [CrossRef]

50. Busam, K.J.; Shah, K.N.; Gerami, P.; Sitzman, T.; Jungbluth, A.A.; Kinsler, V. Reduced H3K27me3 Expression Is Common in Nodular Melanomas of Childhood Associated with Congenital Melanocytic Nevi but Not in Proliferative Nodules. *Am. J. Surg. Pathol.* **2017**, *41*, 396–404. [CrossRef]
51. Bastian, B.C.; Xiong, J.; Frieden, I.J.; Williams, M.L.; Chou, P.; Busam, K. Genetic changes in neoplasms arising in congenital melanocytic nevi: Differences between nodular proliferations and melanomas. *Am. J. Pathol.* **2002**, *161*, 1163–1169. [CrossRef]
52. Fan, Y.; Lee, S.; Wu, G.; Easton, J.; Yergeau, D.; Dummer, R. Telomerase Expression by Aberrant Methylation of the TERT Promoter in Melanoma Arising in Giant Congenital Nevi. *J. Investig. Dermatol.* **2016**, *136*, 339–342. [CrossRef]
53. Busam, K.J.; Barnhill, R.L. Pagetoid Spitz nevus. Intraepidermal Spitz tumor with prominent pagetoid spread. *Am. J. Surg. Pathol.* **1995**, *19*, 1061–1067. [CrossRef] [PubMed]
54. Ferrara, G.; Gianotti, R.; Cavicchini, S.; Salviato, T.; Zalaudek, I.; Argenziano, G. Spitz nevus, Spitz tumor, and spitzoid melanoma: A comprehensive clinicopathologic overview. *Dermatol. Clin.* **2013**, *31*, 589–598. [CrossRef] [PubMed]
55. Barnhill, R.L. The Spitzoid lesion: Rethinking Spitz tumors, atypical variants, "Spitzoid melanoma" and risk assessment. *Mod. Pathol.* **2006**, *19* (Suppl. 2), S21–S33. [CrossRef]
56. Dika, E.; Ravaioli, G.M.; Fanti, P.A.; Neri, I.; Patrizi, A. Spitz Nevi and Other Spitzoid Neoplasms in Children: Overview of Incidence Data and Diagnostic Criteria. *Pediatr. Dermatol.* **2017**, *34*, 25–32. [CrossRef] [PubMed]

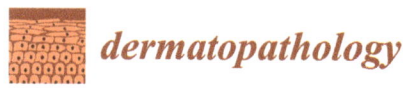 dermatopathology

Article

What to Look Out for in a Newborn with Multiple Papulonodular Skin Lesions at Birth

Sylvie Fraitag [1,*] and Olivia Boccara [2]

1 Department of Pathology, Necker-Enfants Malades Hospital, APHP, 75015 Paris, France
2 Department of Dermatology, Necker-Enfants Malades Hospital, APHP, 75015 Paris, France; olivia.boccara@aphp.fr
* Correspondence: sylvie.fraitag@aphp.fr

Abstract: Multiple papulonodular skin lesions at birth can indicate the presence of various benign and malignant disorders. Although the lesions' clinical aspect (color and consistency, in particular) may steer the clinician towards one disorder or another (infantile myofibromatosis, xanthogranuloma, or metastatic neuroblastoma), the diagnosis can only be confirmed by the histopathologic assessment of a biopsy. In neonates, a rapid but accurate diagnosis is critical because skin lesions may be the first manifestation of a malignant disorder like leukemia cutis or metastatic neuroblastoma. Here, we review the various disorders that may manifest themselves as multiple skin lesions at birth.

Keywords: newborn; blueberry muffin rash; dermal erythropoiesis; leukemia cutis; metastatic neuroblastoma; metastatic rhabdomyosarcoma; metastatic rhabdoid tumor; Langerhans cell histiocytosis; multiple juvenile xanthogranuloma; infantile myofibromatosis; subcutaneous fat necrosis of the newborn; mastocytosis; multiple neonatal hemangiomatosis; lymphangioendotheliomatosis with thrombocytopenia; blue rubber bleb nevus syndrome; glomuveinous malformation

Citation: Fraitag, S.; Boccara, O. What to Look Out for in a Newborn with Multiple Papulonodular Skin Lesions at Birth. *Dermatopathology* **2021**, *8*, 390–417. https://doi.org/10.3390/dermatopathology8030043

Academic Editor: Gürkan Kaya

Received: 4 July 2021
Accepted: 12 August 2021
Published: 17 August 2021

Publisher's Note: MDPI stays neutral with regard to jurisdictional claims in published maps and institutional affiliations.

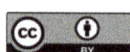

Copyright: © 2021 by the authors. Licensee MDPI, Basel, Switzerland. This article is an open access article distributed under the terms and conditions of the Creative Commons Attribution (CC BY) license (https://creativecommons.org/licenses/by/4.0/).

1. Introduction

Skin lesions that develop at birth or within the first weeks of life (i.e., during the neonatal period) may variously be papular, nodular, ulcerated, or crusted. The lesions color (flesh-colored, pinkish, reddish, brownish, or rather blue or violaceous), aspect (nodular, angiomatous, or that of a white peripheral halo), consistency (hard or soft), and the presence of associated systemic symptoms may steer the clinician towards one diagnosis rather than another. However, the clinical findings alone are usually insufficient for a firm diagnosis, and a skin biopsy is usually necessary. Skin lesions at birth have several possible causes, and it is important to bear in mind that malignant conditions can appear at this early age. Indeed, skin metastases may be the revealing signs of malignant neoplasms in neonates [1]. Hence, when multiple skin lesions are observed, the physician must do everything possible to deliver an accurate diagnosis as soon as possible and rule out malignancy if necessary. The skin biopsy should be as large and deep as possible and should be cut into two pieces, one of which should be frozen in case cytogenetic tests are subsequently needed.

2. Blueberry Muffin Rash

The "blueberry muffin baby" was first described in congenital rubella with thrombocytopenia [2]. It is characterized by bluish-red macules, papules, or nodules of dermal erythropoiesis primarily caused by intra-uterine infections with rubella virus, cytomegalovirus, or *Toxoplasma*. This rash can also be a sign of other serious systemic disorders, including congenital leukemia (Figure 1) (Table 1) [3,4]. A skin biopsy is mandatory for rapid diagnosis of the underlying disease.

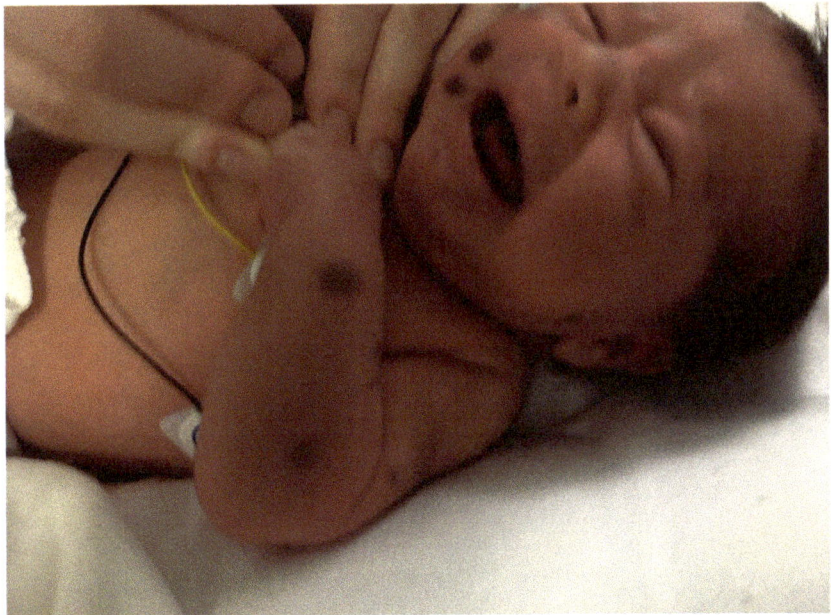

Figure 1. Blueberry muffin rash.

Table 1. Causes of blueberry muffin rash.

Dermal Erythropoiesis
• Congenital infections
Toxoplasmosis
Rubella
Cytomegalovirus
Herpes simplex virus
Coxsackie B2 virus
Syphilis (Figure 2a–d)
• Hemolytic disease of the newborn
Rhesus and ABO incompatibility
Hereditary spherocytosis
Twin-twin transfusion syndrome
Neoplastic Diseases
• Congenital leukemia
• Metastatic neuroblastoma
• Transitory myeloproliferative disease
• Langerhans cell histiocytosis
• Congenital metastatic rhabdomyosarcoma
• Metastatic rhabdoid tumor
• Disseminated juvenile xanthogranuloma
• Multicentric infantile myofibromatosis

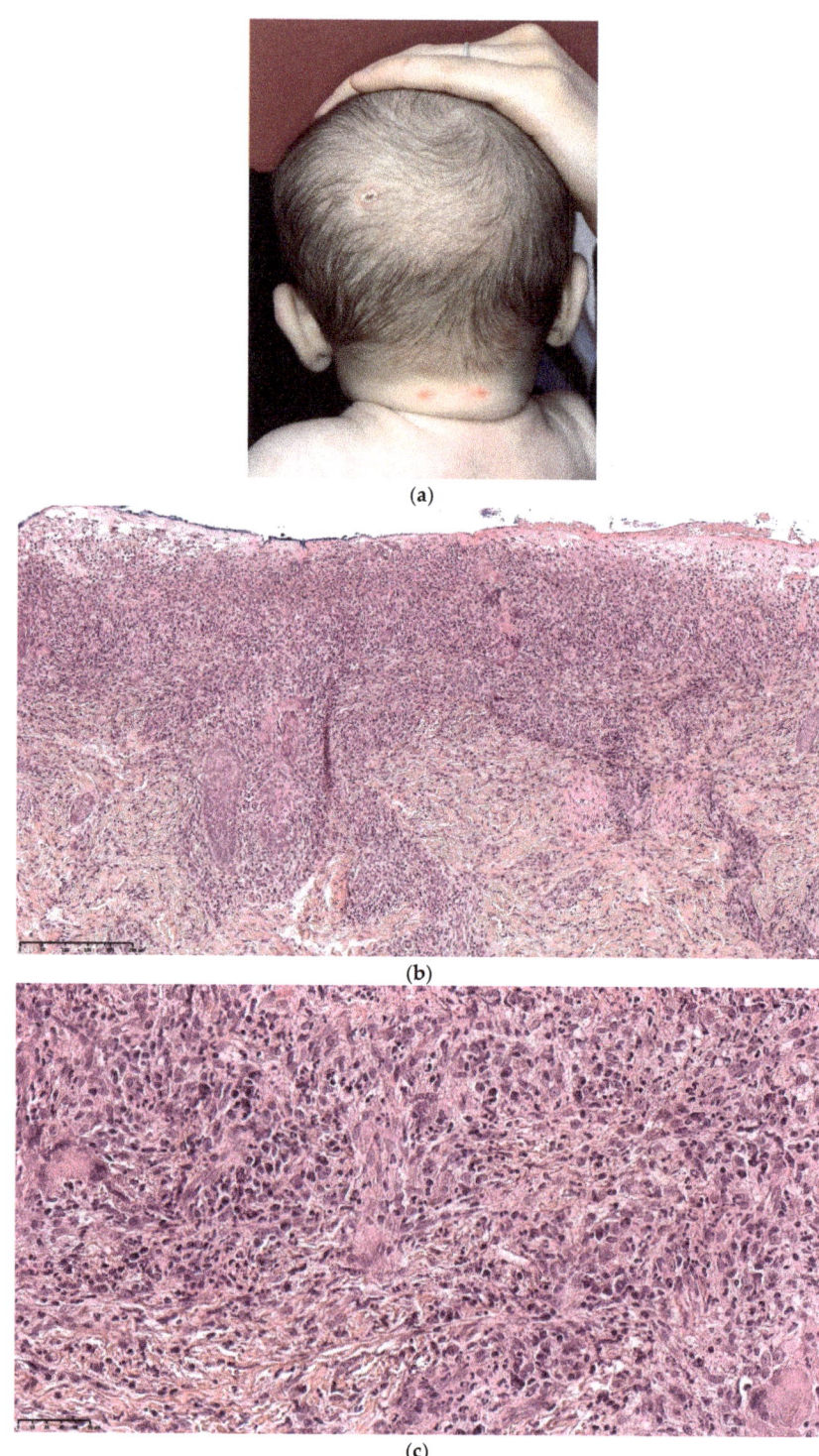

Figure 2. *Cont.*

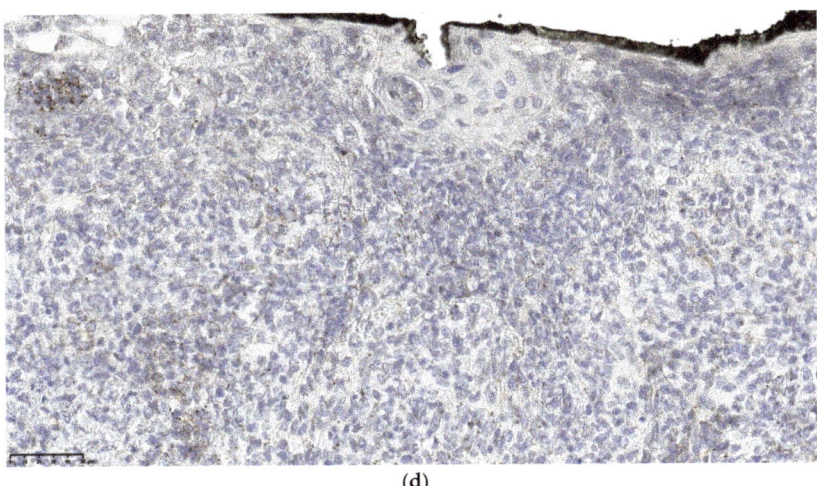

(d)

Figure 2. Congenital syphilis. (**a**) Multiple small erythematous lesions (by courtesy S Mallet). (**b**) 4× superficial and deep cellular infiltrate with ulcerated overlying epidermis (by courtesy N Macagno). (**c**) 25× polymorphic infiltrate containing plasma cells. (**d**) Positivity of anti-treponema showing numerous spirochetes between cells.

2.1. Dermal Erythropoiesis

Dermal erythropoiesis is easy to recognize histologically. It is characterized by the presence of clusters of erythroblasts in the superficial dermis and mid-dermis (Figure 3a–c). The erythroblasts are atypical and, to avoid confusion with leukemic blasts, can be highlighted by immunohistochemical staining with an anti-glycophorin antibody.

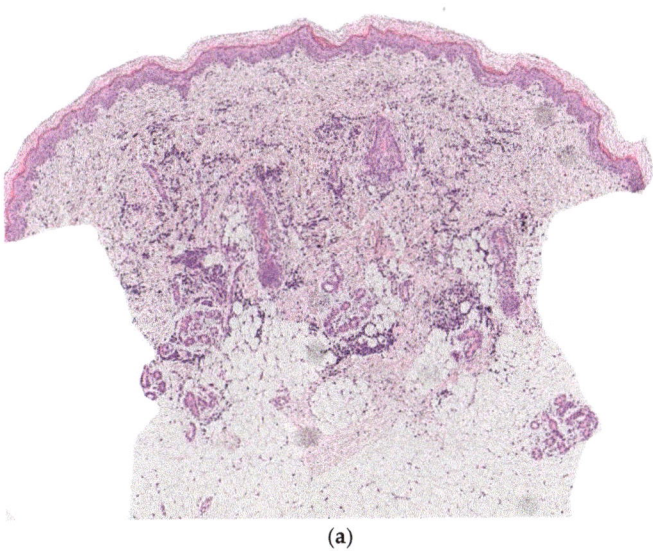

(a)

Figure 3. *Cont.*

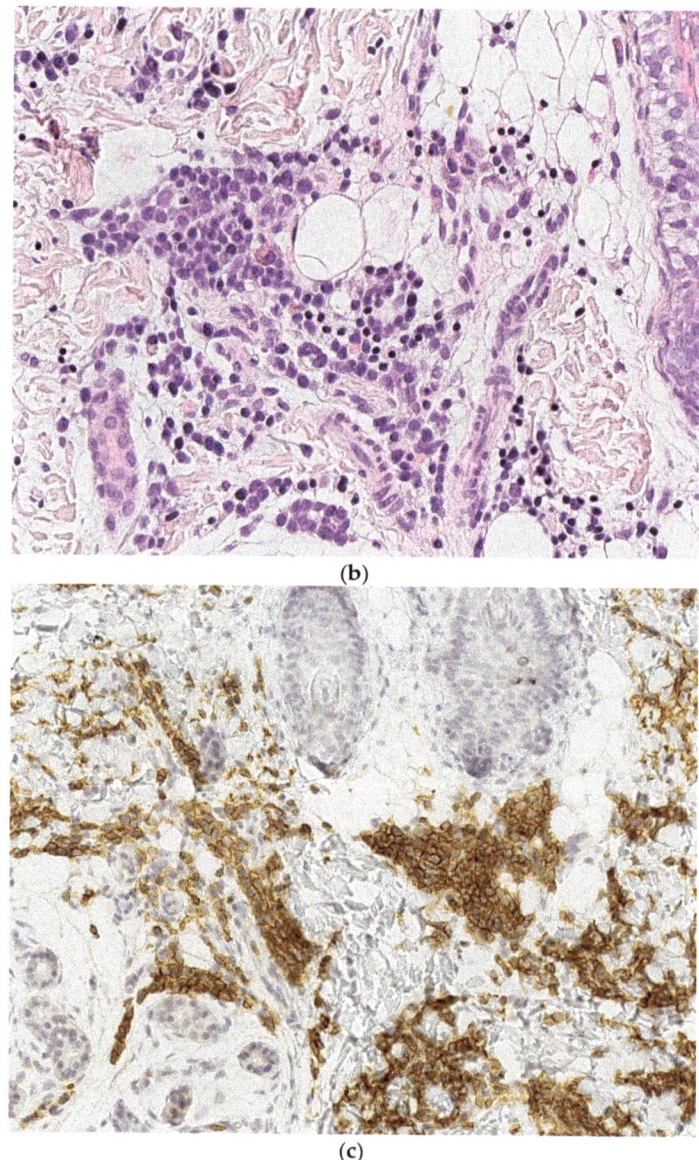

Figure 3. Dermal erythropoiesis (**a**,**b**) 2.5× and 25× clusters of erythroblasts in the dermis. They are highlighted by anti-glycophorin antibody (**c**).

2.2. Neoplastic Diseases

2.2.1. Leukemia Cutis

Acute leukemia is the most common malignancy that presents with specific skin lesions [1]. Most neonates have a high leukocyte count and hepatosplenomegaly. However, aleukemic leukemia cutis (characterized by leukemic cells that invade the skin alone before spreading to the bloodstream) is not rare. Although the skin lesions occur early, the blood cell count and even the bone marrow profile are normal for a while. The lesions may have a nodular, indurated, and bluish appearance (Figure 4a). Early diagnosis and treatment are critical.

Histology

In most cases, the diagnosis is straightforward. A dense dermal infiltrate is separated from the epidermis by a "grenz zone" and extends into the subcutaneous tissue with a perivascular and peri-appendageal arrangement. Cells are arranged in single file between the collagen bundles. They are medium-sized, with a high nuclear-cytoplasmic ratio, nuclear debris (apoptosis), and mitotic figures (Figure 4b–h). A good clue is the very high proportion of tumor cells, and almost no reactive inflammatory cells, in the infiltrate. CD68, lysozyme, and myeloperoxidase are the most sensitive immunohistochemical markers for detecting monoblasts (acute monocytic leukemia 5) or myelomonoblasts (acute monocytic leukemia 4), which account for the vast majority of leukemias at this age. In most cases, 90 to 100% of the cells are positive for KI67. Importantly, these immature monoblasts may lack CD163.

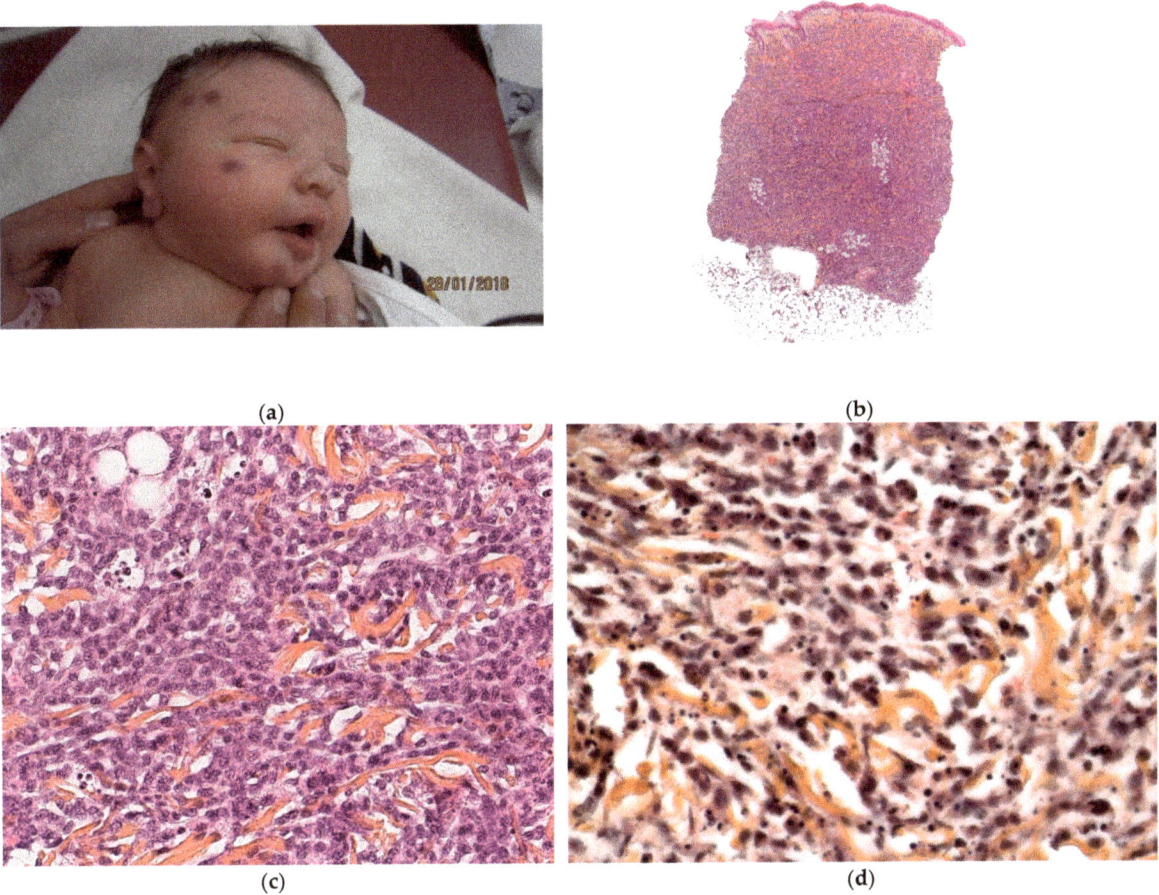

Figure 4. Cont.

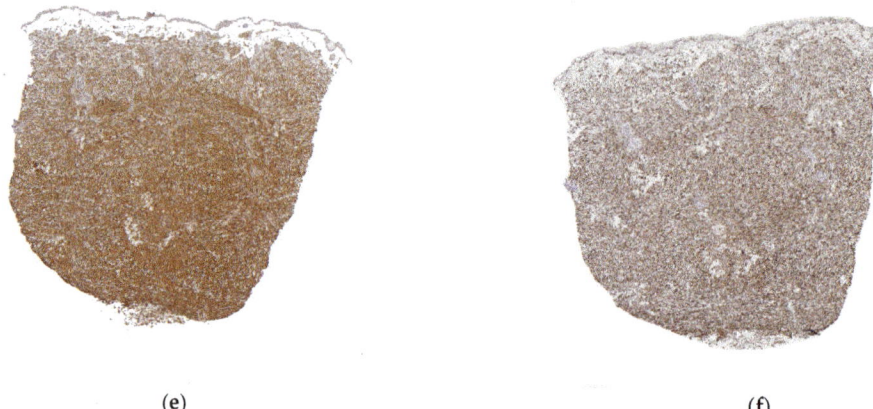

(e)   (f)

Figure 4. Congenital leukemia cutis: (**a**) blueberry muffin rash; (**b**) 4× dense dermal infiltration separated from the epidermis by a grenz-zone; (**c**) 10× medium-sized blastic cells arranged in single-file between collagen bundles and with a peri-vascular and peri-adnexal arrangement as well; (**d**) 25× apoptotic cells and mitotic figures; (**e**) CD68 intense positivity; (**f**) Ki67 immunostaining: almost 100% of nuclei are positive.

Outcome

Infantile leukemia and leukemia cutis can be very severe, lethal conditions but can also resolve spontaneously [5]. These disorders appear to be strongly linked to cytogenetic anomalies. For example, the 11q23 translocation appears to be linked to aggressive acute leukemia. In contrast, t(8;16) tends to be associated with spontaneous regression.

2.2.2. Metastatic Neuroblastoma

Neuroblastoma is the most common tumor of childhood and accounts for 32% of all neonatal tumors (Figure 5a). This tumor is unique because of its distinctive biological behavior and the large number of clinical manifestations. Multiple bluish cutaneous nodules (producing the "blueberry muffin rash") occur in more than a third of patients under 12 months of age and may constitute the initial sign of metastatic neuroblastoma [1]. A vaso-constrictive white halo around the nodules is suggestive of the latter disorder and should prompt the clinician to perform a biopsy without delay. Most infants with this sign are classified as stage IV-S.

Histology

Examination of a cutaneous nodule reveals a uniform, small-cell, malignant tumor and, in some cases, Homer–Wright pseudorosette formations. The tumor cells are positive for Phox2b and synaptophysin (Figure 5b–d).

Outcome

Despite the presence of tumors in the liver, skin, and bone marrow, neonates with stage IV-S disease paradoxically have a relatively good prognosis. The tumor may remit or transform spontaneously into a benign ganglioneuroma.

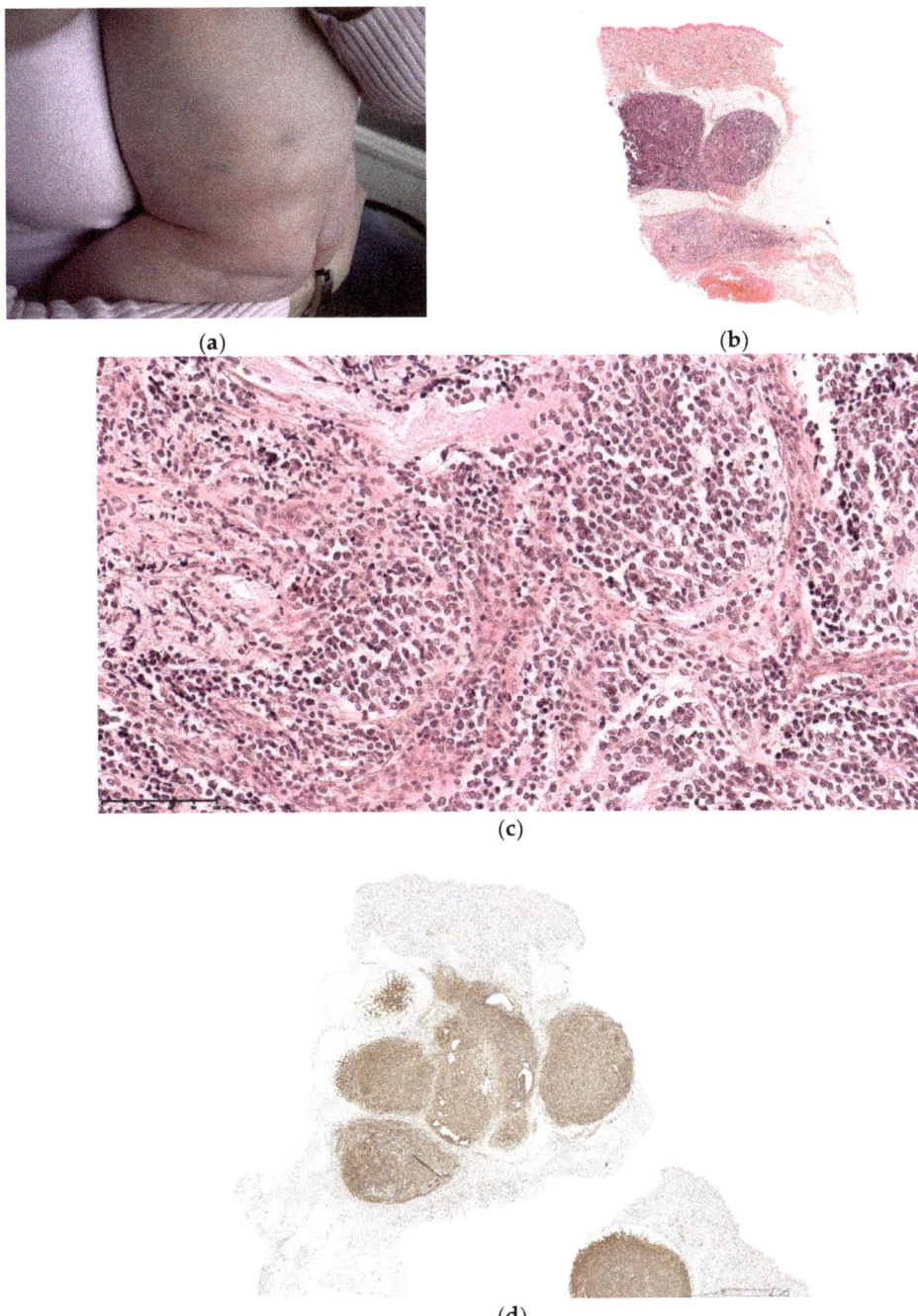

Figure 5. Metastatic neuroblastoma. (**a**) Pink lesion surrounded by a whitish halo. (**b**) 2.5× tumoral nodules in the reticular dermis and the subcutis. (**c**) 25× blue round cells. (**d**) Anti-synaptophysin immunostaining.

2.2.3. Transitory Myeloproliferative Disease

Transient myeloproliferative disorder (TMD) is a Down's syndrome-specific spontaneously regressing neoplasm that affects up to 10% of neonates with the syndrome. In 20–30% of cases, TMD reoccurs as progressive acute megakaryoblastic leukemia (AMKL) at 2–4 years of age. The TMD and AMKL blasts are morphologically and immunophenotypically identical, and have the same acquired mutations in the *GATA1* gene [6].

Metastatic Rhabdomyosarcoma

Rhabdomyosarcoma (RMS) is a highly malignant neoplasm that accounts for most of the soft tissue sarcomas in neonates; it is the second most common after fibrosarcoma [7,8]. Girls outnumber boys by 3.3 to 1. The most frequent disease site is the limb, followed by the neck, the orbit of the eye, and the trunk. RMS accounts for 6% of the malignancies that metastasize into the skin. Although rare, cutaneous metastasis of RMS may be the revealing sign. The cutaneous metastases commonly form bluish cutaneous nodules [9].

Histology

Alveolar rhabdomyosarcoma is the main histological type involving the skin. The tumor comprises small- to medium-sized darkly staining cells with round nuclei and scant cytoplasm arranged in an alveolar pattern. The most diagnostically useful immunohistochemical markers are myogenin and MyoD1, followed by desmin. The diagnosis must be confirmed in a cytogenetic test.

Outcome

In one study, rhabdomyosarcoma had the second lowest survival rate (2 out of 13, 15%) after rhabdoid tumor (4%) [1]. The prognosis has not improved in recent years, despite changes in therapy [10].

Metastatic Rhabdoid Tumor

Metastatic rhabdoid tumor (MRT) is a highly malignant exceedingly rare neoplasm characterized clinically by rapid growth, early metastases, and a high mortality rate among neonates and infants [7]. Rhabdoid tumors rank fourth in order of incidence after leukemia, Langerhans cell histiocytosis, and neuroblastoma. MRT may present in the skin (especially in the head and neck area) as a solitary primary tumor or as one or more metastatic skin nodules [7]. Metastatic disease is present in more than half of fetuses and neonates at the time of diagnosis. The main skin sites for metastases are the limbs, trunk, face, and neck; several sites can be affected simultaneously. Almost all patients present with blue cutaneous nodules.

Histology

Classically, MRT is described as sheets of polygonal cells with abundant acidophilic cytoplasm, eccentric round vesicular nuclei, prominent nucleoli, and periodic acid Schiff-positive hyaline cytoplasmic inclusions (Figure 6). Loss of immunoreactivity for INI1 is a distinguishing (but not pathognomonic) feature of MRT. The disorder is associated with loss of the tumor suppressor SMARCB1/INI1/SNF5/BAF47 on chromosome 22q11 due to either heterozygous germline deletions or somatic mutations.

Outcome

Rhabdoid tumors have the lowest survival rate (1 out of 24, 4%) of all malignancies at this age [7].

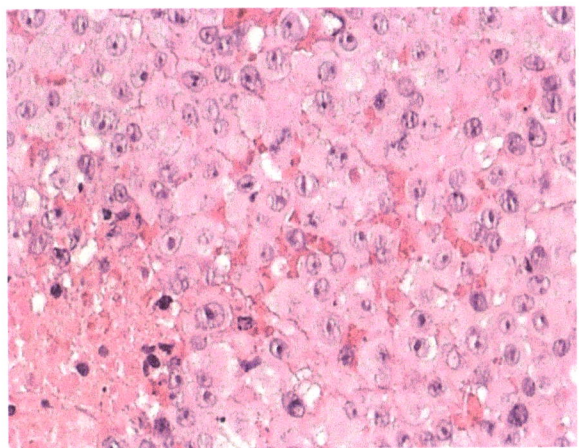

Figure 6. 40× Rhaboid tumor. Very atypical large cells.

2.2.4. Congenital Histiocytosis

Congenital Langerhans Cell Histiocytosis (LCH)

Congenital Langerhans cell histiocytosis (LCH) is rare and, in most cases, regresses spontaneously very quickly, within a few weeks of birth. This self-resolving form of histiocytosis was first described by Hashimoto and Pritzker in 1973. Typically, skin lesions manifest as widespread vesicles, pustules, or both. They are often erosive and purpuric and can be mistaken for neonatal herpes. Purplish, reddish-brown, crusted, papulonodular lesions with central necrosis and ulceration are observed in 25–30% of cases of neonatal LCH (Figure 7a,b). A few nodules may develop [11,12]. Furthermore, some babies with congenital LCH may develop a "blueberry muffin rash" [13].

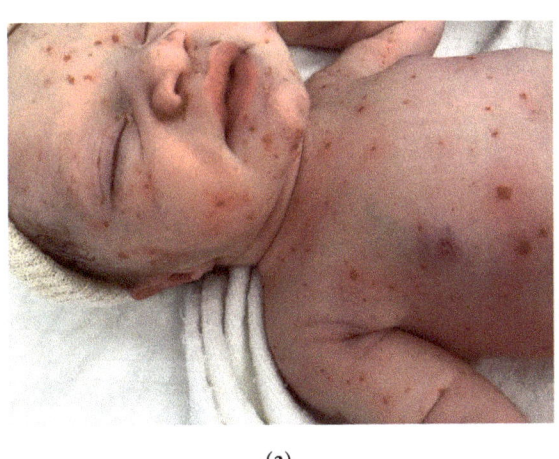

(a)

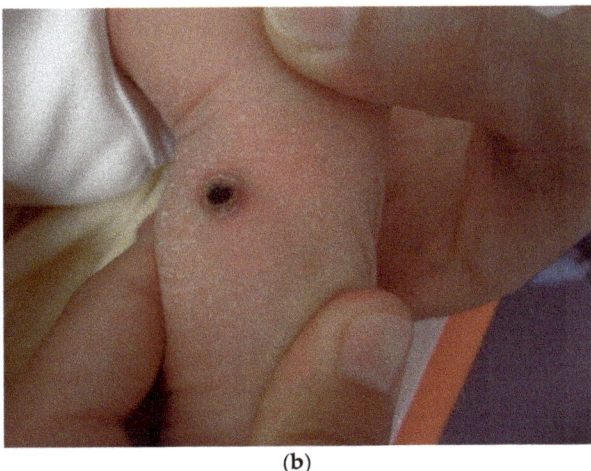

(b)

Figure 7. *Cont.*

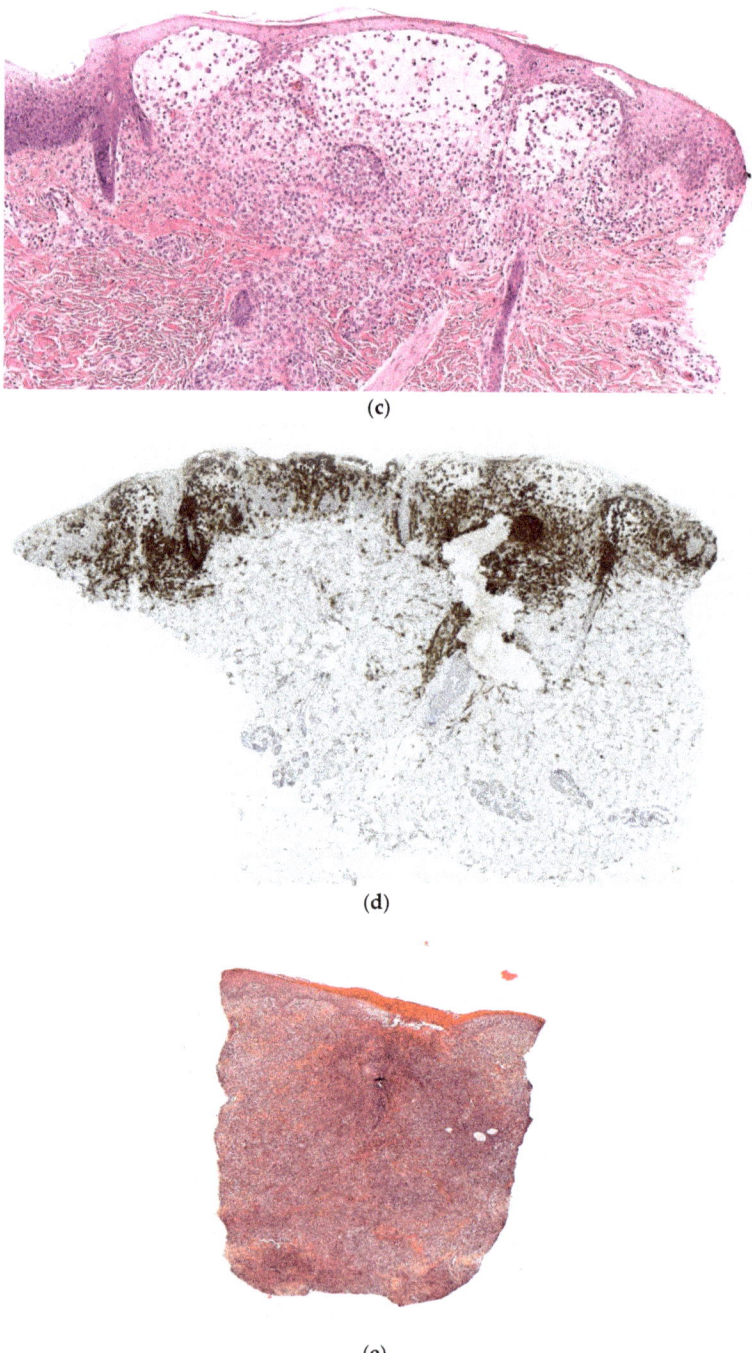

Figure 7. Langerhans cell histiocytosis (**a**) disseminated congenital lesions with erosive and purpuric lesions. (**b**) nodular and crusted lesion (Hashimoto-Pritzker). (**c**) 2.5× usual aspect of LCH with Langerhans cell infiltrate filling the papillary dermis. (**d**) 2.5× anti-CD1a. (**e**) 2.5× Nodular spontaneously regressive lesion. Dense infiltrate throughout the dermis with very few epidermotropism.

Histology

A skin biopsy is always necessary to confirm the diagnosis of LCH. Cutaneous LCH is characterized by an infiltration of the papillary dermis by monomorphous, medium-sized histiocytes with a pink, non-xanthomized cytoplasm and a kidney-shaped, grooved, or folded nucleus. These cells are positive for CD1a and CD207 (Langerin); the latter is specific for Birbeck granules. These cells may be associated with eosinophils, lymphocytes, and/or red blood cells. Epidermotropism results in a spongiform pattern with focal parakeratosis. It is not possible to differentiate between regressing LCH and non-regressing LCH on the sole basis of the histological data. The nodular form of LCH shows a tumoral intradermal infiltration of large histiocytes and commonly ulcerated overlying epidermis. The cells comprise Langerhans cells (CD1a+, CD207+), indeterminate cells (CD1a+, CD207− (Figure 7c–e), and macrophages (CD163+, CD1a−, CD207−) [14]. Most cases harbor mutations in the MAP kinase pathway and especially in the *BRAF* gene.

Outcome

In most cases of LCH, the lesions observed at birth are not accompanied by systemic signs and tend to involute spontaneously within a few weeks or months. Since the original description, however, many cases of extracutaneous involvement, visceral involvement, and/or disease recurrence have been reported. It has not yet been possible to define clinical or histological factors that distinguish between the "self-healing" and progressive multisystem forms of neonatal LCH [15]. Accordingly, careful work-up and close follow-up are necessary in all cases.

Multiple Xanthogranuloma

Juvenile xanthogranuloma (JXG) is a fairly common non-Langerhans cell histiocytosis. It most often affects infants and young children and is characterized by the dermal accumulation of variably xanthomized histiocytes. The skin lesions usually resolve, and most patients have an otherwise unremarkable clinical course. In total, 20% of cases of JXG are congenital, and multiple lesions are observed in 20% of congenital cases. Very rarely, the disorder also affects extracutaneous organs: mostly the eyes but also the liver, spleen, lungs, central nervous system, kidneys, retroperitoneum, or elsewhere in the body. JXG features small, smooth, and dome-shaped papules rather than large nodules. The color depends on the age of the lesions (i.e., the degree of xanthomization): first pink to red-brown, and then yellow (Figure 8a,b). Most lesions resolve spontaneously, albeit over months or even years.

Histology

Typically, the lesions demonstrate a well-demarcated, dense infiltrate of histiocytes within small lesions in the superficial dermis. Larger lesions extend into the deep dermis or subcutis. There is often loss of the rete ridges, and ulceration occurs in rare cases. Early lesions usually contain monomorphous histiocytes with abundant eosinophilic cytoplasm. In mature lesions, an accumulation of lipids in the histiocytes' cytoplasm gives them a foamy "xanthomatous" appearance. Touton giant cells are common at this stage. Lymphocytes and eosinophils are also scattered throughout the infiltrate. In fact, all types and shapes of histiocyte can be present (Figure 8c–e).

These histiocytes may originate from a "dermal dendrocyte"; they are always strongly positive for CD163, sometimes positive for FXIIIa (Figure 8f), and always negative for CD1a and CD207. Although most patients with cutaneous JXG do not carry any mutations, mutations in the MAP kinase pathway have been described in some cases with multiple lesions and organ involvement [16].

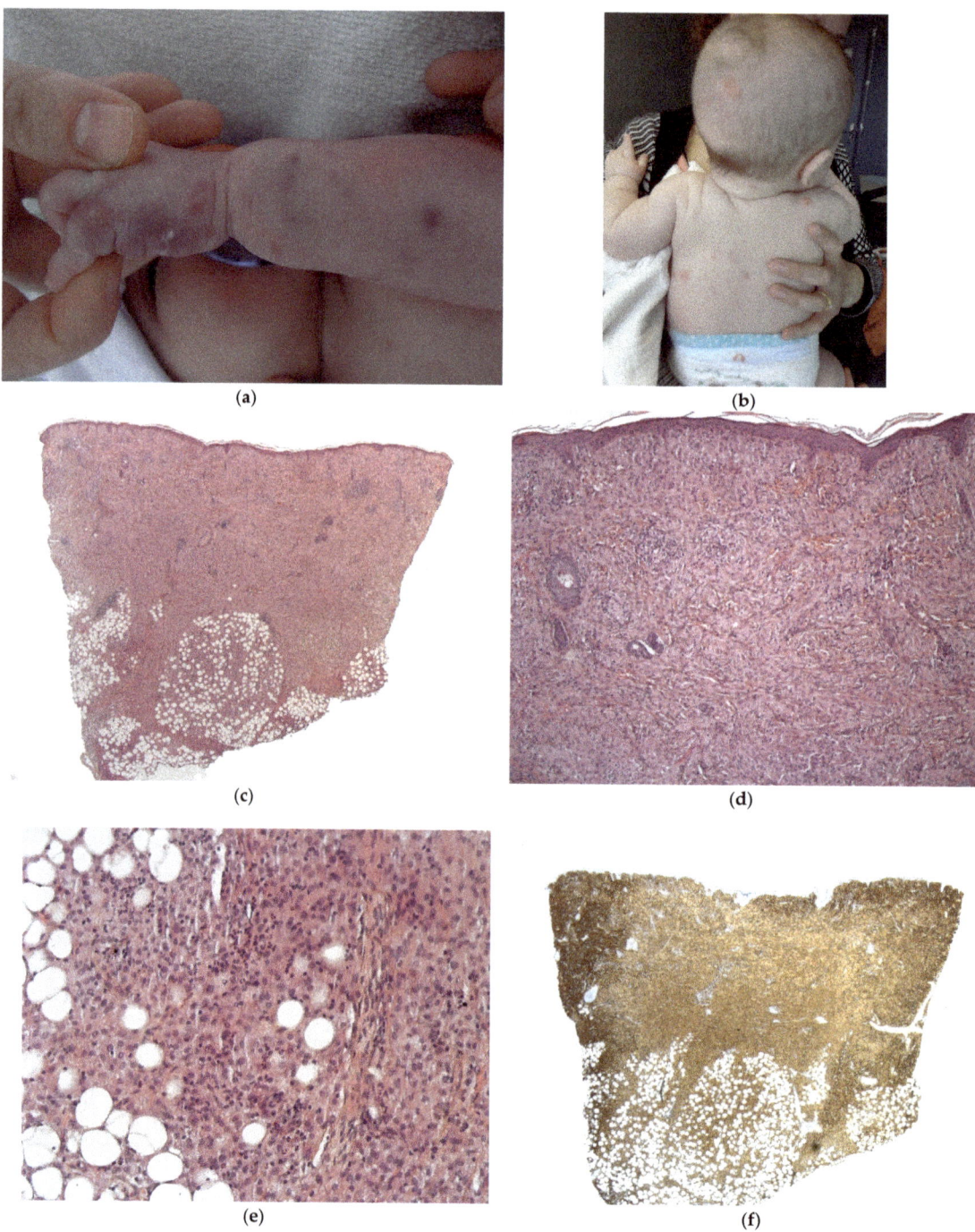

Figure 8. Juvenile xanthogranuloma. (**a**) Presenting as blueberry muffin rash (by courtesy E Puzenat); (**b**) multiple yellowish lesions. (**c**) 4× rather dense infiltrate in the dermis extending into the superficial subcutis. (**d**) 10× non xanthomized histiocytes with no giant cells (mononuclear-vacuolated early variant). (**e**) 25× Histiocytes are accompanied by inflammatory cells, in particular here, neutrophils. (**f**) Anti-Factor XIIIa positivity.

Outcome

In patients with systemic disease, the clinical course can be catastrophic, and spontaneous remission is very rare [17]. The treatment of choice is a combination of vinblastin and dexamethasone. A BRAF inhibitor can be considered in patients with a mutation. Therefore, children with multiple lesions at birth—particularly those involving the eye—should always be screened for systemic involvement [18].

2.2.5. Transplacentally Acquired Tumors

It has been estimated that 1 in every 1000 pregnancies will feature a malignancy, about the same frequency as in age-matched nonpregnant women. Melanoma is one of the least rare.

Transplacental Melanoma

Melanoma is the most common neoplasm with transplacental transmission to the fetus [19]. The estimated incidence of melanoma during pregnancy is 0.1 to 2.8 per 1000. Fetal metastases are rare; around 100 case reports have been published. Although spontaneous regression has very occasionally been reported, most neonates with clinical evidence of maternal metastases at birth have an exceedingly poor prognosis [20].

Histology

In some circumstances, the diagnosis of transplacental melanoma may be confirmed by biopsy. In most cases, the diagnosis is straightforward when pigmentary lesions are seen in a newborn born to a mother with confirmed metastatic melanoma.

Outcome

Death typically occurs before the age of 3 months. Placental involvement appears to be a key risk factor among patients with no clinical evidence of metastasis at birth [21].

Transplacental Choriocarcinoma

Infantile choriocarcinoma is a rare, highly malignant germ cell tumor that arises from the placenta. It is characterized by the secretion of human chorionic gonadotropin (hCG). Simultaneous intraplacental choriocarcinomas involving both the mother and infant are extremely rare, and cutaneous metastasis in infantile choriocarcinoma is even rarer [22,23]: fewer than 30 cases have been described in the literature. About half of these cases arise from a complete hydatidiform mole, a quarter arise after normal pregnancies, and a quarter appear after a spontaneous abortion or an ectopic pregnancy. The cutaneous manifestations of choriocarcinoma are metastatic nodules, subcutaneous masses, and multiple angiomatoid tumors.

Histology

The two-zone tumor has a central core of mononuclear cytotrophoblasts and a peripheral rim of multinucleated syncytiotrophoblasts. Extensive hemorrhage and necrosis are frequent (Figure 9a,b). The trophoblasts show marked cytological atypia, and immunohistochemistry with antibodies against hCG or human placental lactogen confirms the diagnosis [23].

Outcome

The outcome is poor, with a survival rate below 25%. More recently, however, it has been shown that prompt diagnosis (from a biopsy of a metastatic skin nodule) and chemotherapy improve the prognosis significantly [23,24].

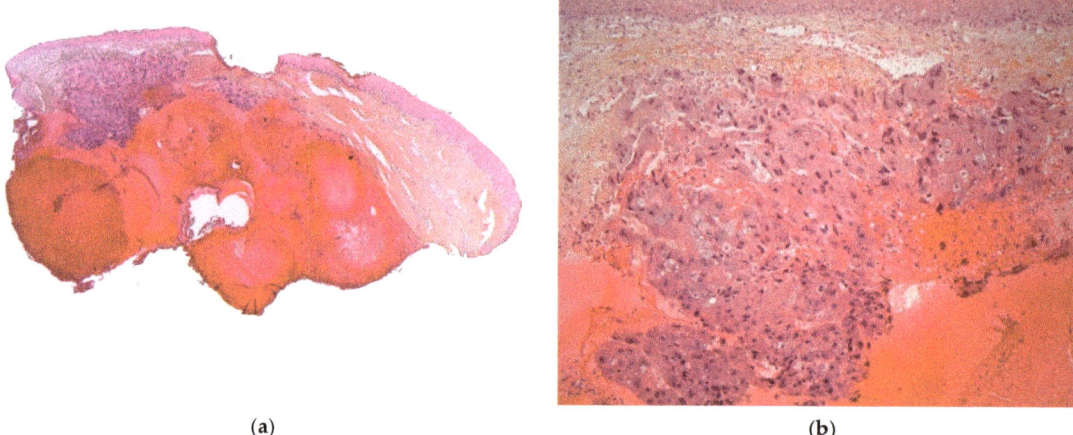

Figure 9. Metastatic choriocarcinoma. (**a**) 4× cellular and hemorrhagic areas in the reticular dermis arranged in lobules. (**b**) 25× very large typical cells of syncytiotrophoblast.

2.2.6. Infantile Myofibromatosis

Infantile myofibromatosis (IM) is a benign mesenchymal tumor from the juvenile fibromatosis group and is commonly encountered by dermatologists. The name "infantile myofibromatosis" reflects the fact that the tumor is composed of myofibroblasts. Infantile myofibromatosis affects children during the first decade of life, and 60% are present at birth.

There are three defined clinical patterns: (i) solitary, self-limiting disease (also called myofibroma); (ii) multicentric disease (involving the skin, subcutaneous tissues, muscles and bones, with a typical benign course and spontaneous resolution); and (iii) a generalized form with visceral involvement and a poor prognosis [25]. The multifocal lesions may be quite numerous (from a few dozen up to 100 or more) and are present at birth. Girls are more commonly affected than boys.

There are many different clinical presentations, depending on the proportion of myofibroblasts and the degree of vascular proliferation. The lesions may present as (i) firm, flesh-colored papulonodules; (ii) crusted or angiomatous infiltrate plaques; (iii) pedunculated, infiltrated, calcified tumors; or (iv) ulcerated, necrotic, pseudo-sarcomatous tumors mimicking cutaneous metastases (neuroblastoma) and leukemia cutis (all causes of multiple nodules at birth) (Figure 10a). Hence, an appropriate biopsy is always necessary.

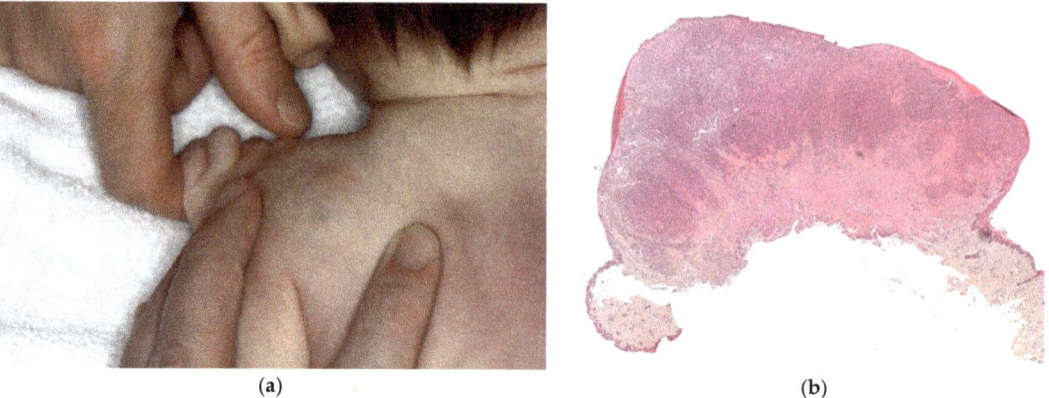

Figure 10. *Cont.*

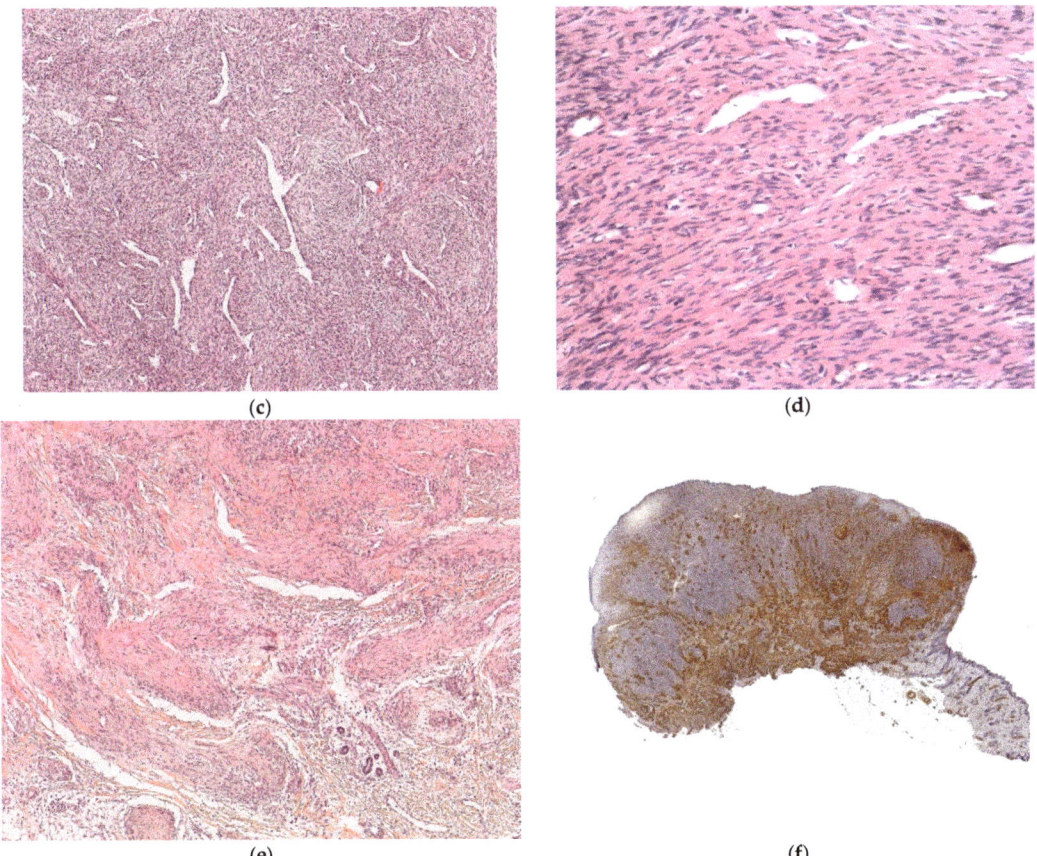

Figure 10. Infantile myofibromatosis. (**a**) This baby presented with multiple small blueish lesions. (**b**) 4× dermal rounded well-circumscribed lesion. (**c**) 10× antler-shaped vascular proliferation associated with spindle-shaped cells in the center of the lesion. (**d**) 25× spindle-shaped cells arranged in fascicles. (**e**) 10× round lobules made up of elongated cells with poorly seen cytoplasmic borders at the periphery of the lesion. (**f**) 4× anti-SMA.

Histology

The lesion is characterized by a two-zone pattern best seen at low power: a central hemangiopericytoma-like area surrounded by a leiomyoma-like area. The relative proportions of the two areas can vary. The periphery of the myofibroma is marked by the proliferation of short bundles of spindle cells with a myoid appearance (i.e., plump nuclei and abundant pale cytoplasm), which are frequently clustered into round aggregates. The tumor's central region is often marked by a proliferation of rather small round-to-oval cells with little cytoplasm. Centrally located round-to-oval cells are often arranged around prominent "antler-shaped" vascular spaces (Figure 10b–e). This central region often develops areas of ischemic necrosis. Mitotic figures are not rare. Spindle cells are strongly positive for smooth muscle actin (Figure 10f) and calponin and, in some cases, desmin [25].

Outcome

Patients with multifocal disease still have an excellent prognosis; most experience spontaneous disease resolution over 12 to 18 months [25]. However, patients with generalized IM typically have severe systemic diseases. Visceral involvement can involve the gastrointestinal tract, lungs, heart, and upper respiratory tract [26]. Death occurs mainly within the first weeks of life and within 4 months at the latest.

Neonates with multiple lesions should undergo a full skin examination and imaging, to determine the extent of the disease. In patients with visceral involvement, systemic treatment may be necessary. The tumor typically responds slowly to conventional chemotherapy, and tumor reduction is usually not observed until after several weeks of treatment. Recently, somatic mutations in the gene coding for platelet-derived growth factor receptor beta polypeptide (PDGFR-β) have been identified in most sporadic multicentric forms of the disease. Hence, PDGFR inhibitors, like imatinib, have been considered for use in life-threatening cases. However, second-line treatment with a targeted therapy should only be considered in the context of life-threatening disease progression [27,28].

2.3. Non-Neoplastic Disorder: Subcutaneous Fat Necrosis of the Newborn

This is a rare condition, characterized by multiple erythematous or skin-colored indurated subcutaneous nodules or plaques that appear during the neonatal period in a large hardened area on the back, buttocks, and limbs.

The lesions are primarily observed on the body areas with the most adipose tissue, such as the shoulders, buttocks, cheeks, and thighs (Figure 11a). The nodules frequently soften and become fluctuant, or occasionally liquefy. At birth, these nodules may mimic the lesions in leukemia cutis or neuroblastoma metastases; a biopsy may then be necessary.

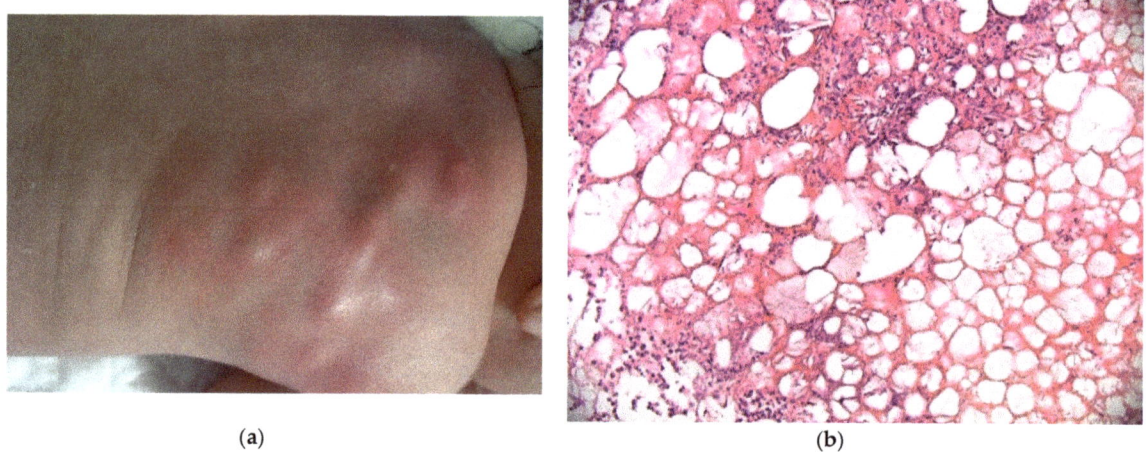

Figure 11. Subcutaneous fat necrosis of the newborn. (**a**) Multiple skin-colored nodular lesions at the upper back. (**b**) 10× lobular panniculitis with inflammatory cells and typical radially arranged needle-shaped cleft into the fatty tissue.

2.3.1. Histology

The biopsy of an early lesion always has a characteristic appearance: a dense, inflammatory, lobular infiltrate in the subcutis is composed of lymphocytes, histiocytes, eosinophils (occasionally), and multinucleated giant cells with fat necrosis. Radially arranged needle-shaped clefts, corresponding to crystallized fatty acids that were dissolved during slide processing, are seen within the adipocytes and giant cells [29] (Figure 11b).

2.3.2. Outcome

The lesions resolve spontaneously within a few weeks or months.

3. Multifocal Vascular Skin Lesions

Multifocal vascular lesions at birth may correspond to different entities of different prognosis and therapeutic management (Table 2).

Table 2. Multifocal neonatal vascular skin lesions.

Multifocal infantile hemangioma
Multifocal lymphangiomatosis with thrombocytopenia
Multiple neonatal pyogenic granuloma
Multiple tufted angioma/kaposiform hemangioendothelioma
Venous malformations:
glomuvenous malformation
blue rubber bleb naevus syndrome (Bean's syndrome)

3.1. Multifocal Infantile Hemangioma

Multifocal infantile hemangiomas develop shortly after birth [30], ranging from several to hundreds. These dome-shaped, bright red papules or nodules vary in size from a few millimeters to centimeters but tend to be small, extraordinarily numerous, spread all over the body, and superficial (Figure 12a).

3.1.1. Histology

The histological features of multifocal infantile hemangioma are identical to those of solitary infantile hemangioma, except that capillaries are well differentiated from the outset and are arranged in lobules within the dermis, usually the superficial dermis (Figure 12b). The lesions are always positive for Glut1 (endothelial staining) (Figure 12c).

3.1.2. Outcome

The lesions regress spontaneously as early as the first year of life and often have involuted completely by 2 years of age. The presence of more than five cutaneous infantile hemangiomas is a potential marker for hepatic involvement, and an abdominal ultrasound assessment is indicated. Depending on their number, density, and severity, the hepatic lesions are usually asymptomatic but can cause serious complications (such as heart failure). Patients with widespread hepatic involvement can be treated with propranolol [31].

3.2. Multifocal Lymphangiomatosis with Thrombocytopenia

Multifocal lymphangiomatosis with thrombocytopenia (MLT) is a vascular disorder affecting several organs. It is associated with thrombocytopenia, the severity of which may vary. Classically, both the skin and the gastrointestinal tract are involved [32]. The skin lesions are present at birth and appear as multifocal, discrete, and red-brown to burgundy papules, plaques, and nodules, ranging from a few millimeters to several centimeters in size (Figure 13a) [33]. The number of lesions ranges from a few to hundreds. The trunk and limbs are more commonly involved. Gastrointestinal tract lesions present with hematemesis and/or melaena, usually early in infancy. Endoscopy reveals a few or many small vascular lesions on the gastrointestinal mucosa. Additional lesion sites include the lung, bone, liver, brain, synovium, and muscle. Thrombocytopenia is most commonly present in the first month of life. It is usually sustained, with a mean platelet count of 50,000–100,000/ mL, and results in gastrointestinal tract bleeding. Fibrinogen levels are normal to low, and D-dimer levels may be elevated.

It is important to distinguish MLT from other multifocal congenital vascular diseases that affect the skin and viscera, such as multifocal venous malformations (e.g., blue rubber bleb nevus syndrome) and multiple congenital pyogenic granulomas. Hence, a biopsy is always required.

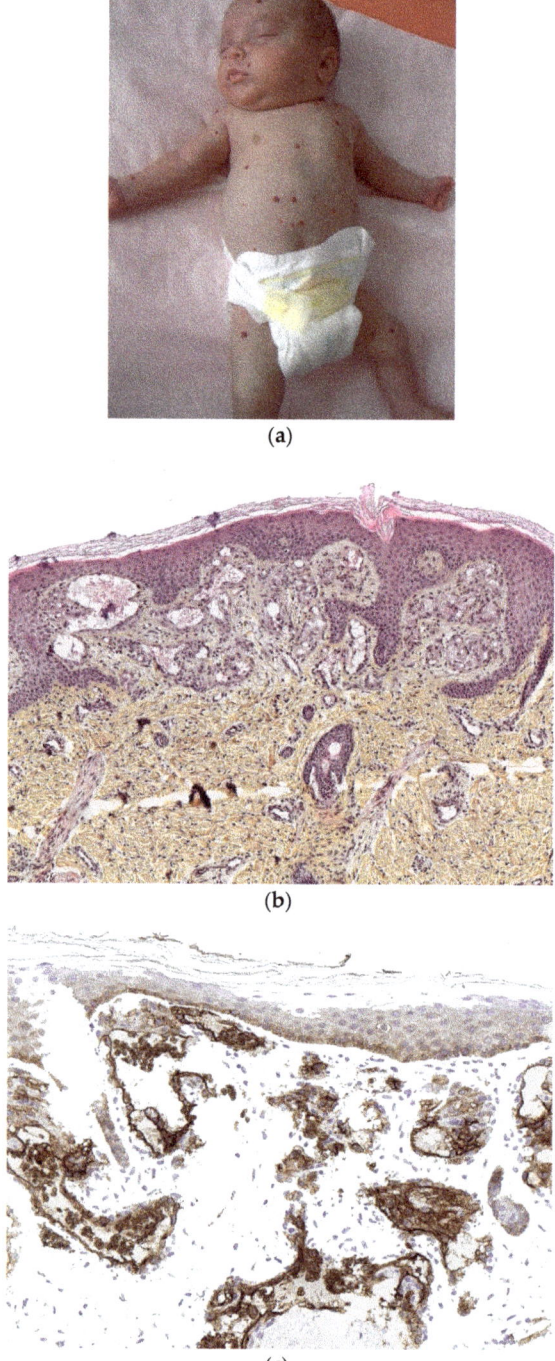

Figure 12. Multifocal infantile hemangioma. (**a**) Multiple small red lesions disseminated over the body. (**b**) 10× Well-differentiated small vessels in the superficial dermis. (**c**) Anti-Glut1 immunostaining showing positivity of all the endothelia.

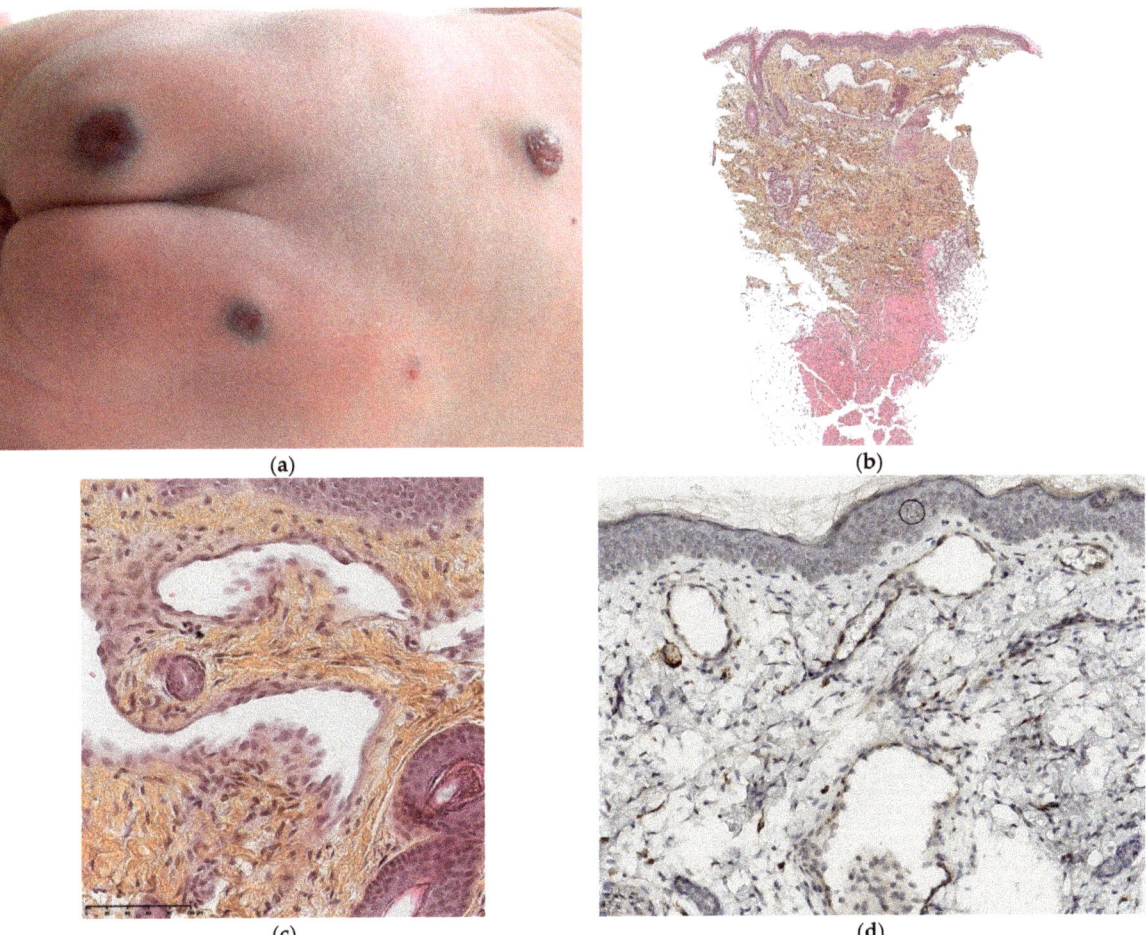

Figure 13. Multifocal lymphangiomatosis with thrombocytopenia. (**a**) Red-brown papules and plaques (by courtesy C Droitcourt). (**b**) 2.5× Thin-walled vascular channels dissecting the superficial and mid-dermis. (**c**) 4× These vessels are lined by endothelial cells with a plump, sometimes hobnail, nucleus. (**d**) These cells are positive for Lyve 1.

3.2.1. Histology

A histologic assessment of MLT will reveal dilated, thin-walled vascular channels and variable endothelial hyperplasia in the dermis and subcutis. Most lesions display intraluminal papillary projections [32,33] (Figure 13b,c). The endothelial nuclei are prominent and sometimes hobnailed. MLT is often positive for the lymphatic marker Lyve-1 but may be negative for podoplanin (using the D2-40 antibody) (Figure 13d).

3.2.2. Outcome

MRI and computed tomography are used to document the extent of the disease in patients with MLT. The lesions may develop progressively throughout the body or may stabilize or regress over time [32,33]. Treatment strategies are not well established because of phenotypic variations and the rarity of this disease. Blood and platelets can be administered. Sirolimus appears to be promising. In one study, the vascular lesions responded fully or partly to treatment, leading to clinical improvement in a small number of patients [34].

3.3. Multiple Neonatal Pyogenic Granulomas

Congenital disseminated pyogenic granuloma is a distinctive, multisystemic aggressive disorder that primarily affects the skin, brain, visceral organs, and musculoskeletal system [35].

The granulomas commonly affect the skin and the epithelia mucosa. Multiple congenital pyogenic granuloma is very rare but must be accounted for as a diagnosis because extracutaneous organs (such as the brain and liver) may be affected. The lesion is typically a bright red, friable papule that grows quickly and is prone to bleeding. A loosely adherent hemorrhagic crust may be seen. Lesions may be pedunculated or sessile (Figure 14a) and most are less than 1 cm in diameter [36]. Differentiation of this entity from other multiple cutaneous vascular lesions is critical because of possible cerebral hemorrhagic involvement. A tissue biopsy is essential for a definitive diagnosis.

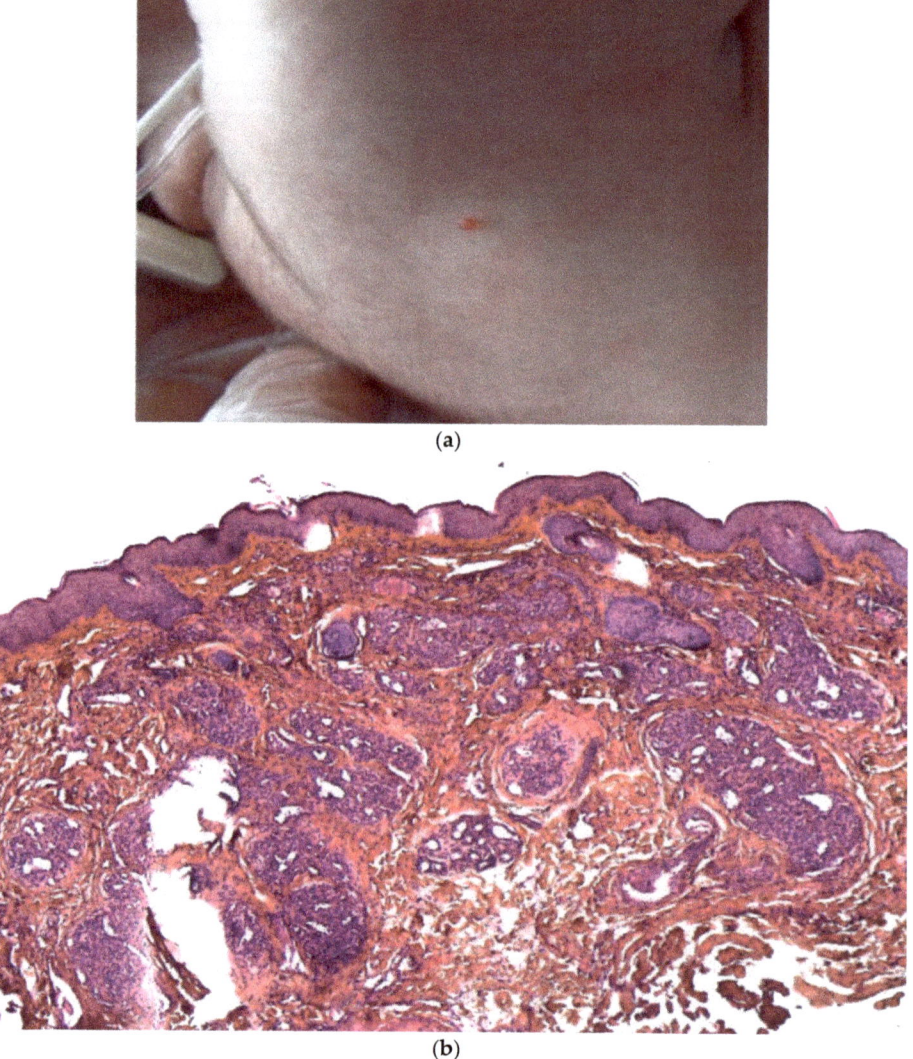

(a)

(b)

Figure 14. *Cont.*

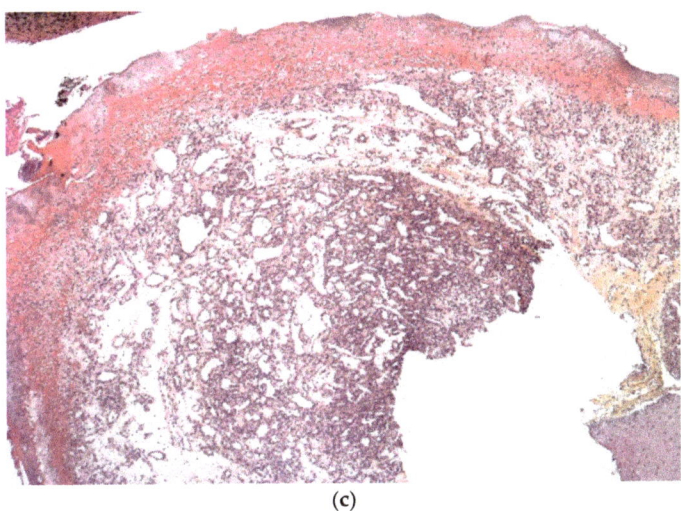

(c)

Figure 14. Neonatal pyogenic granulomas. (**a**) Small red typical pyogenic granuloma. (**b**) 4× lobulated vascular lesion in the dermis. The overlying epidermis is normal whereas in (**c**), it is ulcerated and the lesion contains inflammatory cells.

3.3.1. Histology

A histologic assessment shows a well-circumscribed lobular proliferation of capillaries. The lobules are separated by bands of fibrous stroma. An epidermal collarette, ulceration, and inflammation are additional features (Figure 14b,c). The endothelial cells are always negative for Glut1 and podoplanin.

3.3.2. Outcome

Spontaneous regression is usually observed.

3.4. Multiple Tufted Angiomas/Kaposiform Hemangioendotheliomatosis

Multiple tufted angiomas (TAs) and kaposiform hemangioendotheliomatosis (KHE) are related vascular tumors that present in infancy and childhood. They share histological features (including the proliferation of blood vessels and lymphatic vessels) and are now considered to different clinical expressions along the spectrum of the same vascular anomaly. Multifocal presentation is very rare. Clinically, multiple reddish-blue skin nodules are observed. Histopathologic assessment is mandatory because TA/KHE is a differential diagnosis for other multifocal vascular disorders [37,38].

Histology

A histological assessment of TA shows nodules of densely packed endothelial cells that are scattered throughout the dermis in a "cannonball" pattern. The lobules are surrounded by crescent-shaped vascular spaces. The endothelial cells are only partially canalized, and the vessels have a slit-like appearance reminiscent of Kaposi sarcoma. KHE has more infiltrating sheets and lobules of tightly packed, spindle-shaped endothelial cells associated with microthrombi, hemorrhagic areas, lymphatic-like vascular spaces, and hemosiderin deposits.

TA and KHE have a similar immunophenotype, with a positive staining for CD31, CD34, and, in all cases, the lymphatic marker podoplanin in the lobules and some extralobular vessels (Figure 15a–f).

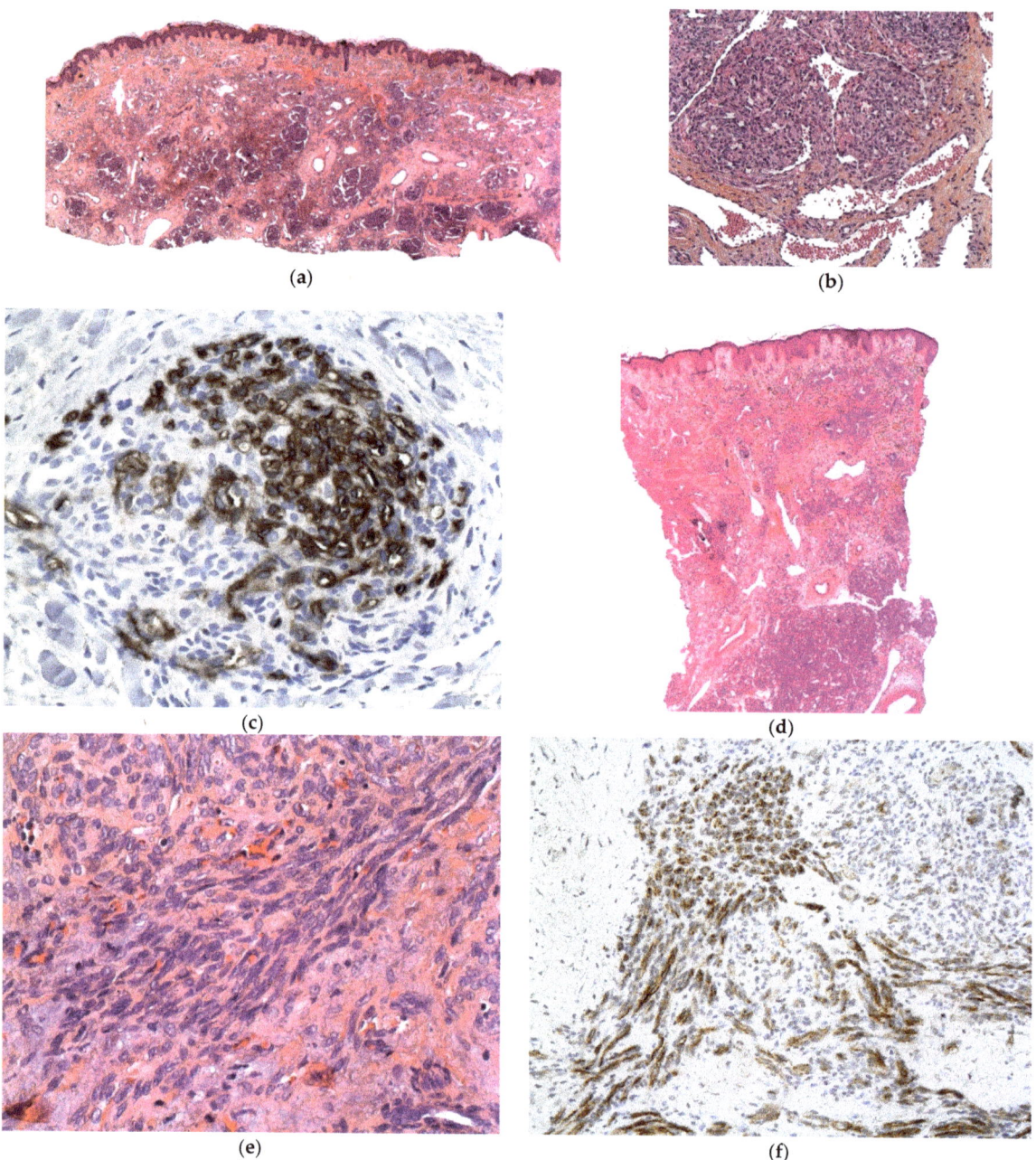

Figure 15. Tufted angioma and kaposiform hemangioendotheliomatosis. (**a**) 25× numerous very small and well-limited lobules throughout the dermis. (**b**) 25× packed small vessels and crescent-shaped vascular channel surrounding it. (**c**) Anti-podoplanin staining the lobules partially. (**d**) Poorly limited and infiltrative vascular tumor in the dermis extending into the subcutis. (**e**) Spindle-shaped cells with red blood cells in between. (**f**) Partial staining of the vessels with anti-podoplanin.

3.5. Venous Malformations

TA and KHE are congenital disorders that can present with multiple deep cutaneous lesions. Multiple venous malformations can be associated with blue rubber bleb nevus syndrome, cutaneomucosal venous malformation, or glomuvenous malformation. The venous malformations are typically bluish, soft, and compressible.

3.5.1. Glomuvenous Malformation

This disorder is inherited in an autosomal dominant fashion. It only affects the skin and never the viscera. Congenital forms are very rare and are difficult to diagnose clinically because the regional or multifocal lesions are pink and not blue [39]. In most cases, new lesions appear after birth (Figure 16a).

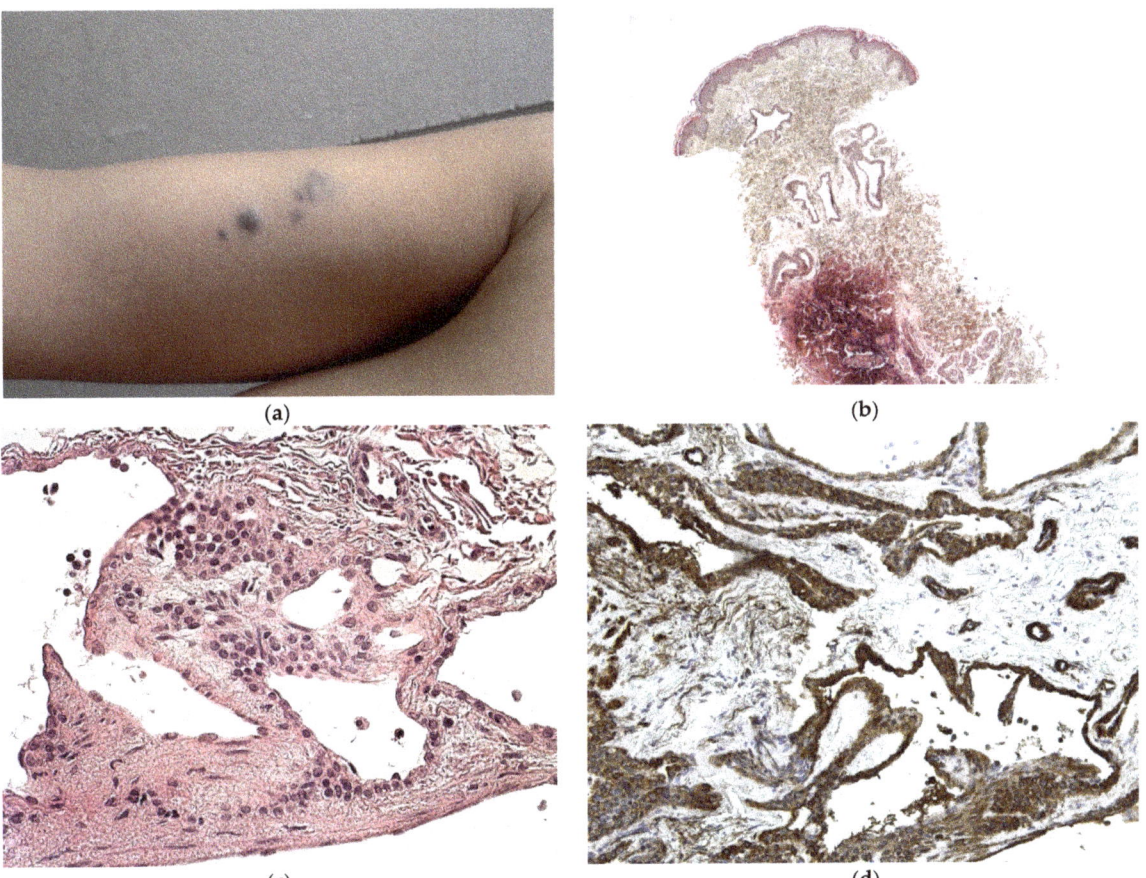

Figure 16. Glomuvenous malformation. (**a**) Bluish to violet small nodules in the arm. (**b**) 10× multiples veinous channels in the dermis. (**c**) 25× these vessels are surrounded by round glomus cells. (**d**) These cells are highlighted by anti-SMA.

Histology

A biopsy is always required for a firm diagnosis. It will typically show clusters of glomus cells situated around dilated vascular structures (Figure 16b–d). Immunohistochemically, the clusters are positive for smooth muscle actin.

3.5.2. Blue Rubber Bleb Naevus Syndrome (Bean's Syndrome)

Blue rubber bleb nevus syndrome is a rare vascular syndrome characterized by the continuous eruption of vascular nodules in the skin, mucous membranes, and solid organs due to somatic activating mutations in the gene coding for the angiopoietin receptor TEK (tunica interna endothelial cell kinase). The gastrointestinal tract, muscles, joints, central nervous system, eyes, parotid gland, spine, kidneys, and lungs may occasionally be affected. Skin lesions consist of soft blue nodules that occasionally aggregate into large masses. The small, colorless, dome-shaped, nipple-like lesions ("rubber blebs") (Figure 17a) are often associated with a large "dominant" venous malformation.

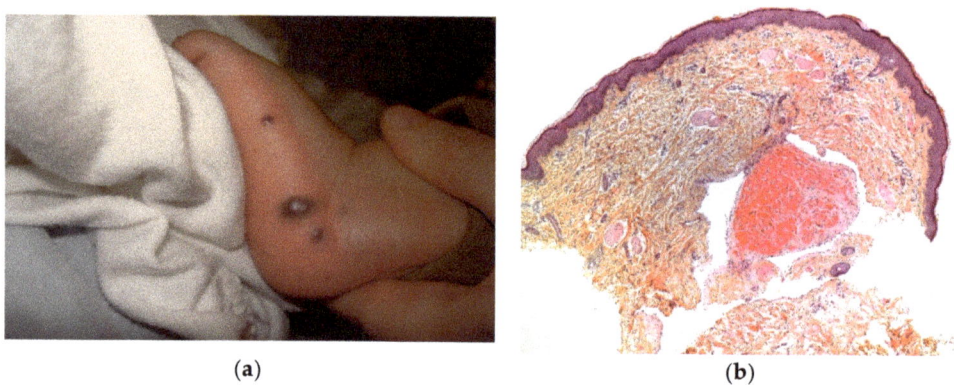

Figure 17. A blue rubber bleb nevus syndrome. (**a**) Blue nodules on the foot. (**b**) 4× dilated venous vessels, some of them containing thrombi.

Histology

A histological assessment shows multiple dilated venous structures in the dermis, with no glomus cells (Figure 17b).

Outcome

Blue rubber bleb nevus syndrome may be complicated by acute, life-threatening hemorrhage and localized intravascular coagulation. Sirolimus may be considered as a first-line treatment, depending on the severity of the disease [40].

4. Cutaneous Mastocytosis

Around 30% of cases of pediatric cutaneous mastocytosis are present at birth. The lesions can be isolated and nodular and so are referred to as mastocytomas. However, other forms, such as maculopapular cutaneous mastocytosis, formerly referred to as urticaria pigmentosa, or diffuse cutaneous mastocytosis, can occur [41]. Maculopapular cutaneous mastocytosis manifests itself as multiple small nodules; this condition is very rare and may be difficult to distinguish from multiple xanthogranulomas, due to its yellowish hue. Darier sign is not always present. A biopsy is often necessary (Figure 18a).

4.1. Histology

Biopsies from neonatal cases of mastocytosis are usually easy to interpret. They show a large number of mast cells in the superficial dermis and mid-dermis that sometimes extend towards the subcutis (mostly surrounding the vessels) (Figure 18b,c). The cells stain positive for CD117 (c-kit) (Figure 18d).

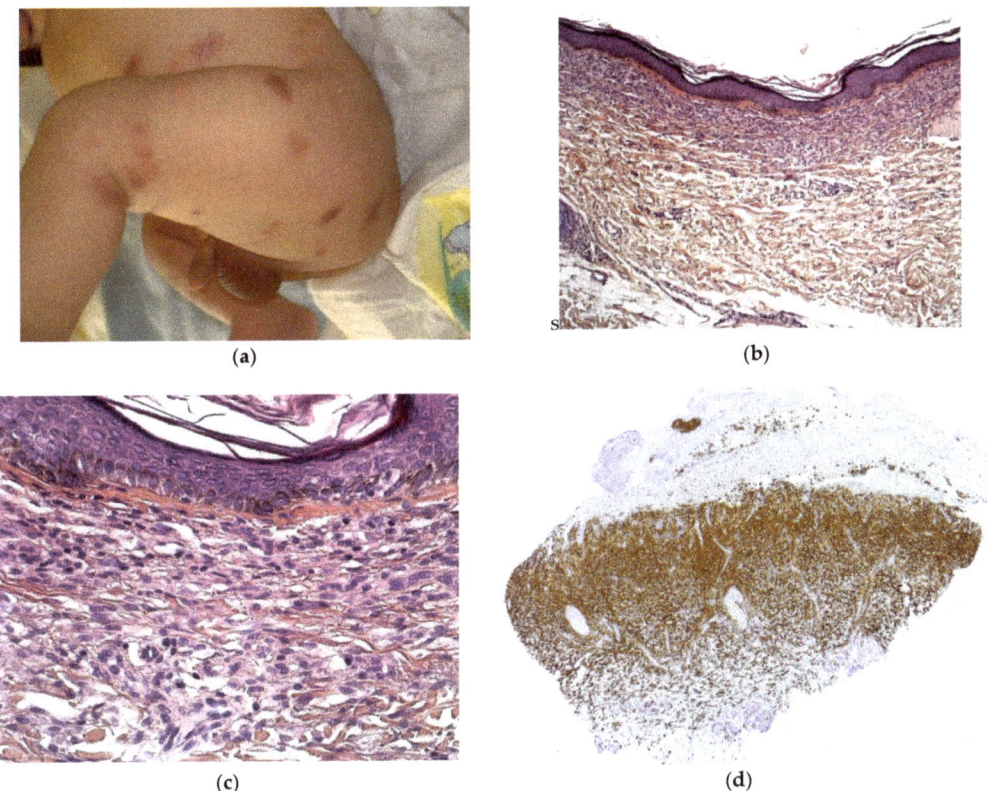

Figure 18. Cutaneous mastocytosis. (**a**) Multiple maculopapular lesions present at birth. (**b**) Rather dense band-like infiltrations at the upper dermis. (**c**) 40× large mast cells containing granules in their cytoplasm. (**d**) anti-CD117 stains mast cells in bullous mastocytosis.

4.2. Outcome

The outcome in neonatal cases is usually favorable, and the lesions regress before puberty [41].

5. Conclusions

Neonatal conditions with multiple cutaneous nodules often have a poor prognosis and thus require prompt diagnosis. A skin biopsy should always be part of the initial examination because the lesion's histology will determine which further diagnostic investigations are required. Given that some congenital skin conditions (neoplastic or not) resolve spontaneously, prompt recognition and diagnosis are required.

Author Contributions: Conceptualization, S.F.; methodology, S.F.; software, S.F.; validation, S.F.; O.B.; formal analysis, S.F.; investigation, S.F.; resources, S.F.; data curation, S.F.; writing—original draft preparation, S.F.; writing—review and editing, S.F.; O.B.; visualization, S.F.; supervision, S.F.; O.B.; project administration, S.F.; funding acquisition, S.F. Both authors have read and agreed to the published version of the manuscript.

Funding: The authors thank the Lions Club de Correze and Nicole Brousse for financial support.

Institutional Review Board Statement: Not applicable.

Informed Consent Statement: Not applicable.

Conflicts of Interest: The authors declare no conflict of interest.

References

1. Isaacs, H., Jr. Cutaneous metastases in neonates: A review. *Pediatr. Dermatol.* **2011**, *28*, 85–93. [CrossRef]
2. Brough, A.J.; Jones, D.; Page, R.H.; Mizukami, I. Dermal erythropoïesis in neonatal infants: A manifestation of intrauterine viral disease. *Pediatrics* **1967**, *40*, 627–635.
3. Bowden, J.B.; Hebert, A.A.; Rapini, R.P. Dermal hematopoiesis in neonates: Report of 5 cases. *J. Am. Acad. Dermatol.* **1989**, *20*, 1104–1110. [CrossRef]
4. Gottesfeld, E.; Silverman, R.A.; Coccia, P.F.; Jacobs, G.; Zaim, M.T. Transient blueberry muffin appearance of a newborn with congenital monoblastic leukemia. *J. Am. Acad. Dermatol.* **1989**, *21*, 347–351. [CrossRef]
5. Eberst, E.; Michel, B.; Stoebner, P.; Dandurand, M.; Meunier, L. Spontaneous remission of congenital leukemia cutis. *Ann. Dermatol. Venereol.* **2011**, *138*, 586–590. [CrossRef] [PubMed]
6. Groet, J.; McElwaine, S.; Spinelli, M.; Rinaldi, A.; Burtscher, I.; Mulligan, C.; Mensah, A.; Cavani, S.; Dagna-Bricarelli, F.; Basso, G.; et al. Acquired mutations in GATA1 in neonates with Down's syndrome with transient myeloid disorder. *Lancet* **2003**, *361*, 1617–1620. [CrossRef]
7. Isaacs, H., Jr. Fetal and neonatal rhabdoid tumor. *J. Pediatr. Surg.* **2010**, *45*, 619–626. [CrossRef] [PubMed]
8. Isaacs, H., Jr. Pathology of skin diseases. In *Potter's Pathology of the Fetus Infant and Child*, 2nd ed.; Gilbert-Barness, E., Ed.; Mosby Elsevier: Philadelphia, PA, USA, 2007; Volume 2, pp. 1743–1795.
9. Grundy, R.; Anderson, J.; Gaze, M.; Gerrard, M.; Glaser, A.; Gordon, A.; Malone, M.; Pritchard-Jones, K.; Michalski, A. Congenital alveolar rhabdomyosarcoma: Clinical and molecular distinction from alveolar rhabdomyosarcoma in older children. *Cancer* **2001**, *91*, 606–612. [CrossRef]
10. Hayes-Jordan, A.; Andrassy, R. Rhabdomyosarcoma in children. *Curr. Opin. Pediatr.* **2009**, *21*, 373–378. [CrossRef]
11. Morren, M.A.; Broecke, K.V.; Vangeebergen, L.; Sillevis-Smitt, J.H.; Van Den Berghe, P.; Hauben, E.; Jacobs, S.; Van Gool, S.W. Diverse Cutaneous Presentations of Langerhans Cell Histiocytosis in Children: A Retrospective Cohort Study. *Pediatr. Blood Cancer* **2016**, *63*, 486–492. [CrossRef] [PubMed]
12. Larralde, M.; Rositto, A.; Giardelli, M.; Gatti, C.F.; Muñoz, A.S. Congenital self-healing histiocytosis (Hashimoto–Pritzker). *Int. J. Dermatol.* **1999**, *38*, 693–696. [CrossRef]
13. Kapur, P.; Erickson, C.; Rakheja, D.; Carder, K.R.; Hoang, M.P. Congenital self-healing reticulohistiocytosis (Hashimoto-Pritzker disease): Ten-year experience at Dallas Children's Medical Center. *J. Am. Acad. Dermatol.* **2007**, *56*, 290–294. [CrossRef]
14. Dupeux, M.; Boccara, O.; Frassati-Biaggi, A.; Hélias-Rodzewicz, Z.; Leclerc-Mercier, S.; Bodemer, C.; Molina, T.J.; Emile, J.F.; Fraitag, S. Langerhans Cell Histiocytoma: A Benign Histiocytic Neoplasm of Diverse Lines of Terminal Differentiation. *Am. J. Dermatopathol.* **2019**, *41*, 29–36. [CrossRef]
15. Battistella, M.; Fraitag, S.; Teillac, D.H.; Brousse, N.; de Prost, Y.; Bodemer, C. Neonatal and early infantile cutaneous Langerhans cell histiocytosis: Comparison of self-regressive and non-self-regressive forms. *Arch. Dermatol.* **2010**, *146*, 149–156. [CrossRef]
16. Haughton, A.M.; Horii, K.A.; Shao, L.; Daniel, J.; Nopper, A.J. Disseminated juvenile xanthogranulomatosis in a newborn resulting in liver transplantation. *J. Am. Acad. Dermatol.* **2008**, *58*, S12–S15. [CrossRef]
17. Paxton, C.N.; O'Malley, D.P.; Bellizzi, A.M.; Alkapalan, D.; Fedoriw, Y.; Hornick, J.L.; Perkins, S.L.; South, S.T.; Andersen, E.F. Genetic evaluation of juvenile xanthogranuloma: Genomic abnormalities are uncommon in solitary lesions, advanced cases may show more complexity. *Mod. Pathol.* **2017**, *30*, 1234–1240. [CrossRef] [PubMed]
18. Dehner, L.P. Juvenile xanthogranulomas in the first two decades of life: A clinicopathologic study of 174 cases with cutaneous and extracutaneous manifestations. *Am. J. Surg. Pathol.* **2003**, *27*, 579–593. [CrossRef] [PubMed]
19. Ferreira, C.M.; Maceira, J.M.; Coelho, J.M. Melanoma and pregnancy with placental metastases. Report of a case. *Am. J. Dermatopathol.* **1998**, *20*, 403–407. [CrossRef] [PubMed]
20. Menada, M.V.; Moioli, M.; Garaventa, A.; Nozza, P.; Foppiano, M.; Trimarchi, N.; Fulcheri, E. Spontaneous regression of transplacental metastases from maternal melanoma in a newborn: Case report and review of the literature. *Melanoma Res.* **2010**, *20*, 443–449. [CrossRef]
21. Alomari, A.K.; Glusac, E.J.; Choi, J.; Hui, P.; Seeley, E.H.; Caprioli, R.M.; Watsky, K.L.; Urban, J.; Lazova, R. Congenital nevi versus metastatic melanoma in a newborn to a mother with malignant melanoma—Diagnosis supported by sex chromosome analysis and Imaging Mass Spectrometry. *J. Cutan. Pathol.* **2015**, *42*, 757–764. [CrossRef] [PubMed]
22. Brooks, T.; Nolting, L. Cutaneous manifestation of metastatic infantile choriocarcinoma.Case reports in pediatrics. *Case Rep. Pediatr.* **2014**, *2014*, 104652.
23. Blohm, M.E.; Göbel, U. Unexplained anaemia and failure to thrive as initial symptoms of infantile choriocarcinoma: A review Unexplained anaemia and failure to thrive as initial symptoms of infantile choriocarcinoma: A review. *Eur. J. Pediatr.* **2004**, *163*, 1–6. [CrossRef]
24. Getrajdman, J.; Kolev, V.; Brody, E.; Chuang, L. Case of maternal and infantile choriocarcinoma following normal pregnancy. *Gynecol. Oncol. Case Rep.* **2012**, *2*, 102–104. [CrossRef] [PubMed]
25. Mashiah, J.; Hadj-Rabia, S.; Dompmartin, A.; Harroche, A.; Laloum-Grynberg, E.; Wolter, M.; Amoric, J.C.; Hamel-Teillac, D.; Guero, S.; Fraitag, S.; et al. Infantile myofibromatosis: A series of 28 cases. *J. Am. Acad. Dermatol.* **2014**, *71*, 264–270. [CrossRef]
26. Wiswell, T.E.; Davis, J.; Cunningham, B.E.; Solenberger, R.; Thomas, P.J. Infantile myofibromatosis: The most common fibrous tumor of infancy. *J. Pediatr. Surg.* **1988**, *23*, 315–318. [CrossRef]

27. Dachy, G.; de Krijger, R.R.; Fraitag, S.; Théate, I.; Brichard, B.; Hoffman, S.B.; Libbrecht, L.; Arts, F.A.; Brouillard, P.; Vikkula, M.; et al. Association of PDGFRB Mutations With Pediatric Myofibroma and Myofibromatosis. *JAMA Dermatol.* **2019**, *155*, 946–950. [CrossRef] [PubMed]
28. Proust, S.; Benchimol, G.; Fraitag, S.; Starck, J.; Giacobbi, V.; Pierron, G.; Bodemer, C.; Orbach, D. Major response to imatinib and chemotherapy in a newborn patient prenatally diagnosed with generalized infantile. *Pediatr. Blood Cancer* **2021**, *68*, e28576. [CrossRef]
29. Mahé, E.; Girszyn, N.; Hadj-Rabia, S.; Bodemer, C.; Hamel-Teillac, D.; De Prost, Y. Subcutaneous fat necrosis of the newborn: A systematic evaluation of risk factors, clinical manifestations, complications and outcome of 16 children. *Br. J. Dermatol.* **2007**, *156*, 709–715. [CrossRef] [PubMed]
30. Wessman, L.L.; Mori, W.S.; Totoraitis, K.; Murati, M.; Maguiness, S. Multifocal infantile hemangiomas associated with concomitant giant hepatic rapidly involuting congenital hemangioma. *Pediatr. Dermatol.* **2020**, *37*, 972–973. [CrossRef]
31. Ferrandiz, L.; Toledo-Pastrana, T.; Moreno-Ramirez, D.; Bardallo-Cruzado, L.; Perez-Bertolez, S.; Luna-Lagares, S.; Rios-Martin, J.J. Diffuse neonatal hemangiomatosis with partial response to propranolol. *Int. J. Dermatol.* **2014**, *53*, e247–e250. [CrossRef]
32. North, P.E.; Kahn, T.; Cordisco, M.R.; Dadras, S.S.; Detmar, M.; Frieden, I.J. Multifocal lymphangioendotheliomatosis with thrombocytopenia: A newly recognized clinicopathological entity. *Arch. Dermatol.* **2004**, *140*, 599–606. [CrossRef]
33. Prasad, V.; Fishman, S.J.; Mulliken, J.B.; Fox, V.L.; Liang, M.G.; Klement, G.; Kieran, M.W.; Burrows, P.E.; Waltz, D.A.; Powell, J.; et al. Cutaneovisceral angiomatosis with thrombocytopenia. *Pediatr. Dev. Pathol.* **2005**, *8*, 407–419. [CrossRef]
34. Droitcourt, C.; Boccara, O.; Fraitag, S.; Favrais, G.; Dupuy, A.; Maruani, A. Multifocal lymphangioendotheliomatosis with thrombocytopenia: Clinical features and response to sirolimus. *Pediatrics* **2015**, *136*, e517–e522. [CrossRef]
35. Alomari, M.H.; Kozakewich, H.P.W.; Kerr, C.L.; Uller, W.; Davis, S.L.; Chaudry, G.; Liang, M.G.; Orbach, D.B.; Mulliken, J.B.; Greene, A.K.; et al. Congenital Disseminated Pyogenic Granuloma: Characterization of an Aggressive Multisystemic Disorder. *J. Pediatr.* **2020**, *2*, 157–166. [CrossRef]
36. Mallet, S.; Rebelle, C.; Ligi, I.; Scavarda, D.; Bouvier, C.; Petit, P.; Fraitag, S.; Wassef, M.; Gaudy-Marqueste, C.; Hesse, S.; et al. Congenital and disseminated pyogenic granuloma-like vascular lesions. *Acta Derm. Venereol.* **2015**, *95*, 860–861. [CrossRef]
37. Maronn, M.; Chamlin, S.; Metry, D. Multifocal tufted angiomas in 2 infants. *Arch. Dermatol.* **2009**, *145*, 847–848. [CrossRef] [PubMed]
38. Gianotti, R.; Gelmetti, C.; Alessi, E. Congenital cutaneous multifocal kaposiform hemangioendothelioma. *Am. J. Dermatopathol.* **1999**, *21*, 557–561. [CrossRef] [PubMed]
39. Mallory, S.B.; Enjolras, O.; Boon, L.M.; Rogers, E.; Berk, D.R.; Blei, F.; Baselga, E.; Ros, A.M.; Vikkula, M. Congenital plaque-type glomuvenous malformations presenting in childhood. *Arch. Dermatol.* **2006**, *142*, 892–896. [CrossRef] [PubMed]
40. Weiss, D.; Teichler, A.; Hoeger, P.H. Long-term sirolimus treatment in blue rubber bleb nevus syndrome: Case report and review of the literature. *Pediatr. Dermatol.* **2021**, *38*, 464–468. [CrossRef]
41. Meni, C.; Georgin-Lavialle, S.; Le Saché de Peufeilhoux, L.; Jais, J.P.; Hadj-Rabia, S.; Bruneau, J.; Fraitag, S.; Hanssens, K.; Dubreuil, P.; Hermine, O.; et al. Paediatric mastocytosis: Long-term follow-up of 53 patients with whole sequencing of KIT. A prospective study. *Br. J. Dermatol.* **2018**, *179*, 925–932. [CrossRef]

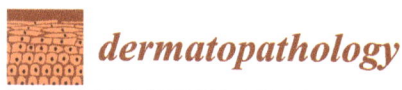 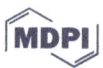

Review

Venous Malformations in Childhood: Clinical, Histopathological and Genetics Update

Isabel Colmenero [1,*] and Nicole Knöpfel [2,3]

[1] Department of Pathology, Hospital Infantil Universitario Niño Jesús, 28009 Madrid, Spain
[2] Department of Dermatology, Great Ormond Street Hospital for Children and UCL GOS Institute of Child Health, London WC1N 3JH, UK; nicole.knoepfel@crick.ac.uk
[3] Mosaicism and Precision Medicine Laboratory, The Francis Crick Institute, London WC1N 3JH, UK
* Correspondence: isabelcolmenero@gmail.com

Abstract: Our knowledge in vascular anomalies has grown tremendously in the past decade with the identification of key molecular pathways and genetic mutations that drive the development of vascular tumors and vascular malformations. This has led us to better understand the pathogenesis of vascular lesions, refine their diagnosis and update their classification while also exploring the opportunity for a targeted molecular treatment. This paper aims to provide an overview of venous malformations (VM) in childhood. Specific entities include common VMs, cutaneo-mucosal VM, blue rubber bleb nevus syndrome or Bean syndrome, glomuvenous malformation, cerebral cavernous malformation, familial intraosseous vascular malformation and verrucous venous malformation. The clinicopathological features and the molecular basis of each entity are reviewed.

Keywords: vascular anomalies; venous malformations; histopathology; genetics; somatic and germline mutations; targeted therapy

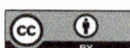

1. Introduction

Venous malformations (VMs) are slow-flow vascular lesions that occur due to a defect in vascular morphogenesis during early embryonic life, sometime between 4 and 10 weeks of gestation. As a result, VMs are composed of ectatic venous channels with a thin or absent muscle wall. VMs are considered the most frequent vascular malformation referred to multidisciplinary centers that specialize in vascular anomalies, with an estimated incidence of 1 to 5 in 10,000 births [1,2]. They typically involve the skin, mucosa and subcutaneous tissue, but may also arise in deeper structures such as muscle, bone and internal organs. Most VMs are sporadic and isolated, but they can be part of complex vascular disorders such as blue rubber bleb nevus syndrome and the spectrum of overgrowth syndromes, among others. Somatic activating mutations in *TEK/TIE2* cause more than half of sporadic unifocal VMs [3,4], and somatic mutations in *PIK3CA* are responsible for around 20% of cases [5]. Mutations in both genes activate the PI3K/AKT/mTOR signalling pathway, underscoring the importance of this pathway in the pathogenesis and the opportunity of targeted molecular inhibitors for the treatment of VMs. However, TEK-mediated venous anomalies include a spectrum of phenotypes of varying severity and models of mutation acquisition that are distinctive to sporadic unifocal VM, inherited cutaneo-mucosal VM, sporadic multifocal VM and blue rubber bleb nevus syndrome [6].

In addition, the increasing advances in genetics uncovering the molecular mechanisms in vascular anomalies have contributed and without question will continue to play an essential role in the classification of vascular anomalies. One example is the identification of a somatic mutation in *MAP3K3* in the previously called "verrucous hemangioma", which has been relocated to the VM group under the term "verrucous venous malformation" [7].

Most patients with VMs are diagnosed clinically, but when diagnosis is uncertain a biopsy for histopathology and genetic testing are recommended.

VMs may still be found in the literature as "cavernous hemangioma" or "cavernoma". This obsolete terminology should be avoided, as the suffix "oma" would suggest that VMs are neoplasms. Following the recommendations of the 2018 International Society for the Study of Vascular Anomalies (ISSVA) classification for vascular anomalies, we provide an outline of the sporadic and inherited conditions that encompass VMs (Table 1), discussing the clinicohistopathological features and molecular basis for each entity.

Table 1. ISSVA classification for vascular anomalies—venous malformations, last revision May 2018.

Venous Malformations (VMs)	Genetics
Common VM	*TEK* (TIE2)/*PIK3CA*
Familial VM cutaneo-mucosal (VMCM)	*TEK* (TIE2)
Blue rubber bleb nevus (Bean) syndrome	*TEK* (TIE2)
Glomuvenous malformation (GVM)	*Glomulin*
Cerebral cavernous malformation (CCM)	CCM1—*KRIT1*, CCM2—*Malcavernin*, CCM3—*PDCD10*
Familial intraosseous vascular malformation (VMOS)	*ELMO2*
Verrucous venous malformation (formerly verrucous hemangioma)	*MAP3K3*
Others	

Available at https://www.issva.org/classification (accessed on 28 March 2021).

2. Common VM

Common VMs are mostly sporadic and unifocal, and account for more than 90% of VMs [2,8].

2.1. Clinical Features

VMs are usually noted at birth, but some cases become clinically evident later. They grow proportionally with the child and exhibit progressive ectasia with age. The most frequent location is the head and neck region (40%), followed by the extremities and trunk. The clinical presentation consists of a bluish-to-purple, soft and compressible nodule or mass, and its size may range from very small to extensive and deep lesions (Figure 1). Skin temperature is normal, and there is no thrill as these are slow-flow vascular malformations. As the dysmorphological features of VMs predispose to stagnant blood flow, these lesions can spontaneously thrombose and thus present with swelling and pain. On palpation, the presence of phleboliths (due to long-standing localized thrombosis) is pathognomonic for VM. A rapid expansion can be observed after trauma or hormonal modulation, typically during puberty or pregnancy when they tend to increase in size and become symptomatic.

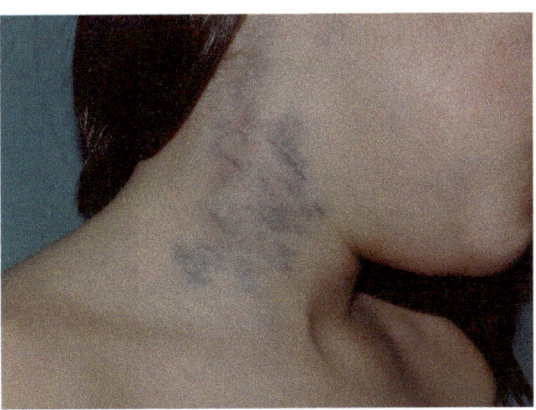

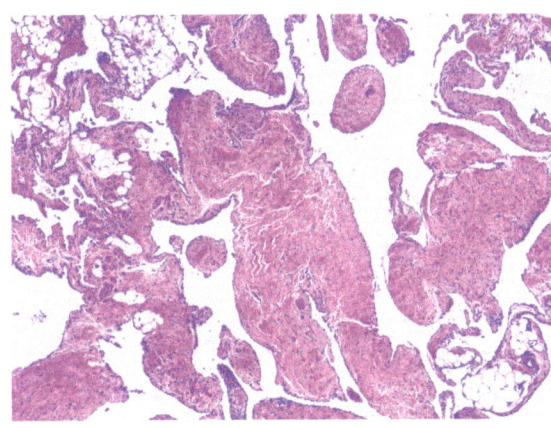

(a)

(b)

Figure 1. *Cont.*

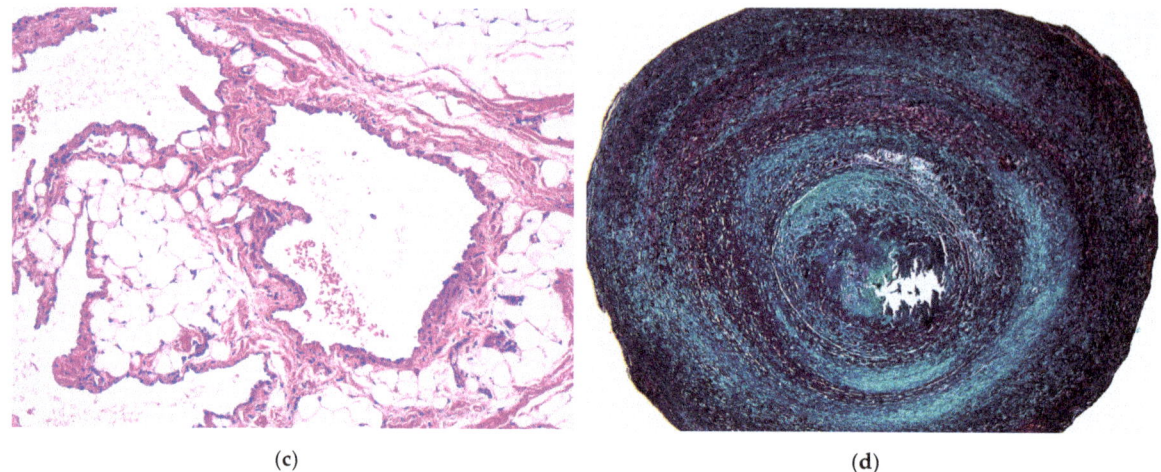

Figure 1. (**a**) Clinical appearance of a VM on the lateral neck. (**b**) A common VM showing large irregular vessels intersecting the tissue in a sponge-like fashion. Floating islands of normal tissue surrounded by endothelium are frequently seen. (**c**) One of the malformed venous channels showing a thin muscle wall and non-atypical endothelial cells lining the inner aspect of the vessel. (**d**) Pheboliths are characteristic of VMs.

2.2. Genetics

Somatic activating mutations in *TEK/TIE2*, the gene encoding endothelial cell tyrosine kinase receptor TIE2, cause 60% of sporadic unifocal VMs [3]. The most frequent mutation found in resected VM tissue is L914F (different from the inherited cutaneo-mucosal VM). Two major pathways involved in mediating the effects of TIE2 on endothelial cell function are the phosphoinositide 3-kinase (PI3K)/AKT and mitogen-activated protein kinase (MAPK) pathway (Figure 2) [9]. An estimated 20% of sporadic VMs are caused by somatic mutations in the *PIK3CA* gene [5]. In both cases, downstream signalling functions via the PI3K/AKT/mTOR pathway are responsible for regulating angiogenesis, proliferation, cell migration and vessel stability. The identification of genetic mutations and key molecular pathways that drive sporadic VMs have had a critical role in the understanding of the pathogenesis and use of targeted therapies in VMs (see prognosis and treatment) [10–12].

2.3. Histopathology

Microscopically, VMs exhibit large, widely dilated venous channels of irregular shape and size, haphazardly arranged in the dermis, subcutis and deep soft tissues. These malformed vessels are lined by a single layer of flat endothelial cells with a concentrical muscle layer that is often focally absent or scant relative to luminal diameter (Figure 1). In some areas, the walls can show irregular strands or nodules of smooth muscle merging with fibromyxoid tissue, which is probably the consequence of organized thrombi. Lumens are empty or contain blood or organizing thrombi that may eventually become calcified (pheboliths). Papillary endothelial hyperplasia (Masson's phenomenon) is a common finding. Vessels are separated by normal background tissue (Figure 2). Endothelial cells are diffusely positive for CD31, but CD34 staining is variable. Negative immunostaining for lymphatic markers such as D2-40 or PROX1 is helpful to differentiate VMs from lymphatic malformations, their main differential diagnosis. Similar to other malformations, WT1 is not expressed and the Ki-67 rate is extremely low [13–15].

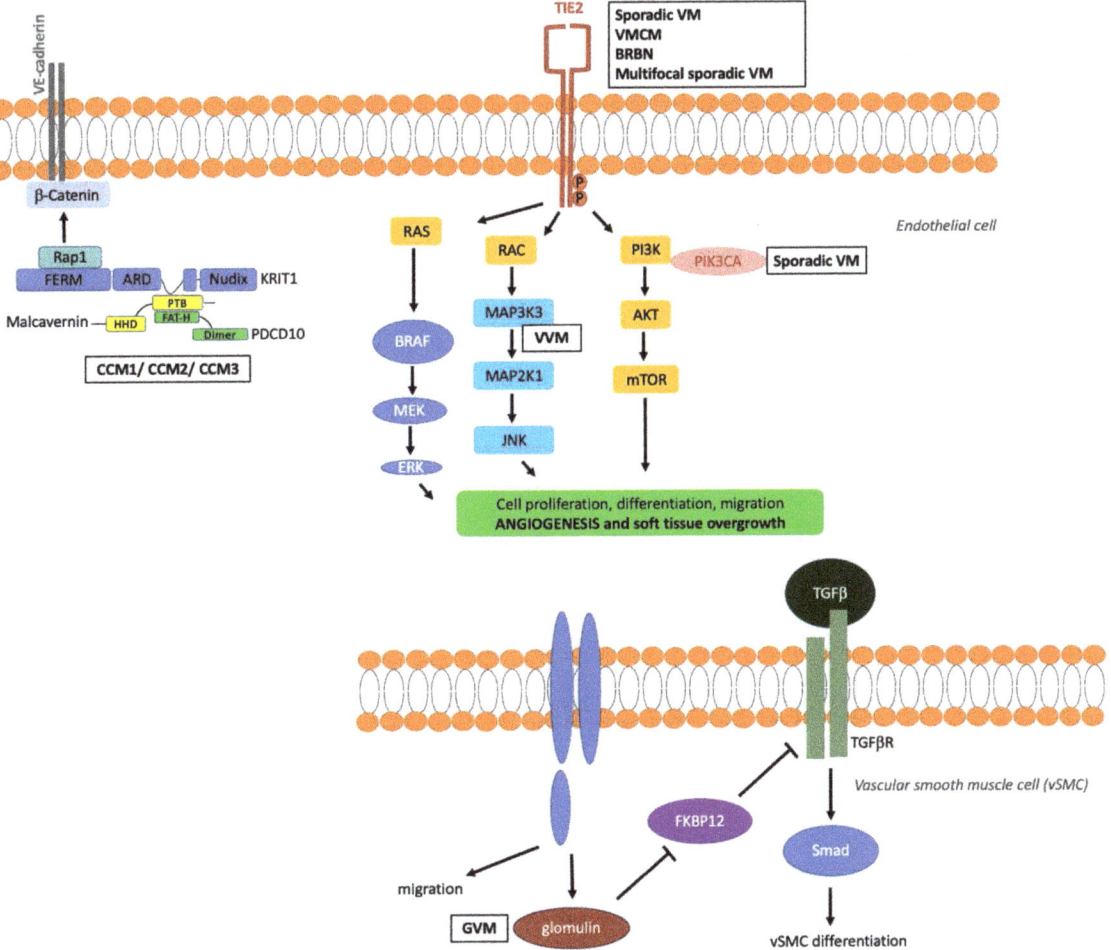

Figure 2. Diagram illustrating the genes and signalling pathways involved in venous malformations. VM, venous malformation; VMCM, cutaneo-mucosal venous malformation; BRBN, blue rubber bleb nevus; CCM, cerebral cavernous malformation; VVM, verrucous venous malformation; GVM, glomuvenous malformation. Adapted from ref. [12].

2.4. Prognosis and Treatment

An estimated 40% of patients with a VM develop a localized intravascular coagulopathy characterized by elevated levels of D-dimers and normal-to-low levels of fibrinogen, which often correlates with the size and depth of lesions and the presence of phleboliths [1]. Depending on the size and location, VMs can be life-threatening because of bleeding, expansion or obstruction of vital structures; for example, when located in the oral mucosa and extending to the oropharynx and larynx, potentially compromising the airway [16]. However, the main complications associated with the slow expansion of VMs are aesthetically related, followed by chronic and significant pain. Regarding management, if patients are asymptomatic and there are no risks or associated complications, it is prudent to delay any therapeutic intervention and continue regular clinical follow-up. When treatment is contemplated, percutaneous intralesional sclerotherapy is the gold standard treatment of VM, alone or combined with surgical resection, to diminish the risk of recurrence. If the lesion is small and complete resection is possible without anatomic or functional consequences, surgical excision should be performed as the first choice. In complex VMs, the caring physicians are advised to take a multidisciplinary approach involving dermatologists, radiology interventionists, and surgeons involved in vascular anomalies, to determine the best treatment approach. However, these classical approaches have their limitations, including inaccessibility to challenging locations, and failure to completely eliminate the VM, therefore accounting for the persistence of the VM and regrowth over time. The identification of *TEK/TIE2* mutations in VMs has led to testing targeted therapy with the mTOR inhibitor rapamycin (sirolimus) [11,12]. Previous animal models of VM overexpressing mutant *TEK/TIE2* have shown that treatment with rapamycin reduced endothelial cell accumulation and development of VMs. Another model generated by injection of PIK3CA (H1047R)-expressing cells into mice led to the formation of highly vascularized and proliferative masses that reduced in size after everolimus treatment, though PI3K inhibitor, alpelisib (BYL719) resulted in a greater response. A prospective multicentric single-arm phase 3 trial (VASE) is currently ongoing to evaluate rapamycin efficacy in pediatric and adult patients with various slow-flow vascular malformations. The preliminary results for VMs suggest that rapamycin has a good effect in reduction of pain and/or in limitation (mobility or organ function), resulting in a general improvement rate of up to 89% [11].

3. Familial Cutaneo-Mucosal Venous Malformation (OMIM 600195)

The presence of multifocal VMs is often a clue to a familial form known as cutaneomucosal venous malformation (VMCM). This form accounts for 1–2% of VMs.

3.1. Clinical Features

Patients with VMCM present a varying phenotype with multiple VMs on the skin and mucous membranes, most of them of small size, dome-shaped and with a bluish hue appearance (Figure 3). Family inspection is essential in this autosomal dominant disease, with an estimated penetrance of 90% by the age of 20 years [17].

3.2. Genetics

VMCM is caused by germline mutations in *TEK/TIE2* that also result in ligand-independent hyperphosphorylation of TIE2 and activation of the downstream PI3K/AKT pathway [18]. These activating mutations are most likely inherited as an autosomal-dominant familial trait. Several families have been found to carry a germline mutation causing a one amino acid substitution, R849W, but a second event (somatic) to the same gene is required to give rise to a VM [18,19].

More recently, a sporadic form of multifocal VM has been reported, which is also caused by *TEK/TIE2* mutations [6]. This newly defined entity termed multifocal sporadic VM (MSVM) appears to present as a milder phenotype of VMCM, without a family history of VMs. In this form, the mutation R915C is most frequently present as a mosaicism in blood, and a somatic Y897C mutation occurs at a different timepoint on the same gene allele [6].

3.3. Histopathology

Features are similar to those of common VMs. Vessels are of small and medium size, and are lined by inconspicuous endothelial cells with flat or round nuclei. The smooth muscle coat is largely absent in most of the channels [20] (Figure 3).

3.4. Prognosis and Treatment

The clinical management of VMs in VMCM does not differ from sporadic VMs, except for the importance on careful family history of vascular lesions consistent with autosomal dominant inheritance. Laboratory findings of D-dimer show elevated levels more often than in common VMs [9].

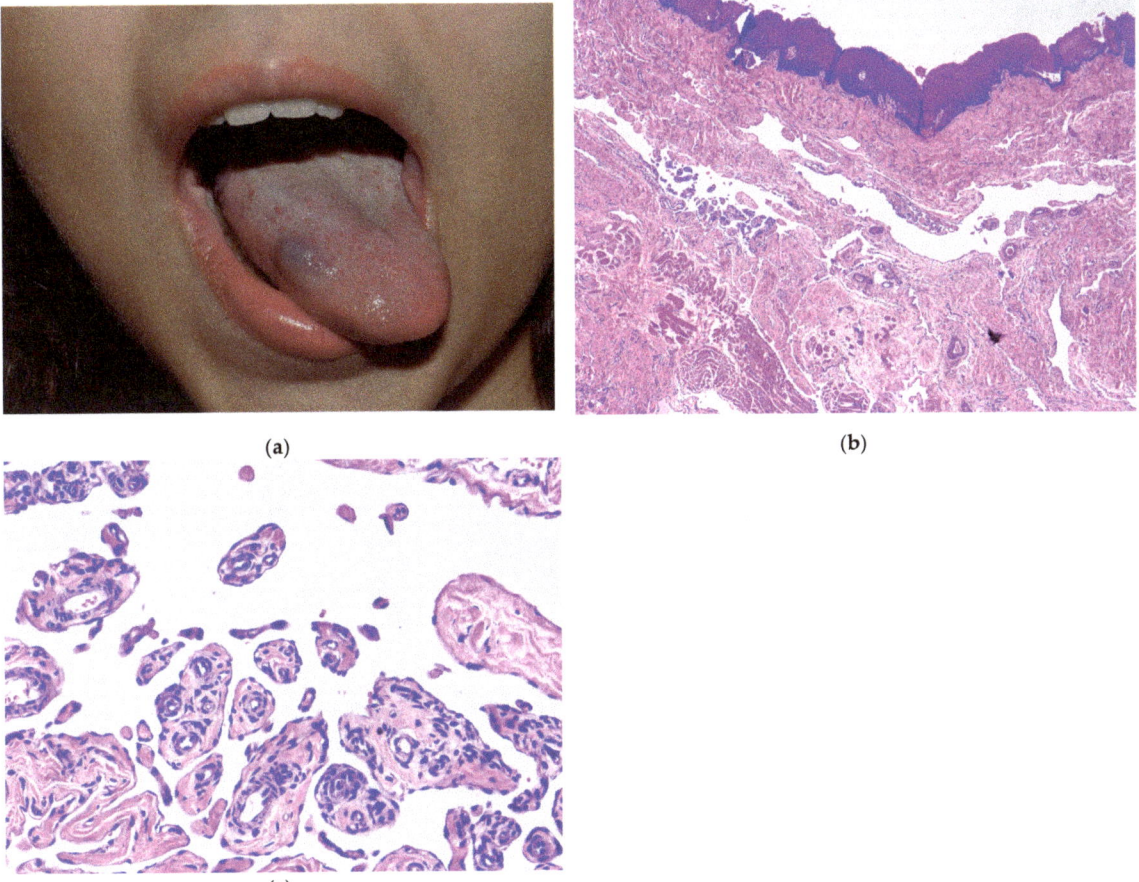

Figure 3. Clinical presentation of a VM in the setting of VMCM as a bluish soft nodule on the lateral tongue. This child also presented with multiple VMs on the skin. (**a**) Clinical presentation of a VM in the setting of VMCM as a bluish soft nodule on the lateral tongue. This child also presented with multiple VMs on the skin. (**b**) Irregular channels with absent muscle next to the mucosal surface. (**c**) Pseudopapillary projections within one of the lumens showing entrapped normal elements.

4. Blue Rubber Bleb Nevus Syndrome (OMIM 112200)

Blue rubber bleb nevus syndrome (BRBN) also known as Bean syndrome, is a rare sporadic disorder characterized by multiple cutaneous and internal VMs [21]. Patients present with a large number of lesions that increase in size and number with age, with a predilection for the skin, mucosae and gastrointestinal (GI) tract, though they can occur in any visceral organ.

4.1. Clinical Features

Cutaneous VMs in BRBN are characterized by small, dome-shaped, nipple-like bluish nodules with a rubbery consistency, hence the term "rubber bleb" (Figure 4). They occur on any surface of the skin and mucosae, and tend to aggregate and become hyperkeratotic on palms and soles. At some point, hundreds of lesions are found on the skin. Patients often exhibit a large VM, a so-called "dominant VM", and in some cases a congenital single large VM with distinguishing features reported as central arborized-pattern or "fern-shaped" represents the first manifestation of BRBN (Figure 4) [22].

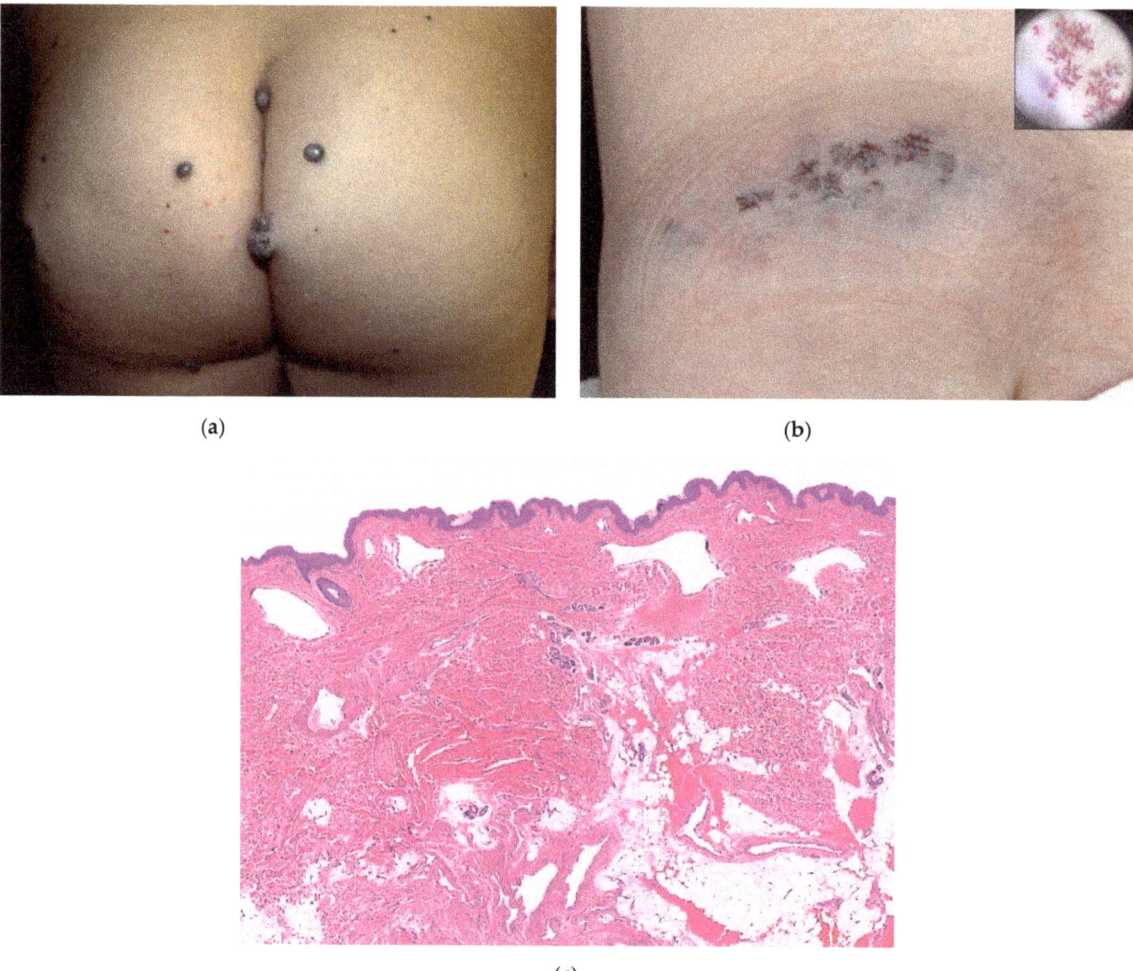

Figure 4. (**a**) Typical clinical presentation of BRBN with multiple small, soft, dome-shaped, bluish nodules. (**b**) Neonate with a large subcutaneous VM with a "fern-shaped" pattern. Dermoscopy (inset) highlights the central arborized pattern. Courtesy of Dr. Lisa Weibel. (**c**) Biopsy from the patient in (**b**) shows large abnormal channels with very thin muscle walls scattered all over the dermis. Note the larger and dilated vessels next to the epidermis, accounting for the fern-shaped appearance on the surface of the lesion. Genetic analysis of affected tissue identified doble *(cis)* mutations (T1105N-T1106P) confirming the diagnosis of BRBN. Courtesy of Dr. Peter Bode.

4.2. Genetics

In 2017, Soblet et al. identified two somatic double mutations (T1105N-T1106P) on the same allele *(cis)* in *TEK/TIE2* as the principal cause of BRBN [6]. In a cohort of 15 out of 17 patients with BRBN, deep sequencing reads from affected-tissue cDNA showed that all lesions from a given patient shared the same double mutations, hence in BRBN the cells are exclusively double mutant or wild-type, but never single mutant [6].

4.3. Histopathology

Similar to other forms of VMs, the histological findings of the cutaneous lesions are large channels with thin walls having remarkably little or no smooth muscle. If a biopsy is taken from the "fern-shaped" areas of a large lesion, the dysmorphic channels can be seen very close to the epidermis (Figure 4). The deeper lesions have dysmorphic vessels with a discontinuous layer of smooth muscle, and the channels are separated by variable amounts of fibrous tissue. The intestinal lesions are mainly located at the submucosa with minimal involvement of the mucosa, and the muscular layer of the channels typically merges with the muscularis mucosa. The muscular layer of the bowel and the mesentery may be involved as well [23].

4.4. Prognosis and Treatment

The prognosis of BRBN is dictated by the extent of intestinal involvement and the presence of other organ involvement. The GI lesions are typically located in the small intestine and exhibit a pathognomonic appearance under endoscopy. These can cause recurrent hemorrhage leading to chronic anemia, but patients may also develop other intestinal complications such as intussusception, volvulus and intestinal infarction [21]. The most common finding is symptomatic microcytic anemia due to chronic GI bleeding, requiring lifelong iron supplementation or repeated blood transfusions. Endoscopic treatment, as well as surgical excision, have proven to be beneficial to treat GI lesions; however, they are both ineffective in the long-term with high rate of lesion recurrence, especially in children [24].

In recent years, medical treatment with sirolimus (rapamycin) has shown an impressive improvement of GI bleeding with fast recovery of hemoglobin levels, and is currently considered the best therapeutic option when there is multi-organ involvement in BRBN [25,26]. The cutaneous lesions do not seem to respond to sirolimus in the same degree as the VMs in the GI tract [27]. Surgical removal of cutaneous lesions may be indicated due to cosmetic reasons or presence of symptoms such as pain.

5. Glomuvenous Malformation (OMIM 138000)

Glomuvenous malformation (GVM), previously considered a variant of glomus tumour, is best regarded as a peculiar type of venous malformation with glomus cells in the wall of the malformed veins.

GVMs represent 5% of the venous anomalies and are familial in more than 60% of the cases [17].

5.1. Clinical Features

GVMs present as multiple purplish-blue macular to papular and nodular lesions that can appear isolated or grouped following a segmental distribution known as plaque-type GVM (Figure 5). They are characterized by being tender on palpation and are not compressible. Paroxysms of pain can occur either spontaneously or evoked by trauma or compression. The congenital extensive GVM presents with a peculiar phenotype in newborns being more pinkish in colour and showing an atrophic appearance that can be misdiagnosed as a capillary malformation. Over time, lesions become more bluish in colour. The number of lesions varies among family members, some having only few lesions while others present hundreds of them.

5.2. Genetics

GVMs can be either sporadic or most commonly autosomal dominant inherited. GVMs are caused by several loss-of-function mutations in the *glomulin* gene, located on chromosome 1p21-22 (OMIM 601749) [28]. The expressivity is variable, and penetrance is incomplete. Somatic second hits explain the wide phenotypic variability of GVMs in patients with inherited GVMs. The most common second hit appears to be an acquired uniparental isodisomy of chromosome 1p [28–30]. Superimposed mosaic (linear or plaque-type) lesions can appear in this setting [31]. Mutations in *glomulin* are not a feature of classic glomus tumors.

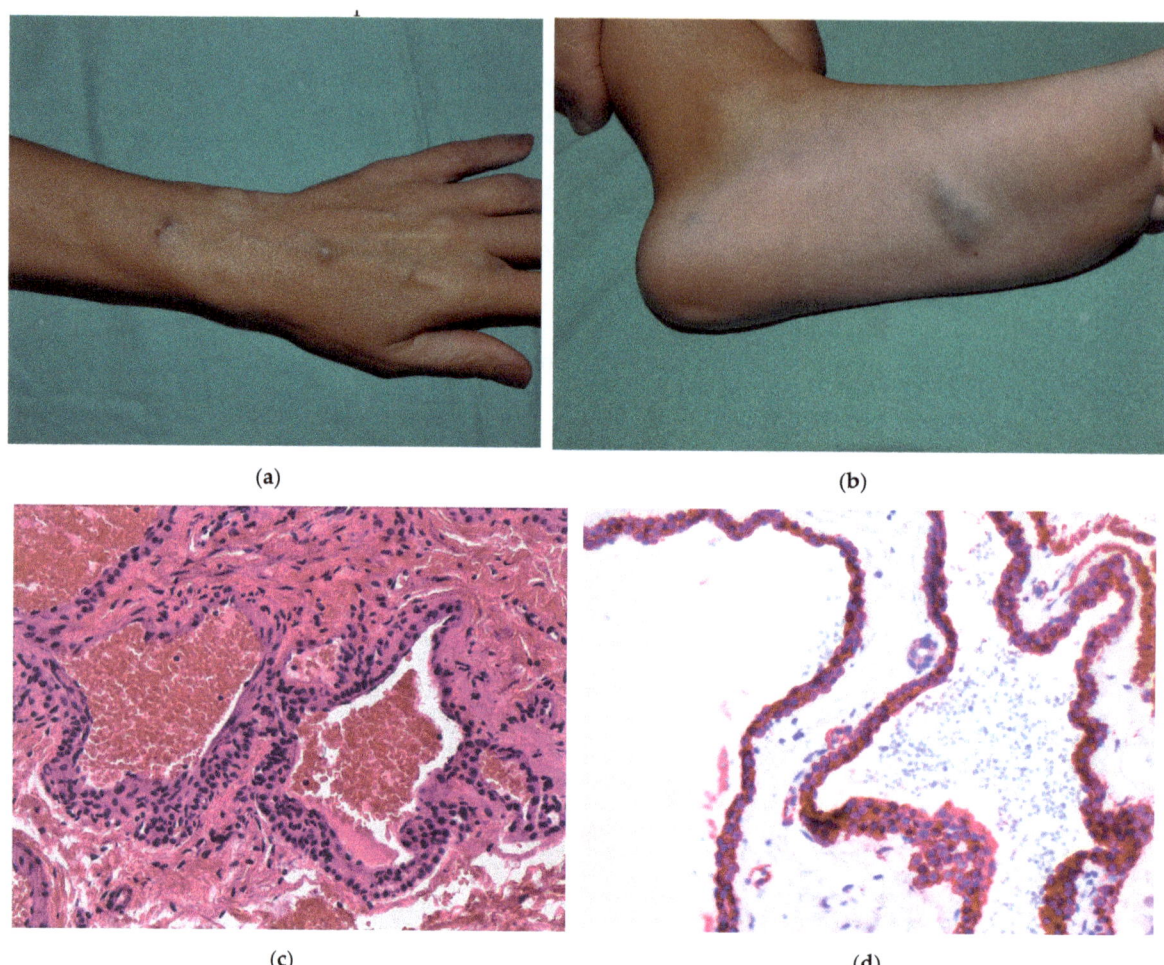

Figure 5. (**a**) Clinical presentation of GVM as multiple bluish-to-purplish papulo-nodular lesions in a mother and (**b**) daughter, as plaque-type GVM. (**c**) A group of dilated vascular channels showing monomorphic glomus cells in the wall. (**d**) Glomus cells are strongly positive for SMA.

5.3. Histopathology

GVMs show venous-like dysplastic channels of variable size lined by flattened endothelium and surrounded by one or more layers of glomus cells. The glomus cell component may vary widely between regions, and some microscopic fields may show only veins devoid of glomus cells. GVMs with smooth muscle cells have been designated as glomangiomyomas [32]. Due to their derivation from vascular smooth-muscle cells, glomus cells in GVMs are positive for smooth muscle α-actin (SMA), muscle specific actin (MSA), h-caldesmon and vimentin (Figure 5).

5.4. Prognosis and Treatment

New lesions may appear over time. Elastic compressive garments often aggravate the pain. Surgery can be considered for cosmetically disturbing solitary lesions. Nd:YAG laser therapy and sclerotherapy have shown to be a successful treatment in some cases [33–36].

6. Cerebral-Cavernous Malformation (OMIM 116860)

Cerebral-cavernous malformation (CCM) is a vascular disorder that affects up to 0.5% of the total population [37]. The vascular lesions encountered in CCM are frequently referred to as "cerebral cavernomas", and they arise primarily in the central nervous system (CNS), though they can affect at a lower frequency the retina, liver, kidney, and skin [38–40].

6.1. Clinical Features

Many affected individuals are clinically asymptomatic during their entire lives, but patients present an increased risk for stroke, seizures, motor and sensory deficits, and headaches [40–42]. CCM usually manifests between 20 to 30 years of age, but clinical manifestations can occur at any age.

Cutaneous vascular malformations are estimated to be present in around 9% of CCM patients. Three distinct major cutaneous vascular malformations phenotypes have been described: hyperkeratotic cutaneous capillary venous malformations (39%), capillary malformations (34%) (Figure 6) and venous malformations (21%) [43].

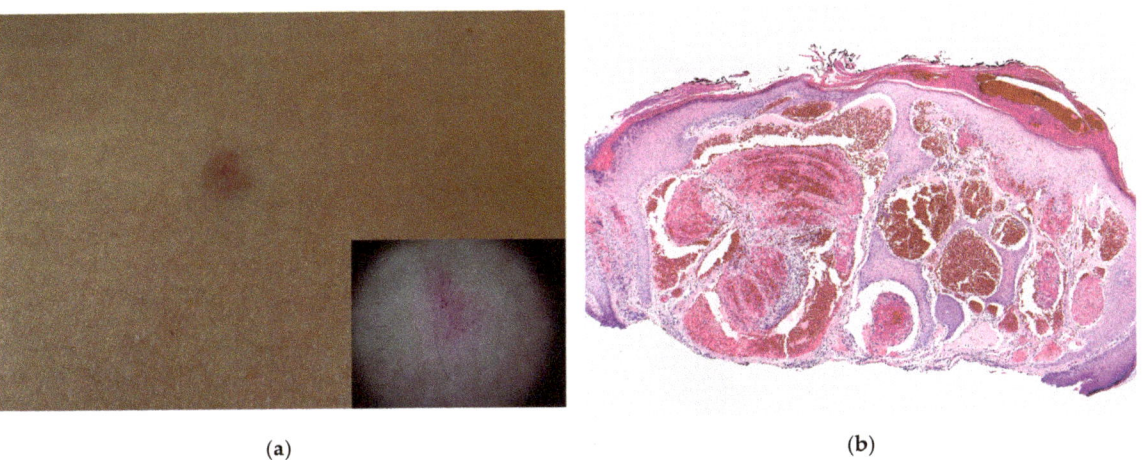

(a) (b)

Figure 6. (**a**) Clinical presentation of a cutaneous vascular lesion in the setting of CCM known as capillary malformation of punctate type. Dermoscopy (inset) highlights a dotted vascular pattern. Courtesy of Dr. Ana Martin-Santiago. (**b**) Dilated thin-walled vessels expand the papillary dermis in this superficial biopsy of a hyperkeratotic lesion in a patient with CCM. The epidermis shows acanthosis and elongation of the rete ridges, together with hyperkeratosis. Thrombi are frequently seen within the lumens. Courtesy of Carles Saus.

Hyperkeratotic cutaneous capillary venous malformations are congenital and mostly located on the limbs. They are plaque-like, more or less thick, irregularly shaped, and black or crimson coloured with bluish discolouration of the peripheral skin [43].

Capillary malformations are usually congenital and appear as a port wine stain or so called "punctate" capillary malformation [43].

Venous malformations in patients with CCM may appear as single or multiple nodules. Single lesions are frequently located on a limb, and multiple lesions affect the head and neck, trunk and limbs. Most lesions are not present at birth, and new lesions may emerge into adulthood. Depending on the depth of cutaneous involvement, some large subcutaneous nodules are colourless. Lesions range from a few millimeters (superficial lesions) to 5 cm (subcutaneous nodules).

6.2. Genetics

About 20% of CCMs are inherited because of familial mutations in CCM genes while 80% of CCMs occur without a positive family history. CCM is transmitted as an autosomal dominant trait with incomplete penetrance. Mutations in *CCM1/KRIT1* (krev interaction trapped 1, OMIM: 604214), *CCM2/MGC4607* (encoding a protein named malcavernin, OMIM: 607929), and *CCM3/PDCD10* (programmed cell death 10, OMIM: 609118) cause cerebral cavernous malformations type 1 (OMIM: 116860), type 2 (OMIM: 603284), and type 3 (OMIM: 603285), respectively. All the mutations identified in these genes cause a loss of function and compromise the protein functions needed for maintaining the vascular barrier integrity. Loss of function of CCM proteins causes molecular disorganization and dysfunction of endothelial adherens junctions [44]. CCM1 is the most frequently mutated gene in CCM patients with cutaneous vascular malformations [43]. Recently, somatic mutations of *MAP3K3*, *PIK3CA*, *MAP2K7*, and CCM genes have been identified in cerebral CCM lesions, suggesting that CCM may also present as a mosaic disorder [37].

6.3. Histopathology

CNS lesions are usually small and composed of compact masses of large thin-walled blood vessels with collagenous walls lacking smooth muscle, often in a back-to-back arrangement. Organizing thrombi are common. Lesions are surrounded by a rim of brain parenchyma with gliosis and hemosiderin deposition [45].

Histological examination of hyperkeratotic cutaneous capillary venous malformations shows one superficial component with acanthosis and hyperkeratosis of the epidermis, associated with dilated vessels in the upper dermis. A second deeper component is characterized by dilated capillaries and veins in the deep dermis and hypodermis (Figure 6). The walls of the venous vessels contain two to several layers of smooth-muscle cells, readily visible on haematoxylin–eosin stained sections [43].

The venous malformations in patients with CCM are well-circumscribed lesions in the dermis, made of closely packed, enlarged, thin-walled vessels, without intervening normal cutaneous components. This nodular histological pattern is the same in CNS lesions [43].

6.4. Prognosis and Treatment

A comparison between the 3 CCM genes has revealed that CCM3 patients have an increased risk of hemorrhage, particularly during childhood. In fact, germline mutations in *PDCD10* predispose patients to a more severe form of CCM disease [41,46]. Treatment strategies fall into 2 categories: surgical removal and symptom relief. Lesions causing disabling seizures and/or focal neurologic deficits and/or cerebral hemorrhages need to be removed whenever possible. Medical treatment is recommended in case of seizures and headaches. Acetylsalicylic acid, heparin and warfarin may increase the risk of hemorrhage. Regarding the management of cutaneous vascular lesions in the setting of CCM, surgical removal or laser treatment may be indicated in case of cosmetic concerns.

7. Familial Intraosseous Vascular Malformation (OMIM 606893)

Familial intraosseous vascular malformation (VMOS) is a biologically aggressive intraosseous form of VM associated with ELMO-2 gene mutations. Abnormally enlarged blood vessels specifically involve membranous bone, resulting in dysregulated bone remodeling [47,48].

7.1. Clinical Features

Patients with VMOS present with life-threatening progressive expansion of the mandible, maxilla or other craniofacial bones. Clavicle, ribs, and vertebrae can also be affected. In some cases, bone lesions are accompanied by midline abnormalities such as diastasis recti and supraumbilical raphe.

Prior to the onset of puberty, the lesion is restricted to the mandibular and maxillary region; thereafter, rapid expansion occurs, and lesions extend to all cranial bones, causing an increase in intracranial pressure or massive bleeding that can be life threatening.

7.2. Genetics

VMOS is an autosomal-recessive condition caused by loss of function homozygous mutations in the Engulfment and cell motility protein 2 (*ELMO2*) gene located in chromosome 20. Absence of *ELMO2* correlates with a significant downregulation of binding partner DOCK1, resulting in deficient RAC1-dependent cell migration [47].

7.3. Histopathology

As no pathognomonic radiographic findings have been reported, pathological findings are critical for diagnosis of VMOS. The abnormally dilated blood vessels that expand and destroy the bone are lined by bland endothelial cells (CD31+, Ki67-) and surrounded by a thin smooth muscle layer demonstrating an immature phenotype. Abundant mature fatty tissue is present between the abnormal venous channels. On immunohistochemistry, the muscle cells are positive for smooth muscle actin (SMA); however, desmin and h-caldesmon—considered markers for mature vascular smooth muscle cells—are negative. Given that h-caldesmon tethers actin and myosin in smooth muscle cells for regulation of muscle tone [49], it has been hypothesised that the h-caldesmon negative immature smooth muscle cells in VMOS are incapable of withstanding blood pressure, causing dilatation [50].

7.4. Prognosis and Treatment

VMOS is a type of intraosseous vascular malformation with aggressive biological and challenging management. As the disease rapidly progresses as the affected individual grows, surgical interventions should be taken into consideration before the initiation of complications. Close follow-up is necessary for determining intracranial and orbital involvement to prevent complications such as exophthalmos, dystopia, and vision loss. Total or near-total surgical resection should be taken into consideration, following endovascular embolization, before orbital and cranial base involvement takes place.

Early placement of a ventriculoperitoneal shunt to prevent intracranial pressure elevation may be lifesaving. Full-mouth tooth extraction should be taken into consideration to prevent life-threatening recurrent gingival episodes. Percutaneous administration of 99% ethyl alcohol may be used to prevent postoperative bleeding in the surgical site [50].

8. Verrucous Venous Malformation (Formerly Verrucous Hemangioma)

The term verrucous venous malformation (VVM) refers to vascular lesions consisting of a dermal and subcutaneous vascular component associated with an overlying verrucous surface. The nature of VVM has been controversial. Based on the clinical features, Imperial and Helwig [51] initially considered VVM to be a vascular malformation involving the subcutaneous tissue associated with reactive epidermal acanthosis and hyperkeratosis. Based on histopathological findings such as thick-walled vessels, multilamellated basement membrane, positive staining for Wilms tumour 1 protein (WT1) and glucose transporter 1 protein (GLUT1), some authors have found it difficult to exclude a neoplastic nature [52–56]. The recent identification of a genetic mutation in *MAP3K3*, downstream of the ANG1-TIE2 pathway supports the classification of this lesion as a VM [7].

8.1. Clinical Features

VVMs are present at birth or appear early during infancy. The most common locations are the limbs, especially lower limbs [52]. As most vascular malformations, they exhibit proportional growth with the child. The typical clinical presentation of VVM consists of well-circumscribed purple and hyperkeratotic linear plaques ranging in size from 2.5 to 20 cm in diameter (Figure 7). In young patients, lesions are non-keratotic, soft, and bluish-red, but they become increasingly hyperkeratotic over time. A subcutaneous variant of VVM has been recently reported, presenting as deep-seated bluish nodules [57].

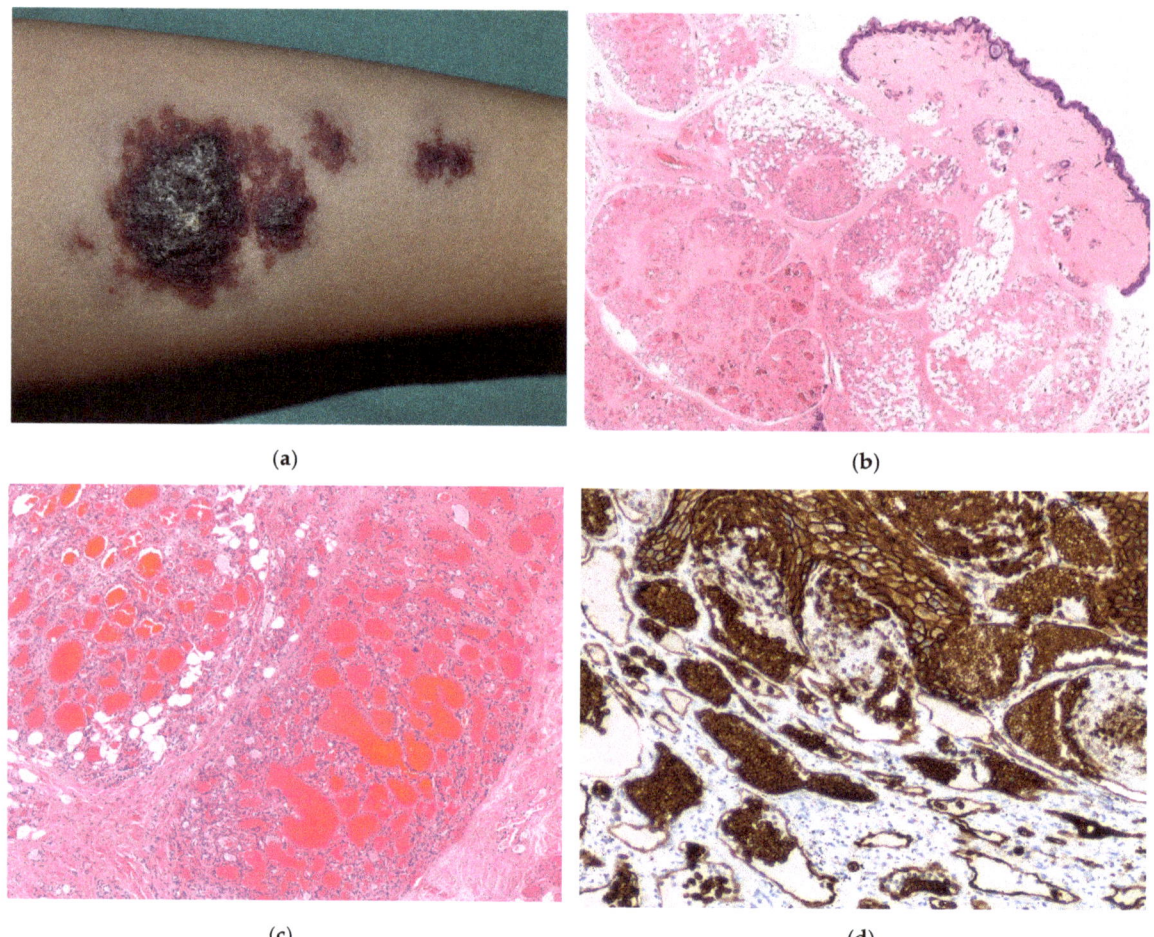

Figure 7. (**a**) Clinical presentation of VVM as grouped hyperkeratotic violaceous plaques on the lower limb. (**b**) Low power view of a VVM showing a superficial vascular component associated with verrucous hyperplasia and hyperkeratosis. The deep portion of the lesions is composed of vessels organized in lobules. (**c**) The lobules show variably dilated vessels and fibrosis. (**d**) GLUT1 positivity is a feature of VVM.

8.2. Genetics

VVM is a non-hereditary venous malformation caused by mosaic missense mutations in mitogen-activated protein kinase kinase kinase (*MAP3K3*), which is involved in the angiopoietin 1 (ANG1) and tunica internal endothelial cell kinase (TIE2) signalling pathway [7].

8.3. Histopathology

A typical case of VVM shows compact hyperkeratosis, papillomatosis and irregular acanthosis overlying dilated vessels that involve the superficial dermis, extending to the deep dermis and subcutaneous tissue. In the deep part of the lesion, the vessels are organized in lobules (Figure 7). Thick-walled round capillaries/venules with a multilayered basement membrane, closely resembling those seen in IH in its involutive phase, are frequently observed. Endothelial cells of VVM are reactive for panendothelial markers and WT1, and show cytoplasmic immunoreactivity for GLUT1, which is usually focal in contrast to the diffuse staining seeing in IH. The lymphatic endothelial marker D2-40 can be focally positive.

VVM can be clinically confused with "angiokeratoma", a vascular anomaly of uncertain nature, that lacks the deep vascular components present in VVM. Lymphatic malformations can also show varying degrees of hyperkeratosis and acanthosis, but they lack the lobular arrangement of the vessels seen in most VVMs and are negative for GLUT1 and WT1 [58].

8.4. Prognosis and Treatment

Treatment of VVM is mainly surgical, in a single procedure or in stages. VVM requires wide excision because it usually extends deep into the subcutis and slightly beyond its verrucous surface. Treatment can be quite challenging in lesions involving an extensive anatomic area as recurrence is very common when surgical resection is incomplete. Laser treatment has also been used with good results [59].

9. Others

VMs can be part of complex vascular disorders, such as the Klippel–Trenaunay (OMIM 149000), Servelle–Martorell, Maffucci (OMIM 614569), CLOVES (OMIM 612918), Proteus (OMIM 176920) and Bannayan–Riley–Ruvalcaba (OMIM 158350) syndrome. Table 2 summarizes the associated anomalies and genetics for each syndrome.

Table 2. Other syndromes associated with venous malformations.

	Associated Anomalies	Genetics
Klippel–Trenaunay syndrome	CM + VM +/− LM + limb overgrowth	PIK3CA
Servelle–Martorell syndrome	Limb VM + bone undergrowth	
Maffucci syndrome	VM +/− spindle-cell hemangioma + enchondroma	IDH1 /IDH2
CLOVES syndrome	LM + VM + CM +/− AVM + lipomatous overgrowth	PIK3CA
Proteus syndrome	CM, VM and/or LM + asymmetric somatic overgrowth	AKT1
Bannayan–Riley–Ruvalcaba syndrome	AVM + VM + macrocephaly, lipomatous overgrowth	PTEN

CM, capillary malformation; LM, lymphatic malformation; AVM; arteriovenous malformation; CLOVES, Congenital, Lipomatous, Overgrowth, Vascular malformations, Epidermal nevi and Spinal/skeletal anomalies and/or Scoliosis.

10. Conclusions

Venous malformations represent a heterogenous group of lesions presenting in the skin, soft tissues and sometimes in viscerae. Some histopathological features and the clinicopathological correlation are essential to properly classify the lesions, as they have distinctive features, genetic background, prognosis and treatment. Genetic testing is a helpful tool in the diagnosis of challenging cases where clinicopathological features are not typical.

Author Contributions: Writing—original draft preparation, I.C. and N.K.; Writing—review and editing, I.C. and N.K.; Supervision, I.C. All authors have read and agreed to the published version of the manuscript.

Funding: This research received no external funding.

Institutional Review Board Statement: Not applicable.

Informed Consent Statement: Not applicable.

Conflicts of Interest: The authors declare no conflict of interest.

References

1. Dompmartin, A.; Vikkula, M.; Boon, L.M. Venous malformation: Update on aetiopathogenesis, diagnosis and management. *Phlebol. J. Venous Dis.* **2010**, *25*, 224–235. [CrossRef] [PubMed]
2. Eifert, S.; Villavicencio, J.; Kao, T.-C.; Taute, B.M.; Rich, N.M. Prevalence of deep venous anomalies in congenital vascular malformations of venous predominance. *J. Vasc. Surg.* **2000**, *31*, 462–471. [CrossRef] [PubMed]

3. Limaye, N.; Wouters, V.; Uebelhoer, M.; Tuominen, M.; Wirkkala, R.; Mulliken, J.B.; Eklund, L.; Boon, L.M.; Vikkula, M. Somatic mutations in angiopoietin receptor gene TEK cause solitary and multiple sporadic venous malformations. *Nat. Genet.* **2008**, *41*, 118–124. [CrossRef] [PubMed]
4. Soblet, J.; Limaye, N.; Uebelhoer, M.; Boon, L.; Vikkula, M. Variable SomaticTIE2Mutations in Half of Sporadic Venous Malformations. *Mol. Syndr.* **2013**, *4*, 179–183. [CrossRef]
5. Limaye, N.; Kangas, J.; Mendola, A.; Godfraind, C.; Schlögel, M.J.; Helaers, R.; Eklund, L.; Boon, L.M.; Vikkula, M. Somatic Activating PIK3CA Mutations Cause Venous Malformation. *Am. J. Hum. Genet.* **2015**, *97*, 914–921. [CrossRef]
6. Soblet, J.; Kangas, J.; Nätynki, M.; Mendola, A.; Helaers, R.; Uebelhoer, M.; Kaakinen, M.; Cordisco, M.; Dompmartin, A.; Enjolras, O.; et al. Blue Rubber Bleb Nevus (BRBN) Syndrome Is Caused by Somatic TEK (TIE2) Mutations. *J. Investig. Dermatol.* **2017**, *137*, 207–216. [CrossRef]
7. Couto, J.A.; Vivero, M.P.; Kozakewich, H.P.; Taghinia, A.H.; Mulliken, J.B.; Warman, M.L.; Greene, A.K. A Somatic MAP3K3 Mutation Is Associated with Verrucous Venous Malformation. *Am. J. Hum. Genet.* **2015**, *96*, 480–486. [CrossRef]
8. Vikkula, M.; Boon, L.M.; Mulliken, J.B. Molecular genetics of vascular malformations. *Matrix Biol.* **2001**, *20*, 327–335. [CrossRef]
9. Erickson, R.P.; Wynshaw-Boris, A.J. (Eds.) *Epstein's Inborn Errors of Development*; Oxford University Press: New York, NY, USA, 2016. [CrossRef]
10. Nguyen, H.-L.; Boon, L.M.; Vikkula, M. Genetics of Vascular Anomalies. *Semin. Pediatr. Surg.* **2020**, *29*, 150967. [CrossRef]
11. Seront, E.; Van Damme, A.; Boon, L.M.; Vikkula, M. Rapamycin and treatment of venous malformations. *Curr. Opin. Hematol.* **2019**, *26*, 185–192. [CrossRef]
12. Dekeuleneer, V.; Seront, E.; Van Damme, A.; Boon, L.M.; Vikkula, M. Theranostic Advances in Vascular Malformations. *J. Investig. Dermatol.* **2020**, *140*, 756–763. [CrossRef]
13. Wassef, M. Tumeurs et pseudotumeurs vasculaires. Cas no6. Malformation veineuse commune. *Ann. de Pathol.* **2011**, *31*, 281–286. [CrossRef]
14. Miller, D.D.; Gupta, A. Histopathology of vascular anomalies: Update based on the revised 2014 ISSVA classification. *Semin. Cutan. Med. Surg.* **2016**, *35*, 137–146. [CrossRef]
15. Trindade, F.; Tellechea, O.; Torrelo, A.; Requena, L.; Colmenero, I. Wilms Tumor 1 Expression in Vascular Neoplasms and Vascular Malformations. *Am. J. Dermatopathol.* **2011**, *33*, 569–572. [CrossRef]
16. Ohlms, L.A.; Forsen, J.; Burrows, P.E. Venous malformation of the pediatric airway. *Int. J. Pediatr. Otorhinolaryngol.* **1996**, *37*, 99–114. [CrossRef]
17. Boon, L.M.; Mulliken, J.B.; Enjolras, O.; Vikkula, M. Glomuvenous Malformation (Glomangioma) and Venous Malformation. *Arch. Dermatol.* **2004**, *140*, 971–976. [CrossRef] [PubMed]
18. Wouters, V.; Limaye, N.; Uebelhoer, M.; Irrthum, A.; Boon, L.M.; Mulliken, J.B.; Enjolras, O.; Baselga, E.; Berg, J.; Dompmartin, A.; et al. Hereditary cutaneomucosal venous malformations are caused by TIE2 mutations with widely variable hyperphosphorylating effects. *Eur. J. Hum. Genet.* **2009**, *18*, 414–420. [CrossRef] [PubMed]
19. Nätynki, M.; Kangas, J.; Miinalainen, I.; Sormunen, R.; Pietilä, R.; Soblet, J.; Boon, L.M.; Vikkula, M.; Limaye, N.; Eklund, L. Common and specific effects of TIE2 mutations causing venous malformations. *Hum. Mol. Genet.* **2015**, *24*, 6374–6389. [CrossRef]
20. Vikkula, M.; Boon, L.M.; Iii, K.L.; Calvert, J.T.; Diamonti, A.; Goumnerov, B.; Pasyk, K.A.; Marchuk, D.; Warman, M.L.; Cantley, L.; et al. Vascular Dysmorphogenesis Caused by an Activating Mutation in the Receptor Tyrosine Kinase TIE2. *Cell* **1996**, *87*, 1181–1190. [CrossRef]
21. Bean, B.W. Blue Rubber Bleb Nevi of the Skin and Gastrointestinal Tract. In *Vascular Spiders and Related Lesions of the Skin*; Bean, W.B., Ed.; Charles C Thomas: Springfield, IL, USA, 1958; pp. 178–185.
22. Ivars, M.; Martin-Santiago, A.; Baselga, E.; Guibaud, L.; Lopez-Gutierrez, J.C. Fern-shaped patch as a hallmark of blue rubber bleb nevus syndrome in neonatal venous malformations. *Eur. J. Pediatr.* **2018**, *177*, 1395–1398. [CrossRef] [PubMed]
23. Mulliken, J.B.; Fishman, S.J.; Burrows, P.E. Vascular anomalies. *Curr. Probl. Surg.* **2000**, *37*, 517–584. [CrossRef]
24. Isoldi, S.; Belsha, D.; Yeop, I.; Uc, A.; Zevit, N.; Mamula, P.; Loizides, A.M.; Tabbers, M.; Cameron, D.; Day, A.S.; et al. Diagnosis and management of children with Blue Rubber Bleb Nevus Syndrome: A multi-center case series. *Dig. Liver Dis.* **2019**, *51*, 1537–1546. [CrossRef] [PubMed]
25. Yuksekkaya, H.; Ozbek, O.; Keser, M.; Toy, H. Blue Rubber Bleb Nevus Syndrome: Successful Treatment With Sirolimus. *Pediatrics* **2012**, *129*, e1080–e1084. [CrossRef] [PubMed]
26. Wong, X.L.; Phan, K.; Bandera, A.I.R.; Sebaratnam, D.F. Sirolimus in blue rubber bleb naevus syndrome: A systematic review. *J. Paediatr. Child. Health* **2019**, *55*, 152–155. [CrossRef]
27. Ferrés-Ramis, L.; Knöpfel, N.; Salinas-Sanz, J.; Martín-Santiago, A. Rapamicina para el tratamiento del síndrome del nevus azul en tetina de goma. *Actas Dermo-Sifiliogr.* **2015**, *106*, 137–138. [CrossRef]
28. Brouillard, P.; Boon, L.M.; Mulliken, J.B.; Enjolras, O.; Ghassibe-Sabbagh, M.; Warman, M.L.; Tan, O.; Olsen, B.R.; Vikkula, M. Mutations in a Novel Factor, Glomulin, Are Responsible for Glomuvenous Malformations ("Glomangiomas"). *Am. J. Hum. Genet.* **2002**, *70*, 866–874. [CrossRef] [PubMed]
29. Brouillard, P.; Boon, L.; Revencu, N.; Berg, J.; Dompmartin, A.; Dubois, J.; Garzon, M.; Holden, S.; Kangesu, L.; Labreze, C.; et al. Genotypes and Phenotypes of 162 Families with a Glomulin Mutation. *Mol. Syndr.* **2013**, *4*, 157–164. [CrossRef]

30. Amyere, M.; Aerts, V.; Brouillard, P.; McIntyre, B.A.; Duhoux, F.; Wassef, M.; Enjolras, O.; Mulliken, J.B.; Devuyst, O.; Antoine-Poirel, H.; et al. Somatic Uniparental Isodisomy Explains Multifocality of Glomuvenous Malformations. *Am. J. Hum. Genet.* **2013**, *92*, 188–196. [CrossRef]
31. Mallory, S.B.; Enjolras, O.; Boon, L.M.; Rogers, E.; Berk, D.R.; Blei, F.; Baselga, E.; Ros, A.-M.; Vikkula, M. Congenital Plaque-Type Glomuvenous Malformations Presenting in Childhood. *Arch. Dermatol.* **2006**, *142*, 892–896. [CrossRef]
32. Calduch, L.; Monteagudo, C.; Martínez-Ruiz, E.; Ramón, D.; Pinazo, I.; Cardá, C.; Jordá, E. Familial Generalized Multiple Glomangiomyoma: Report of a New Family, with Immunohistochemical and Ultrastructural Studies and Review of the Literature. *Pediatr. Dermatol.* **2002**, *19*, 402–408. [CrossRef]
33. Moreno-Arrones, O.M.; Jimenez, N.; Alegre-Sánchez, A.; Fonda, P.; Boixeda, P. Glomuvenous malformations: Dual PDL-Nd:YAG laser approach. *Lasers Med. Sci.* **2018**, *33*, 2007–2010. [CrossRef]
34. Murthy, A.S.; Dawson, A.; Gupta, D.; Spring, S.; Cordoro, K.M. Utility and tolerability of the long-pulsed 1064-nm neodymium:yttrium-aluminum-garnet (LP Nd:YAG) laser for treatment of symptomatic or disfiguring vascular malformations in children and adolescents. *J. Am. Acad. Dermatol.* **2017**, *77*, 473–479. [CrossRef] [PubMed]
35. Phillips, C.; Guerrero, C.; Theos, A. Nd:YAG laser offers promising treatment option for familial glomuvenous malformation. *Dermatol. Online J.* **2015**, *21*. [CrossRef]
36. Khunger, N.; Jha, A.; Malarvizhi, K.; Ramesh, V.; Singh, A. Familial disseminated cutaneous glomuvenous malformation: Treatment with polidocanol sclerotherapy. *J. Cutan. Aesthetic Surg.* **2016**, *9*, 266–269. [CrossRef] [PubMed]
37. Weng, J.; Yang, Y.; Song, D.; Huo, R.; Li, H.; Chen, Y.; Nam, Y.; Zhou, Q.; Jiao, Y.; Fu, W.; et al. Somatic MAP3K3 mutation defines a subclass of cerebral cavernous malformation. *Am. J. Hum. Genet.* **2021**, *108*, 942–950. [CrossRef] [PubMed]
38. Del Curling, O.; Kelly, D.L.; Elster, A.D.; Craven, T.E. An analysis of the natural history of cavernous angiomas. *J. Neurosurg.* **1991**, *75*, 702–708. [CrossRef] [PubMed]
39. Scimone, C.; Donato, L.; Katsarou, Z.; Bostantjopoulou, S.; D'Angelo, R.; Sidoti, A. Two Novel KRIT1 and CCM2 Mutations in Patients Affected by Cerebral Cavernous Malformations: New Information on CCM2 Penetrance. *Front. Neurol.* **2018**, *9*, 953. [CrossRef]
40. Feldmeyer, L.; Baumann-Vogel, H.; Tournier-Lasserve, E.; Riant, F.; Jung, H.H.; French, L.; Kamarashev, J. Hyperkeratotic cutaneous vascular malformation associated with familial cerebral cavernous malformations (FCCM) with KRIT1/CCM1 mutation. *Eur. J. Dermatol. EJD* **2014**, *24*, 255–257. [CrossRef]
41. Gault, J.; Sain, S.; Hu, L.-J.; Awad, I.A. Spectrum of Genotype and Clinical Manifestations in Cerebral Cavernous Malformations. *Neurosurgery* **2006**, *59*, 1278–1285. [CrossRef]
42. Faurobert, E.; Albiges-Rizo, C. Recent insights into cerebral cavernous malformations: A complex jigsaw puzzle under construction. *FEBS J.* **2010**, *277*, 1084–1096. [CrossRef]
43. Sirvente, J.; Enjolras, O.; Wassef, M.; Tournier-Lasserve, E.; Labauge, P. Frequency and phenotypes of cutaneous vascular malformations in a consecutive series of 417 patients with familial cerebral cavernous malformations. *J. Eur. Acad. Dermatol. Venereol.* **2009**, *23*, 1066–1072. [CrossRef] [PubMed]
44. Riolo, G.; Ricci, C.; Battistini, S. Molecular Genetic Features of Cerebral Cavernous Malformations (CCM) Patients: An Overall View from Genes to Endothelial Cells. *Cells* **2021**, *10*, 704. [CrossRef] [PubMed]
45. Tomlinson, F.H.; Houser, O.W.; Scheithauer, B.W.; Sundt, T.M.; Okazaki, H.; Parisi, J.E. Angiographically Occult Vascular Malformations. *Neurosurgery* **1994**, *34*, 792–800. [CrossRef] [PubMed]
46. Denier, C.; Labauge, P.; Bergametti, F.; Marchelli, F.; Riant, F.; Arnoult, M.; Maciazek, J.; Vicaut, E.; Brunereau, L.; Tournier-Lasserve, E.; et al. Genotype-phenotype correlations in cerebral cavernous malformations patients. *Ann. Neurol.* **2006**, *60*, 550–556. [CrossRef]
47. Cetinkaya, A.; Xiong, J.R.; Vargel, I.; Kösemehmetoğlu, K.; Canter, H.I.; Gerdan, F.; Longo, N.; Alzahrani, A.; Camps, M.P.; Taskiran, E.Z.; et al. Loss-of-Function Mutations in ELMO2 Cause Intraosseous Vascular Malformation by Impeding RAC1 Signaling. *Am. J. Hum. Genet.* **2016**, *99*, 299–317. [CrossRef]
48. Vargel, I.; Cil, B.E.; Er, N.; Ruacan, S.; Akarsu, A.N.; Erk, Y. Hereditary intraosseous vascular malformation of the craniofacial region: An apparently novel disorder. *Am. J. Med. Genet.* **2002**, *109*, 22–35. [CrossRef]
49. Lee, Y.-H.; Gallant, C.; Guo, H.; Li, Y.; Wang, C.-L.A.; Morgan, K.G. Regulation of Vascular Smooth Muscle Tone by N-terminal Region of Caldesmon. *J. Biol. Chem.* **2000**, *275*, 3213–3220. [CrossRef]
50. Vargel, I.; Calis, M.; Canter, H.I.; Cil, B.E. Clinical and Molecular Study of ELMO-2–Related Massive Intraosseous Vascular Malformations. *Ann. Plast. Surg.* **2019**, *83*, 293–299. [CrossRef]
51. Imperial, R.; Helwig, E.B. Verrucous Hemangioma. *Arch. Dermatol.* **1967**, *96*, 247–253. [CrossRef]
52. Trindade, F.; Torrelo, A.; Requena, L.; Tellechea, Ó.; Del Pozo, J.; Sacristán, F.; Esteve-Martínez, A.; De Unamuno, B.; De Miquel, V.A.; Colmenero, I. An immunohistochemical study of verrucous hemangiomas. *J. Cutan. Pathol.* **2013**, *40*, 472–476. [CrossRef]
53. Laing, E.; Brasch, H.D.; Steel, R.; Jia, J.; Itinteang, T.; Tan, S.T.; Day, D.J. Verrucous hemangioma expresses primitive markers. *J. Cutan. Pathol.* **2013**, *40*, 391–396. [CrossRef]
54. Lara-Corrales, I.; Somers, G.R.; Ho, N. Verrucous Hemangioma: A Challenging Vascular Lesion. *J. Cutan. Med. Surg.* **2010**, *14*, 144–146. [CrossRef]
55. Koc, M.; Kavala, M.; Kocatürk, E.; Zemheri, E.; Zindanci, I.; Sudogan, S.; Kural, E. An unusual vascular tumor: Verrucous hemangioma. *Dermatol. Online J.* **2009**, *15*. [CrossRef]

56. Tennant, L.B.; Mulliken, J.B.; Perez-Atayde, A.R.; Kozakewich, H.P.W. Verrucous Hemangioma Revisited. *Pediatr. Dermatol.* **2006**, *23*, 208–215. [CrossRef] [PubMed]
57. Schmidt, B.A.; El Zein, S.; Cuoto, J.; Al-Ibraheemi, A.; Liang, M.G.; Paltiel, H.J.; Anderson, M.E.; Labow, B.I.; Upton, J.; Fishman, S.J.; et al. Verrucous Venous Malformation—Subcutaneous Variant. *Am. J. Dermatopathol.* **2021**. [CrossRef] [PubMed]
58. Boccara, O.; Ariche-Maman, S.; Hadj-Rabia, S.; Chrétien-Marquet, B.; Frassati-Biaggi, A.; Zazurca, F.; Brunelle, F.; Soupre, V.; Bodemer, C.; Fraitag, S. Verrucous hemangioma (also known as verrucous venous malformation): A vascular anomaly frequently misdiagnosed as a lymphatic malformation. *Pediatr. Dermatol.* **2018**, *35*, e378–e381. [CrossRef] [PubMed]
59. Palacios, J.M.S.; Boixeda, P.; Rocha, J.; González, J.A.; Castro, L.A.; Rodríguez, C.D.D. Laser treatment for verrucous hemangioma. *Lasers Med. Sci.* **2011**, *27*, 681–684. [CrossRef] [PubMed]

MDPI AG
Grosspeteranlage 5
4052 Basel
Switzerland
Tel.: +41 61 683 77 34

Dermatopathology Editorial Office
E-mail: dermatopathology@mdpi.com
www.mdpi.com/journal/dermatopathology

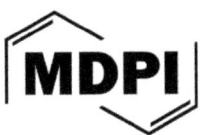

Disclaimer/Publisher's Note: The statements, opinions and data contained in all publications are solely those of the individual author(s) and contributor(s) and not of MDPI and/or the editor(s). MDPI and/or the editor(s) disclaim responsibility for any injury to people or property resulting from any ideas, methods, instructions or products referred to in the content.

www.ingramcontent.com/pod-product-compliance
Lightning Source LLC
LaVergne TN
LVHW070738100526
838202LV00013B/1263